First Copyright 2005 Kerin Webb.

Published by Best Buddy Books (a Seminars Ltd), Jasmine House, 2 Lechlade Gardens, Bournemouth, Dorset, UK, BH7 7JD.   Phone: 01202 424991. Web: www.eosseminars.com

(Authors please note: Best Buddy Books regretfully does not review unsolicited manuscripts or proposals.)

Cover designed by: www.ecdesignltd.co.uk .
Cover © Kerin Webb 2005.

British Library Cataloguing in Publication Data

Webb, Kerin
  The Language Pattern Bible
    Indirect Hypnotherapy Patterns of Influence

  1. Hypnotherapy
  2. Neuro Linguistic Programming
  3. Hypnosis
  4. Psychotherapy

ISBN: 0-9550374-1-7

Disclaimer:

Testimonials

'I am writing to say how very impressed I am with your book, The Language Pattern Bible. I am currently studying hypnotherapy, and will be recommending it to my classmates, and my tutor (if he doesn't own a copy already!). Thank you for sharing your knowledge - your content is generous, accessible, enjoyable and enlightening... I can tell already that this is one of those rare books that I will refer to regularly in my future practice.' Christine.

'This is a must for any professional hypnotherapist and anyone looking to use hypnotic language patterns skilfully and actually understand them too. This book represents the most comprehensive, in-depth and exhaustive work in the hypnotic language field. It is easy to read and understand and fills you with many "oh..yeah.." moments. The hypnotherapist who does not own a copy of the hypnotic language pattern Bible by Kerin Webb is going to lag behind those of us that do! I wish I had this book years ago!' Adam Eason MHA, Author and Hypnosis Trainer.

'The Language Pattern Bible is an extremely well-researched and user friendly resource for the hypnotherapist or trainer. Kerin has done a superb job in creating a thorough and accurate volume with excellent examples and cogent explanations of the Ericksonian model. I recommend this book to all my advanced hypnosis students!' Dr. Mike Mandel, Advanced Ericksonian Hypnosis Instructor, NLP Canada.

'Recently, I purchased your book the Language Pattern Bible and was significantly impressed by the quantity, quality and presentation of the various language patterns and suggestions. It has fast become one of my favourite books... I see exceptional value in your book and would love to see it used as a reference guide in most if not all hypnotherapy and NLP training organizations in Australia.' Paul Mischel, Dip CHt, P.Grad Dip Psychotherapy, Cert Ideo-Ego Dynamics - NLP Trainer and Clinical Hypnotherapist, Australia.

'Excellent and very readable...' Dr. Emma Sainsbury.

Other books by Kerin Webb:

Making Your Dreams Your Reality

www.makingyourdreamsyourreality.com

Contents

Note to the Reader for the 2008 Version

Having made a couple of previous revisions, in 2008 I took the opportunity to make some further alterations and clarifications to several of the explanations given for a number of the indirect hypnosis language patterns that are covered in the main body of this book. I expect we've all probably experienced a situation when, having written something in the past, upon re-reading what was written, years later, we've concluded that we would write things a little bit differently in the present moment than we did 'back then'? But when does the process stop? That's a question I asked myself during this process and I've concluded that having made the revisions I have, as much as I love this book, there are other books to be written too and as a result I believe that this should be the final up-date that will be made. I respectfully ask the reader to bear this issue in mind, particularly with reference to Appendix 2. I've elected to continue to include Appendix 2 (which was originally written by me as 'home work' when I was myself in training) in the pages of this book, for the benefit it affords by way of the examples it contains of the indirect language patterns being covered. During the revision process I considered rewriting some of the explanations provided for the language patterns expounded in this section, however, I've decided against doing so because I don't believe that more <u>understanding</u> would be achieved by way of a revision of this section that isn't already conveyed by what has been written. Therefore, having made the 2008 amendments I've elected to let this work stand as it is now and trust that the reader will be forgiving in those instances where the potential for further improvement is found. Kerin Webb 2008.

About The Author

Kerin Webb MA is a director of Eos Seminars Ltd, a leading UK training company specialising in delivering accredited Indirect Hypnotherapy, NLP and Coaching training programmes. He is widely qualified in the field and continues to maintain a practice as a Registered Hypnotherapist in Bournemouth, UK. His students have included psychiatrists, medical doctors and nurses. Kerin is also the author of Making Your Dreams Your Reality, a self-help book which includes hypnosis and NLP. With his wife, Gill Webb and sister, Andrea Lindsay, Kerin formed Ultra Hypnosis Ltd, a company which creates state-of-the-art hypnotherapy CDs and MP3 downloads. www.eosseminars.com

About The Editors

Gill Webb BA is a Registered Hypnotherapist and a joint director of Eos Seminars Ltd. Together with Kerin she delivers a range of accredited professional courses at Eos. She has over 20 years' experience in the field of holistic care and continues to maintain her own practice in Bournemouth. Gill has appeared on TV, radio and in the local and national press demonstrating her professional work. www.eosseminars.com

Andrea Lindsay HDIH is a director of Halo Hypnotherapy through which she maintains her own practice as a professional hypnotherapist. She has appeared several times on both 2 Counties Radio (2CR) and Fire FM in Wiltshire and Dorset successfully demonstrating live hypnotherapy principles. www.halohypnotherapy.com

'If you want to know how to untie a knot, you must first discover how the knot was tied.'

Gautama Buddha

The 'Knot Sermon'

Dedication:

I dedicate this book to my family. You are all mentioned elsewhere, indirectly, in this book.

Special Acknowledgements:

With great respect I salute the genius of **Milton Erickson** MD, from whose innovative mind the field of Indirect Hypnotherapy developed, which in turn directly influenced my writing of this book.

In admiration of **Frank Farrelly** ACSW, the developer of Provocative Therapy. Your special approach and personal contribution to the field of psychotherapy is revolutionary and an inspiration to us all.

With thanks to Drs **Richard Bandler** and **John Grinder** for developing the field of NLP. To **Virginia Satir** PhD for the pivotal role you played in building the field of modern psychotherapy. To **Ernest Rossi** PhD, **Stephen Gilligan** PhD, **Herbert Lustig** MD, **Jeffrey K. Zeig** PhD, **Jay Haley** MA, **Sidney Rosen** MD, **Michael Yapko** PhD and the **Erickson** family for continuing to relay the torch that Milton lit so well. To **Robert Dilts** and **Judith DeLozier** for your fundamental contribution to the field of NLP psychotherapy. To **Steve Andreas** MA and **Connirae Andreas** PhD for your wonderful expositions. To **Anthony Robbins** for your unbounded enthusiasm and for making NLP principles accessible to us all. To **L. Michael Hall** PhD, **Bob G. Bodenhamer**, DMin**, John Burton** EdD and **Tad James** MS, PhD, for the very significant contribution that you have all made. To **Carol Lankton** MA and **Stephen Lankton** MSW, DHAB, for your excellent work. To **William Hudson O'Hanlon** MS and **Michele Weiner-Davis** PhD for your solution-focussed examples. To **David Groves** and to **Penny Tompkins** and **James Lawley** for sharing 'Clean Language' with us all (sometimes when I hear the expression 'Clean Language' I smile and think of Frank Farrelly!). To **Julie Silverthorne** and **John Overdurf** for Training Trances. To **Stephen Brooks**, for being one of the first to introduce Indirect Hypnotherapy to the UK. To **Paul McKenna** PhD, **Joseph O'Connor, John Seymour, Ian McDermott** and **Judith Lowe** for helping to popularise the field of NLP in the UK. To Dr **Jaap Hollander** for your work with the Farrelly Factors. To **Dick Sutphen** and **Robert Farago** for your hypnotherapy CDs. To **Steven Hassan** for your much needed contribution to this field. And to **all** of the other people who have helped to positively promote Indirect Hypnotherapy / NLP around the world.

Having surveyed the territory that these pioneers have mapped out, I'm reminded of the saying: 'There are some clever people out there!'

Kerin Webb, 2005.

Introduction: How This Book Developed.

The Language Pattern Bible has developed in content and scale over many years. Its first incarnation was as a course manual for the Advanced Ericksonian Hypnotherapy Master Class that we've been delivering over the years at Eos Seminars Ltd (www.eosseminars.com). We (my wife Gill and I) have been happily encouraged by delegates' reactions to the language pattern manual and, as manuals usually do, it naturally developed with the inclusion of new material – in tandem with the course programme. So we decided to use it as the foundation for this book; which has been, slowly but surely, developing in shape and content until it reached its current, comprehensive form.

Since first writing the original manual we've had the opportunity to host a number of experts in the field of psychotherapy. These have included Stephen Brooks, who, I believe, was one of the first people to introduce Ericksonian Hypnotherapy principles into the UK, back in the 1970s/1980s. In 2005 we presented Carol Lankton MA, someone who trained directly with Dr Milton Erickson and who has herself presented at the annual Erickson Congress on many occasions (Carol co-authored the well-known book on Ericksonian Hypnotherapy called: 'The Answer Within'). And we also hosted Frank Farrelly ACSW, the developer of Provocative Therapy, who I've affectionately called 'The Wizard of Wisconsin.' Frank's psychotherapeutic genius is outstanding and his book (co-written with Jeff Brandsma) should, in my opinion, be required reading for everyone who works in the field of psychotherapy.

Along with having had the opportunity to host Frank, Carol and Steve I furthermore took the occasion to attend a five-day hypnosis seminar hosted by Dr Richard Bandler and Paul McKenna Ph.D. which was an enlightening and uplifting experience. Also of relevance to this work; on a couple of occasions, Gill and I attended Anthony Robbins' Unleash The Power Within seminar. Tony Robbins is exceptional for the way he's been able to inspire so many people around the world and, in particular, his seminars specifically provided a remarkable insight for us, as psychotherapists, into the mass communication skills principles that he employs.

It was therefore natural in the developing of this more comprehensive volume that the learnings I gained during these programmes would also be woven into my own interpretations of the principles being shared herein.

I'd also like to acknowledge some other talented people with whom I've had the opportunity to train, whose tuition has helped to positively influence my work. These include:

Caitlin Walker
(NLP Northeast)

Colin Saunders
(Changes)

Cricket Kemp
(NLP Northeast)

Derek Parker
(Bournemouth Adult Education Centre)

Elizabeth (Libby) **Whittaker**
(Bournemouth Adult Education Centre)

Graham Morris
(Training Changes)

Guy Barron
(The NLP Learning Company)

Ian Berry
(NLP Northeast)

Mike Treasure
(NLP Northeast)

Robin Jones
(Spokesman Club)

Steve Howard
(West Mercia Institute of Counselling & Psychotherapy)

Wilf Proudfoot
(Proudfoot School of Clinical Hypnosis & Psychotherapy)

In completing The Language Pattern Bible I've maintained the format of our original manual, in which we sought to demonstrate how the patterns included were constructed (and could be deconstructed for review), because, in-so-doing, I believe, this helps the reader to both 'get the feel' of the pattern in the form of 'the big picture', as it can be utilised therapeutically, when working in the moment, 'in the flow', while also providing a sound analytical basis with which to explore the <u>detailed</u> elements of each example. So, in effect, in most cases, you'll find each language pattern explained, disassembled/reassembled - with examples included of how the patterns can each be used in real-time trancework, in the form of 'mini-scripts.' The overall format that I've chosen for this book (which differed from the original manual) is to sequence each pattern in an alphabetical, dictionary-like arrangement. This, I believe, works better for detection purposes, particularly with the level of new material now included. In fact the word 'dictionary' had originally formed a part of the working title of this project. But, one day, about a year ago, when talking with my mother about how things were developing, she said something like: 'It sounds like it's more than just a dictionary... it sounds more of a hypnotherapy bible!' And so the title: 'The Language Pattern Bible' was born (thanks mum!). In some instances some patterns are known by more than one designation and references are therefore included under both headings... and there are other patterns, such as the 'And' pattern and the 'Contingent Suggestion' pattern which, technically are examples of the same pattern (the 'And' pattern being a type of the class 'Contingent Suggestion') which have nevertheless been, in most cases, listed with definitive descriptions of <u>each example.</u> This means that, in most situations of this nature I've included the class and the type. Readers with existing technical knowledge of this subject will then, in effect, notice 'parallel examples', which, it is my intention, will contribute to greater understanding. Also, as you read further you'll notice that while the focus of this book is on delineating language patterns, in a few instances I've included some 'techniques' (such as Arm Levitation, for instance) which are generated, in the examples given, <u>by</u> language patterns.

The Farrelly Factor

A special appendix called 'The Wizard of Wisconsin' has been added to highlight another form of indirect hypnotherapy which I've observed utilised by Frank Farrelly the developer of Provocative Therapy (whom I mentioned earlier). Frank rapidly generates up-time trance states in his clients which are, in effect, trances that take place at the other end of the Altered State of Consciousness (ASC) spectrum from the downtime (usually eyes-closed) trances that are traditionally associated with hypnotherapy. Frank's trances are more akin to the ASCs generated by whirling dervishes – whereas those that we usually observe which occur at the other end of the spectrum (the more widely experienced form of hypnotherapy) are of the more 'meditative' type of trance phenomena. This demonstrates that hypnotherapy, particularly indirect hypnotherapy, is a flexible method with wide-ranging applications. Here, we'll be exploring some of the methods that Frank, so expertly uses, in his Provocative Therapy approach (patterns which are now known as 'Farrelly Factors'). While these additional examples are not, technically speaking, specifically about language patterns (although there is room in the field for a book exclusively delineating Frank's psychotherapeutic language patterns) they do nevertheless demonstrate therapeutic principles which are a part of the uptime trances Frank generates and which enable him to hypnotically help his clients. On this basis, with Frank's 'blessing and benediction' (thanks Frank) and with the kind permission of Dr Jaap Hollander (who first delineated the Farrelly Factors) I have included them in this work.

Kerin Webb, Director, Eos Seminars Ltd.

A word fitly spoken is like...

Proverbs 25:11.

A

Adverbial Clauses

<u>The Pattern</u>:

This language pattern is very useful for introducing indirect suggestions which include a powerful presupposition element within the meaning being conveyed. This occurs in the form of a focus of attention being drawn to an event taking place which is tied to a temporal element that's also suggested. [See also Implied Causative and Contingent Suggestion.]

1) 'After the situation changes...'

2) 'As things start to improve...'

3) 'Before you go into trance...'

4) 'During the changes...'

5) 'While you get ready to improve things...'

6) 'Since you're getting ready to do something different...'

<u>The Structure</u>:

The emboldened words in the following explanatory examples demonstrate how these suggestions convey the implicit message of <u>a cause in motion</u>.

The implication of this is that <u>whatever follows the Adverbial Clause is a certainty</u>.

1) '**After** the situation changes...' [The situation will change.]

2) '**As** things start to improve...' [Things will improve.]

3) '**Before** you go into trance...' [He/she will be going into trance.]

4) '**During** the changes...' [There will be changes.]

5) '**While** you get ready to improve things...' [He/she will improve things.]

6) '**Since** you're getting ready to do something different...' [He/she is getting ready to do something different.]

[See also Implied Causative and Contingent Suggestion]

Affect Effect

This is a term used to describe the effect that affect can have on a client's perceptions of how well a hypnotherapy session is progressing. Often, with the application of Indirect Hypnosis principles, because they (the principles) are so outside of a client's day-to-day range of 'normal' experiences they will, by their very nature, result in a positive affective event for the client. For instance the client may positively comment, after experiencing hypnosis: 'I've never experienced anything like that before...', or 'Wow! That was different'; and 'That's amazing I feel so relaxed. I haven't relaxed like that in ages.' This <u>affective</u> response can actively enhance the perceptions of how <u>effective</u> the trancework has been and elicit something of a Self Fulfilling Prophesy Affect Effect. It feels like something powerful has happened – so therefore something powerful 'must' be about to happen (maybe it's already started?) the client reasons.

Age Regression Suggestion (1)

<u>The Pattern</u>:

'You can gently drift back into a pleasant memory without having to know how it happens or sense that you've already remembered it without knowing how you recalled it.'

<u>The Structure</u>:

This follows the pattern of a Conscious Unconscious Double Bind (explained below) with the focus on a regression experience taking place. You will notice that it repeats the idea in several different ways, in close succession: 'back into a pleasant memory... you've already remembered it... you recalled it.'

Age Regression Suggestion (2)

<u>The Pattern</u>:

'And you can slowly return to a pleasant memory and forget the future as it passes or find yourself already in the memory knowing that the future hasn't happened yet but recalling a time past when you forgot the future.'

The Structure:

This is one I heard Stephen Brooks use on one of our seminars. You'll notice that it contains Double Dissociated Double Bind principles (explained below). It also suggests a regression in several ways: 'return to a pleasant memory... already in the memory... recalling a time past...'

Age Regression Suggestion Including Anchoring And Future Pacing (1)

The Pattern:

'You can think of a happy memory from your past and forget the future as it becomes the present or find yourself already in the happy memory now in the present excited to discover what your new future is about to become.'

The Structure:

This uses Indirect Suggestion in a number of ways. It quickly creates a **temporal reorientation**: '...a happy memory from your past and forget the future as it becomes the present...'; **some confusion**: '...forget the future...' (you can only forget something which you've experienced in some way); **regression**: '...happy memory from your past... in the happy memory now' and **future pacing**: '...your new future is about to become...'. **Anchoring** also occurs in a number of ways, including by suggesting a '**happy** memory', a '**happy** memory now', and 'present **excited**.' A purpose of this pattern is to help the client draw upon experienced resources and then project similar attributes into his/her future. By accessing a positive state it's more likely that he/she will be able to recreate such frames of reference for future pacing.

For instance:

'...**because**... there is a part of you which knows how to **remember** and it can let you recall how good it can **feel** to **re-experience positive feelings**. And **because**... you know that there **is** a part of you which can **remember**... **because**... there are **many** useful things that you **sense** you could **recall** if you needed to, which means that there is a part of you which knows how to let you **re-experience good feelings**, so that, whenever you need to **feel better now and in the future** that part can let this happen **for you** spontaneously... **remembering... for you** how good it can be to **recall positive experiences** like this, just by letting it happen...**whenever** you need to.'

Age Regression Suggestion Including Anchoring And Future Pacing (2)

The Pattern:

'You may recall a special memory from times past spontaneously or selectively choose the pleasant memory knowing that as you forget the future that hasn't yet happened while experiencing the present memory you can wonder about your wonderful future opportunities which are even now waiting for you.'

The Structure:

This example starts by quickly suggesting a **regressive** experience: '...recall a special memory...', and then **replays** that theme: '...choose the pleasant memory...', it creates some **temporal reorientation** and **confusion**: '...as you forget the future that hasn't yet happened...', with a further **associated temporal reorientation**: '...experiencing the present memory...', by having located the memory in the **present moment**: with the words: '...present memory...', as the **resource development** and **future pacing** begins: '...you can wonder about your wonderful future...', while **anchoring** the expectation, in the present moment, indicating that the resources will be available when needed: 'which are even now waiting for you...'

Age Regression Suggestion With Resource Location: Photo Album Technique

The Pattern:

'It can be a wonderful thing to look back through a photo album and recall pleasant memories of times in the past and re-experience those memories as pleasant feelings again.'

The Structure:

The metaphor of a photo album is employed to elicit a temporal frame of perspective within the client, with the purpose of recollecting pleasant memories and transforming the dissociated memory resources into current **associated feeling resources**: '...re-experience those memories as pleasant feelings again...' This photo album theme can be extended to become a significant component of the trancework experience, which creates continuity and an ongoing frame of reference for the client. Memories can be elicited by the suggestion of 'turning the page', and, likewise, re-dissociated from again by similarly suggesting the metaphor of a page turning over.

Agreement Structure Reorientation

The Pattern:

'The reason that we all call stairs 'stairs' is because we've all agreed to do so. That can be a good thing in many instances – however have you ever wondered about what you may have agreed to believe, without giving it much thought, which isn't helpful for you? Like, perhaps, what ABC kept telling you about your XYZ? Maybe it's time to rethink that belief? Maybe it's time to move to a different level and choose what beliefs you want to agree to utilise and which ones are unreliable?'

The Structure:

This starts with a Truism (see below) about the fact that we've all collectively agreed to call stairs 'stairs.' It then begins to elicit a question in the mind of the client about other 'agreements' he/she has made, which are not as useful. It then refers to a specific situation: 'what ABC kept telling you about your XYZ...' The implication is, of course, that what 'ABC' has been suggesting may be something which the client may want to consider re-evaluating. Two further questions are asked ('Maybe it's time to rethink that belief? Maybe it's time to move to a different level...'), with the intention of helping the client to re-examine, hitherto, automatically accepted beliefs which were, perhaps unwittingly influenced by and in agreement with someone else's unhelpful comments. It further suggests that the client now becomes an observer of his/her own beliefs, thereby choosing which are useful and which could do with a re-appraisal.

All Good Things

The Pattern:

1) 'Isn't it great to know that now that your inner self is helping you more you can get ready to experience changes...and all good things...which help you help yourself improve your life beginning now...which means it has already started...which means that things are already changing for the better...'

2) 'Now... whenever you press that forefinger and thumb together with the intention of feeling more positive it will activate those positivity feelings from that special place really deep inside and you'll find that those nice feelings begin to radiate throughout every level of your body and mind... and the more often you do this with the intention of activating positivity the more powerful it becomes and the

more all good things continue to become a part of your day-to-day life...'

3) 'That's it. Well done. Well done! And as you make that image bigger, brighter, more vibrant, just like that... that's it like this... you've got it... you're doing really well... you can notice how much more you can feel all good things starting to happen and as you turn those feelings up... and all good things happen even more... you can always remember just how easy it is for you now to step into confidence like this as often as you like and you know you like this often...'

The Structure:

This is a nice saying that my mum (Pam Webb) often says and I've found that it fits well in indirect hypnotherapy sessions because it's open ended (in the sense that it allows the client to fit his/her own interpretation to the message) and by its very nature it suggests good, positive, helpful 'things' are happening.

1) 'Isn't it great to know that now that your inner self is helping you more you can get ready to experience changes...**and all good things**...which help you help yourself improve your life beginning now...which means it has already started...which means that things are already changing for the better...'

2) 'Now... whenever you press that forefinger and thumb together with the intention of feeling more positive it will activate those positivity feelings from that special place really deep inside and you'll find that those nice feelings begin to radiate throughout

every level of your body and mind... and the more often you do this with the intention of activating positivity the more powerful it becomes and the more **all good things** continue to become a part of your day-to-day life...'

3) 'That's it. Well done. Well done! And as you make that image bigger, brighter, more vibrant, just like that... that's it like this... you've got it... you're doing really well... you can notice how much more you can feel **all good things** starting to happen and as you turn those feelings up... and **all good things happen** even more... you can always remember just how easy it is for you now to step into confidence like this as often as you like and you know you like this often...'

Alliteration

Rhythm can be employed as a powerful component when working with Indirect Hypnotherapy. And the inclusion of rhyme is known to aid the learning process. Most people are aware of the maxim which states: 'Red sky at night, Shepherd's delight. Red sky in the morning, Shepherd's warning'. Notice: the reason for the existence of the rhyme is to help us to learn something about reading the weather signs. In order to help us to do so the originator of the saying employed both rhythm and rhyme. 'Red sky at **night**, Shepherd's **delight**. Red sky in the **morning**, Shepherd's **warning**'. Alliteration works in the same kind of way. Newspaper publishers understand this and as a result they often use alliteration to get a point across. How can this principle be employed in trancework?

1) 'Those **consciously created capabilities** that your **unconscious unconsciously uses**...'

2) 'Using **powerful positive principles** which let you let yourself **feel fabulously free** and easy about life...'

3) 'Since you now know how you can do this why not **get good grades** in a **calm, comfortable, carefree** way...'

You'll notice that the alliteration effect helps to compound the points being made, thereby enhancing the overall results of the hypnotherapy. When coupled with an appropriate amount of repetition within the trancework the results are ever more firmly embedded.

Altered State of Awareness Suggestion (To Facilitate Hypnosis)

The Pattern:

'Hypnosis is a pleasant experience in which you can gently alter your awareness to a most comfortable perception. And as you do this, in your own special way, you may like to learn how you can create the right kind of altered state of awareness, the right kind of trance, as you continue to explore the possibilities of hypnosis. Because that's what it's all about...hypnosis is a pleasant way to alter your awareness to make some special changes which are most beneficial for you...which means you are in control...and you can let yourself gently choose the best ways to alter your awareness and improve your life as you do this now...'

The Structure:

This approach can be employed, for instance, in situations which may involve a client's first experience of trance. He/she may have concerns about 'awareness' and 'control' so it gently incorporates the words 'hypnosis', 'trance' and 'altered states of awareness', used synonymously, in ways which are designed to reassure the client that he/she is personally involved in the process of helping to create his/her own trance experience (with the added reminder-suggestion that he/she is in control). This can be expanded upon if necessary throughout the trance induction. If a person has questions about whether or not he/she will be 'aware' or 'in control', it's useful to address them before any trancework takes place and then reiterate them in a supportive way (as in the above examples) almost as soon as the trancework begins, during the induction stages. This has the effect of creating a double layer of reassurance for the client, which helps him/her to enjoy the trancework, in a proactive frame of mind.

Ambiguity Suggestion

The Pattern:

'**Your unconscious** mind can **make <u>changes</u> <u>within</u>** without you having to **notice them <u>now</u> <u>that you</u>** do it's easier...'

The Structure:

'**Your unconscious...**' This 'your' is a Phonological Ambiguity, meaning that the words 'your unconscious' can become, in effect, 'you're unconscious', which itself means <u>you are unconscious</u>. It is also, when used with emphasis, an Embedded Command, suggesting that the client goes into a trance. Similarly, the words '**changes within'** can also mean 'change is within', which is both another Phonological Ambiguity and another Embedded Command suggesting, effectively, that changes are taking place 'within'. This is followed by the phrase: '...without you having to **notice them now** <u>that you</u> do it's easier...'. This is an example of a Punctuation Ambiguity. Is the hypnotherapist saying: '...without you having to notice them now', or '...now that you do ...', or both of these things at the same time? (Thanks and recognition go to Colin Saunders who first introduced me to the above patterns.) Richard Bandler utilises these principles very adeptly. [More specific examples of ambiguities can be found below, under the following headings: Phonological Ambiguity, Scope Ambiguity, Punctuation Ambiguity, Temporal Ambiguity, Syntactical Ambiguity and Resource Ambiguity.]

Ambiguous Deletions:

(A type of 'Simple Deletion')

<u>The Pattern</u>:

1) 'That thing that you intuitively sense that you want to improve at an unconscious level.' [An ambiguous form of a Simple Deletion.]

2) 'By tuning into the kind of inner ideas that work for you when you don't even have to consciously

think about them.' [An ambiguous form of a Simple Deletion.]

3) 'Knowing that as you develop more of what you need, knowing that you always understood what it was...' [An ambiguous form of a Comparative Deletion.]

The Structure:

An Ambiguous Deletion, is, in effect, a 'Milton Model' deletion pattern (Simple or Comparative) that's been developed in such a way that makes it more ambiguous – which, in principle, assists unconscious processing and minimises conscious 'interference'.

1) 'That thing [What thing?] that you intuitively sense that you want to improve at an unconscious level [Practically everyone wants to improve something. So this is likely to be a Truism. However, it is so ambiguous that it could rightly refer to any area of personal development. The client can add meaning to it as is appropriate].'

2) 'By tuning into the kind of inner ideas that work for you [Everyone has inner ideas. After all, all ideas, by their very nature – being thoughts – are a part of a person's inner experience. But, what they might be is not directly referred to here. Everyone also has experience of having had ideas that 'work', so, again, in this example, the client is left to add the appropriate meaning to the suggestion] when you don't even have to consciously think about them [this element adds further hypnotic affect].'

3) 'Knowing that as you develop more of what you need [Most everyone feels that they need 'more' of 'something', so this phrase relates to a Truism of general human experience] knowing that you always understood what it was [Most people will have a sense of 'knowing' that they have 'known', for a long time, what it was that was needed, so this too relates to human experience, and is therefore a Truism]...'

Ambiguous Tasking

This is a principle whereby the therapist can suggest that the client undertakes a certain predetermined (by the therapist) task for therapeutic purposes. This can take place before, during or after any Eyes-closed Trance (see below for more details) work takes place. For instance: a client dealing with conflict in a relationship could be invited to research the history of the Arab-Israeli conflict (as a lesson in how unchecked hostility can spiral out of control, demonstrating that in such situations no one really wins, but everyone loses). A friend of mine, when working with a client who obsessively researched disease and then 'developed' the symptoms she'd researched gave her the task of researching spontaneous remission (almost unambiguously and with a certain sense of humour). A person wishing to improve/develop a relationship could be invited to buy some plant seeds, plant them, place them in the right kind of environment, with the right kind of nutrients, amount of sunlight and water (thereby ambiguously suggesting that relationships need time, patience, care and attention to develop). Someone having difficulty with letting go of emotional ties to a partner, after the end of a relationship, could be invited to look through his/her wardrobe and find an item of clothing that used to fit, or that was once in fashion but no longer is, acknowledge that it was right for its time, and equally acknowledge that that time has passed and then discard the item of clothing. He or she could then be invited to go shopping and buy something new – without any pre-determined thoughts as to what that new item of apparel will be until he/she spontaneously discovers it. Thereby suggesting that it is possible to move on, that some things have a time-span to their presence and that, equally it's possible to find something (someone) more apt for the times (and to let it happen without trying).

Amnesia Suggestion (A)

The Pattern:

1) 'You can forget to remember the things you forgot or remember to forget the things you remember.' (I believe I first heard this example used by Stephen Brooks – but I can't remember for sure! ☺)

The Structure:

1) Amnesia is suggested by the phrase: 'you can forget...'. It is reinforced because it's placed in the context of: 'You can forget to remember', which ties forgetting to an inability to remember. It then creates a further amnesic affect by adding: '...the things you forgot', which presupposes forgotten 'things', and then further binds amnesia to the suggestions by concluding that the client would in

fact actually remember something; they would: 'remember to forget the things they remember.' So whether or not they 'forget' or 'remember to forget' the result is the same. Why would someone suggest amnesia in trance? It can be helpful in the context of asking the unconscious mind to create desired change without the conscious mind becoming involved or excessively analysing the process. Another way of doing this that I use often is by saying something along the lines of: '...and your unconscious mind can remember everything that takes place in your trance and your conscious mind can remember whatever it needs to...', which implies that while conscious recollection is possible (if 'needed'), all ('everything') of the recall will be left to the unconscious.

Some further examples of this class of language pattern:

2) 'You can remember how much you forgot without knowing how you forgot it or know that you don't remember it when you sense you've forgotten it.'

3) 'You may forget what you've remembered that you've forgotten without knowing when you forgot it or remember when you forgot it without knowing what it was.'

4) 'You can try hard to remember what your unconscious causes you to consciously forget so that the more you try the less you remember.'

5) 'The less you remember the more you forget and the more you forget the less you remember.'

6) 'And sometimes the learnings of trance can happen in many ways. And I wonder how many you will consciously remember? After all - how much of yesterday have you already forgotten?'

7) 'When you start to notice how much you don't remember you won't remember how much you don't recall.'

Amnesia Suggestion (B)

The Pattern:

1) 'You can think thoughts but you don't have to think them.'

The Structure:

1) This is a form of Conscious Unconscious Dissociated Double Bind. The first part is a Truism: 'You can think thoughts', which relates to the unconscious mind; followed by: 'but you (the conscious mind) don't have to think them.' Which by suggestion is implying amnesia at the conscious level. I've heard Paul McKenna use this form of suggestion. It's employed usually early on in the trancework session, probably because, by it's very nature, it is very open ended, thereby also suggesting to the client that they can think thoughts, but they don't have to, which means that, whether they do or whether they don't, they will be doing the right thing either way. It's a classic win-win suggestion (for all concerned).

Anaesthesia Suggestion

<u>The Pattern</u>:

1) 'Maybe your unconscious can remember a time when you slept on your arm and it became numb or when you held cold snow in your hand and lost the feeling in your fingers...'

<u>The Structure</u>:

1) This pattern uses **universal experience** with which to **revivify** past situations in which numbness/anaesthesia occurred naturally, from which to generate a range of suggestions to facilitate hypnotic anaesthesia.

<u>The Pattern</u>:

2) 'You're wearing a watch on your wrist now, but it's quite likely that although, at some level, you know that it's there, you don't consciously notice it's there until it's time to do so. This means that your unconscious mind can moment-by-moment cause you to not notice certain feelings until the right time to do so. Watch what happens now when you think about your toes, do you notice that a part of you was already aware of them before you were (Conversational Postulate)? That's how easy it can be for your unconscious to turn your awareness up and down (Recalibration), at a moment's notice, so you don't have to consciously notice sensations which are unhelpful, you don't even have to notice much, or anything at all, of that old sensation in your ABC. You can trust in your unconscious mind's ability to only let you notice what is helpful, healthful and appropriate and, just as it can

monitor that watch on your wrist and only let you notice it when you need to, similarly it can monitor whether or not there comes a time that you need to notice that ABC, which, by then, you may not have noticed for a while, perhaps even starting to not notice it quite soon, and if you don't need to notice it much any more you can find that a minute level of awareness of what you no longer need to be aware of can remain, to let you know that it's there, for helpful, healthful and appropriate reasons, without it interfering in the way that it used to.'

The Structure:

2) Using an example of a person wearing a watch (as most people do) most of us will have had the experience of noticing that we don't consciously feel the watch on our wrist until we 'tune into it'. This theme is employed throughout the change-work example used above, similarly utilising the client's awareness of their toes (and this theme could be expanded) to reiterate the same point, that they probably didn't notice them until their attention was drawn to them. A play on words is used around 'watch', 'time' and 'minute' – as in small. Importantly, woven into the suggestion is the directive that the unconscious will monitor the situation so that if ever the client needs to become more aware of the feeling again they will do so. In fact the suggestion is given that they will continue to notice it in a minute way, that no longer interferes 'in the way that it used to', which, by changing the temporal perspective, linguistically, places the pain in the past.

For additional affect rather than saying 'your hands', or 'your foot' you can also say 'those hands' or 'that foot', which can further dissociate the client from the area in which anaesthesia is being developed.

Analogue Marking

The Pattern:

Analogue Marking is a special technique which allows you to highlight certain words that you want people to notice. It's very similar to the principle of embedded commands... the only technical difference being that analogue marking always occurs with embedded commands but not all analogue marking takes the form of a command. It may simply be highlighting a particular word or phrase.

The Structure:

'Analogue marking is a **special technique** which allows you to **highlight** certain words that you want people to **notice**. It's very similar to the principle of **embedded commands**... the only **technical** difference being that analogue marking **always** occurs with embedded commands but not all analogue marking takes the form of a command. It may simply be **highlighting** a particular **word** or **phrase**.'

Analogy

The Pattern:

An analogy is an example of something which has a similar, parallel, resemblance to a topic or theme. In a therapeutic context it can be used to convey information in an indirect, non-threatening way. For instance, in a situation involving a client who was reluctant to become fully involved in life, amongst other examples, I talked about a time when I'd watched one of my dogs sniffing the scent of some plants and of how his whole body was involved in the process. It wasn't just a little 'sniff', his torso was involved, he angled his body to get the best 'sniffing position' and then he became fully involved in sniffing. This offered the client a parallel example, from the natural world, of the fully involved nature of one of my dogs, in relation to his own life. And (on a deeper level) of my own involvement with life in the sense that I noticed the fine detail of my dog's experience, which would otherwise have gone unnoticed.

Analogy (Sleight Of Mouth)

Sleight of Mouth principles were first delineated by Robert Dilts as he himself modelled Richard Bandler's language patterns. Additional contributions have been made by Steve and Connirae Andreas. A number of Sleight of Mouth patterns now exist, which are covered in this book. Sleight of Mouth patterns are utilised to unravel and in the process depotentiate adverse Complex Equivalence and/or Cause and Effect statements made by the client. [See: Analogy, Another

Outcome, Apply To Self, Challenge, Change Of Reference Frame Size, Chunk Size, Consequences, Counter Example, Hierarchy Of Criteria, Intention, Meta Frame, Model Of The World, Reality Strategy, Redefine, Switch Referential Index.]   In this example the principle of Analogy is employed.

<u>Client statement</u>: 'I don't know what to do next...this makes me feel like a failure.'

'(A) I don't know what to do next... (B) this makes me feel like a failure.'

A) 'A river can flow without knowing exactly how it's moving forward.'

This statement uses an analogy that works on the cause and effect relationship in the client's statement. Implicitly it suggests that 'knowing' and 'not knowing' need not be equated with 'failure', in fact success can occur when 'not knowing' is taking place. In this example there is a hint of a 'Zen-like' quality about things.

B) 'Maybe the Beatles felt like they'd failed when they were first turned down by Decca records. But then look what happened.'

This analogy draws on popular culture and raises a rhetorical question regarding the most successful pop group in history to-date. The embedded question says in effect:

'Maybe the Beatles felt like failures too – when Decca turned them down – but that doesn't mean they were failures. In fact, after the setback and related feelings of the moment, they moved forward and became incredibly successful. This means that (Complex Equivalence) you can emulate their approach and in so doing change the way you're feeling and responding.'

It 'says' all of the above without having to say all of the above.

A/B) 'Imagine – if the sun felt like a failure because it doesn't understand the physics involved in sending its light and warmth to our world. Sometimes it's better just to get on with it and leave the rest of nature to work itself out.'

A comparable relationship is presented between the client and the sun (by analogy). In the example a question is implied regarding the sun and its need (or lack of need) to know how it does what it does. It does it quite well without having to know how. This means that (Complex Equivalence) in the terms of the analogy the client need not necessarily 'know' what to do next in order to start to move forward. Sometimes just doing what you don't know can lead to the outcome that you want (like the sun). This example also has a 'Zen like' theme within it.

Here's another example:

The Structure:

Client statement:

'I'm shy so I'll never achieve much in life.'

(A) 'I'm shy (B) so I'll never achieve much in life.'

Therapist:

A) 'I'm shy sometimes too – lots of people are.'

B) 'My friend Sally always seems to achieve the things she sets out to do just by getting on with them.'

A/B) 'Elvis was shy and look how much he achieved.'

Anchoring (Linguistically):

Anchoring (also known as Triggers) is a naturally occurring phenomenon. Most people can think of a certain song from their formative years and by remembering the song, also begin to remember where they were, who they were with and what they were doing at the time the song was popular. We can think of past situations and begin to feel feelings associated with that past situation. A certain scent can elicit memories and feelings tied to the significant times when we were introduced to the scent, along with related experiences of those times. Most of these associations, take place without our conscious choice in the matter. Anchoring however is a method in which we can choose to create powerful associations for therapeutic results.

The Pattern:

1) 'And as you find that you are discovering new ways to let yourself take it easy as you hear my voice you can gently let yourself relax. And as you listen to what I say comfortably at many levels you

can pleasantly enjoy the comfortable experience of going into trance. As I talk to you now and you relax easily, you can listen to what I say comfortably at a conscious level or just be at ease and unconsciously hear whatever you know you need to in order to be totally at ease now.'

The Structure:

1) 'And as you find that you are discovering new ways to let yourself **take it easy** as you <u>hear my voice</u> you can gently let yourself **relax**. And as you <u>listen to what I say comfortably</u> at many levels you can **pleasantly enjoy** the **comfortable experience** of going into trance. <u>As I talk to you</u> now and **you relax easily**, you can <u>listen to what I say</u> **comfortably** at a conscious level or just **be at ease** and unconsciously <u>hear</u> whatever you know you need to in order to **be totally at ease** now.'

You will notice that emphasis is given to words and phrases that suggest an **emotional content** of comfort, along with suggestions related to hearing the therapist's voice. This will create an association, in this example, of comfort and relaxation being linked to the therapist's voice. Here's another example:

The Pattern:

2) '...That's right! And there is a part of you which knows how to feel really confident...and as you start to feel empowered...what will you notice which pleasantly surprises you first when you start to make that presentation? Will it be a wave of unconscious confidence as soon as you start to speak easily and calmly, will it be a sense of self-

esteem as you begin to convey your message? Maybe it will be a kind of inner knowing that you have something really worthwhile to share with the others that let's you feel good about sharing what you have to say in a vibrant and empowered way.'

The Structure:

2) '...That's right! And there is a part of you which knows how to **feel really confident**...and as you start to **feel empowered**...what will you notice which pleasantly surprises you first when you start to <u>make that presentation</u>? Will it be a wave of **unconscious confidence** as soon as you <u>start to speak easily</u> and **calmly**, will it be a sense of **self-esteem** as you <u>begin to convey your message</u>? Maybe it will be a kind of **inner knowing** that you have **something really worthwhile to share** with the others that let's you **feel good about sharing** what <u>you have to say</u> in a **vibrant** and **empowered** way.'

You'll notice here, in this example referring to someone making a presentation, words with a different kind of Emotional Content, this time focussed on the client being self-empowered. And direct <u>associations</u> are made between these <u>positive emotions</u> and <u>speaking</u> to a group of people so that they become associated (meaning that the empowered feelings are linked to the act of presenting).

And

The word 'and' is a very useful word in hypnotherapy. It's a Linking Word that can help to generate the hypnotic state **and** be utilised to convey suggestions.

<u>The Pattern</u>:

'**And** as you wonder when you will start to notice how much easier things are...**and** when you will start to feel more comfortable...you can notice more resources becoming available to you **and** as you do this your unconscious can help you relax **and** enjoy the process of change now.'

<u>The Structure</u>:

You'll notice here that the word 'and' links the phrases very nicely and allows for the suggestions to be accepted in a cooperative way. [See also Contingent Suggestion/Dependent Suggestion.]

A pause can also be used in place of the word 'and'.

<u>The Pattern</u>:

'...As you wonder when you will start to notice how much easier things are...when you will start to feel more comfortable...you can notice more resources becoming available to you ... as you do this your unconscious can help you relax ... enjoy the process of change now.'

<u>The Structure</u>:

The above example is almost identical to the one which preceded it, except for the fact that the word 'and' has been replaced with a pause to create the same kind of linking effect.

Utilising 'And' and ... 'Pauses'.

The Pattern:

'**And** as you wonder when you will start to notice how much easier things are... when you will start to feel more comfortable...you can notice more resources becoming available to you **and** as you do this your unconscious can help you relax ...enjoy the process of change now.'

The Structure:

This illustration is a mixed version of the two preceding examples in which, in some instances the word 'and' has been applied while in others it has been replaced with a pause to create the same kind of linking effect.

Another Outcome (Sleight Of Mouth)

Sleight of Mouth principles were first delineated by Robert Dilts as he himself modelled Richard Bandler's language patterns. Additional contributions have been made by Steve and Connirae Andreas. A number of Sleight of Mouth patterns now exist, which are covered in this book. Sleight of Mouth patterns are utilised to unravel and in the process depotentiate adverse Complex Equivalence and/or Cause and Effect statements made by the client. [See: Analogy, Another Outcome, Apply To Self, Challenge, Change Of Reference Frame Size, Chunk Size, Consequences, Counter Example, Hierarchy Of Criteria, Intention, Meta Frame, Model Of The World, Reality Strategy, Redefine, Switch Referential Index.] In this example the principle of Another Outcome is employed.

The Pattern:

1) 'It's not how uncomfortable you feel now about facing this issue it's about how much more freedom you'll have by dealing with it.'

2) 'Whether or not you believe him is not what's important it's about whether or not you trust yourself to make the right decision.'

3) 'Don't kid yourself, you know it isn't about money...it's about integrity.'

4) 'You know really that it isn't only about a job it's about your vocation.'

The Structure:

In the above examples the Another Outcome pattern is employed to help shift the client's focus from a less relevant (or even spurious) issue to the required area of focus.

Apply To Self (Sleight Of Mouth)

Sleight of Mouth principles were first delineated by Robert Dilts as he himself modelled Richard Bandler's language patterns. Additional contributions have been made by Steve and Connirae Andreas. A number of Sleight of Mouth patterns now exist, which are covered in this book. Sleight of Mouth patterns are utilised to unravel and in the process depotentiate adverse Complex

Equivalence and/or Cause and Effect statements made by the client. [See: Analogy, Another Outcome, Apply To Self, Challenge, Change Of Reference Frame Size, Chunk Size, Consequences, Counter Example, Hierarchy Of Criteria, Intention, Meta Frame, Model Of The World, Reality Strategy, Redefine, Switch Referential Index.] In this example the principle of Apply To Self is employed.

The Pattern:

(A)

1) 'The **feelings** that you've been having in relation to the problem at hand are not worth **feeling** are they?'

2) 'The **trouble** that being involved with this person is causing isn't really worth the **trouble** is it?'

3) 'The **flexibility** that you will gain by making these new choices is worth being **flexible** to attain.'

4) 'The **plans** that you're making about the solutions that you're creating are worth **planning** for.'

The Structure:

The second word spoken in the above examples (which we call the Operative Word) is the word that is applied to itself (using either the exact same word or a word of identical derivation). The focus of the message hinges on that word being reapplied to itself. It is useful in therapy for a number of reasons, including: 1) it's quite hypnotic and: 2) it helps to pack the message quite tightly into a short space of words: 3) there's a certain soporific flow and rhythm that's generated by using this pattern, which makes for a relaxing trance experience.

(B)

The Pattern:

1) 'The **results** that you're **contemplating** in relation to the changes you're avoiding are **results** that are not worth **contemplating**.'

2) 'The **positive** feelings that you'll **experience** by being true to yourself you can be **positive** will be worth the **experience**.'

3) 'The **change** that you'll **make** will start to **change** the way you **make** things happen all by themselves.'

4) 'That **thought** that you're having **within** – what's the **thought** behind it **within** the context of the situation?'

The Structure:

In these examples, the second spoken word plus another relevant word become Operative Words and are themselves reapplied to themselves in the context of the suggestions being made.

(C)

The Pattern:

1) 'You can **notice noticing**...'

2) 'As you **discover discovering**...'

3) 'As you **play playfully...**'

4) 'As you **create creative** new ways...'

<u>The Structure</u>:

In these examples the Operative Word is immediately reapplied, in the form of a word of similar meaning, in order to generate the trance affect and embed the suggestions being made.

(D)

<u>The Pattern</u>:

1) 'You won't **start** this until you're ready to **start** this to make the changes at just the right time...'

2) 'You can't **wait** for this moment to **wait** to be over in order to get started...'

3) 'You won't **consider** what to do until you **consider** what needs to be done...'

4) 'Don't you **think** about changing until you **think** about what needs to happen first...'

<u>The Structure</u>:

In the above examples the third word becomes the Operative Word (because it's where the focus of the statement hinges) and it's then reapplied to itself.

(E)

<u>The Pattern</u>:

1) 'The things that you'll **lose** by not taking action you won't want to **lose**.'

2) 'So the choices that you'll **gain** by doing things differently are really worth the **gain**.'

<u>The Structure</u>:

The Operative Word falls within the sentence at an indeterminate place and is then reapplied to itself.

(F)

Therapist to Client

<u>The Pattern</u>:

1)

Client: 'I need to be **imaginative**.'

Therapist: 'That's an **imaginative** thing to say.'

2)

Client: 'ABC is really **hurtful**, he never cares for anyone.'

Therapist: 'That's a **hurtful** thing to say.'

3)

Client: 'I like feeling **happy**'.

Therapist: 'That's a **happy** thought to have.'

4)

Client: 'I'm feeling **curious** about what to do next.'

Therapist: 'That's a **curious** place to be.'

The Structure:

In these examples the Operative Word that the client used is reapplied, by the therapist, to the context of the statement being made by the client.

Apposition Of Opposites

The Pattern:

1) 'As you listen to sounds outside inside you can be making changes.'

2) 'The deeper into trance you go the higher the thoughts you think.'

3) 'The more you slow down and relax into trance the faster you can find new solutions inside.'

4) 'The heaviness in your body can create a lightness in your mind.'

5) 'The warmth of the coolness can let you relax even more.'

6) 'The dark of the night can herald the light of a new dawn.'

The Structure:

1) 'As you listen to sounds **outside inside** you can be making changes.'

2) 'The **deeper** into trance you go the **higher** the thoughts you think.'

3) 'The more you **slow down** and relax into trance the **faster** you can find new solutions inside.'

4) 'The **heaviness** in your body can create a **lightness** in your mind.'

5) 'The **warmth** of the **coolness** can let you relax even more.'

6) 'The **dark** of the **night** can herald the **light** of a new **dawn**.'

In the above examples a word(s) is employed which is followed soon after by a word(s) with an opposite meaning. This can be utilised to further generate an Affect Effect in trance while also delivering relevant suggestions.

Approach Binds

The Pattern:

1) 'Would you like to consider ways to feel more confident or more positive?'

2) 'It's your choice. Would you rather go to France or Spain for your next holiday?'

3) 'Have you considered whether you'd prefer a new career in hypnotherapy working for yourself or working for a large organisation?'

4) 'What would you rather do first - learn new ways to be calmer or new ways to be more comfortable?'

<u>The Structure</u>:

In the above examples two choices are given, each of which, based on information previously gathered are known by the therapist to be potentially inviting, thereby eliciting an **approach response** (meaning to move in the direction of the choices) towards one or other of the options, in the person being offered the choices. The 'Bind' [see Binds] occurs in the sense that whichever choice the person makes it will be in the direction of the suggestions being offered. Therefore, whatever choice is made of the two options proffered fits in with the therapeutic outcome of the person delivering the suggestions, based, of course, on a detailed understanding of the client's expressed desired outcomes.

Arm Levitation (1)

<u>The Pattern</u>:

1) 'Some people find that their arms begin to lift spontaneously in trance. And what's that happening to your arm now!?'

2) 'I don't know whether you will discover your right arm lifting by itself or your left arm moving before you notice it.'

The Structure:

1) A suggestion is made about how 'other people' experience arm levitation in trance, which seeds the idea in the client's mind. This is then followed by the exclaimed question: 'What's that happening to that arm now!?', which suggests that something is being observed to be happening, which itself, can cause the levitation to begin to occur. This is an example of one of Stephen Brooks' methods.

2)

A) **'I don't know'** = only they can know (**Truism**).

B) **Embedded command** = an arm will lift.

C) An arm will lift by itself = they don't have to lift it consciously (= **Conscious Unconscious Double Bind**).

D) 'before you notice it' (= **Double Dissociated Double Bind**).

Contingent Addition (to the above)

'...As you discover something NOW.' [And if the arm doesn't levitate the therapist can follow up with, for example...] Isn't that curious about how maybe you wondered about that heaviness that you may not have noticed until now?'

(The above example is based on a demonstration that Stephen Brooks delivered.)

Arm Levitation (2)

The Pattern:

'There have been times in the past when you've lifted your arm up and thought about it and other times when you just did it without really thinking that much about raising it. In trance sometimes people find that their unconscious mind likes to give them a sign that changes are taking place by letting their arm begin to lift, it may be the lift arm [a pseudo phonological ambiguity for 'left arm'] or the right arm, and the more it lifts the more your unconscious can signal to us that something wonderful is taking place for you. [And... If the arm doesn't lift...] And other people find that their unconscious mind prefers to let those arms rest and relax there in order to show you and me that you are comfortable about making changes without having to do anything about it. And whether your unconscious chooses to let one of those arms lift up now...or whether it just wants those arms to rest and relax where they are as you make the changes the choice is yours – unconsciously of course.'

The Structure:

'There have been times in the past when you've **lifted** your arm **up** and thought about it and other times when you just did it without really thinking that much about **raising** it. In trance sometimes people find that their unconscious mind likes to give them a sign that changes are taking place by letting their **arm begin to lift**, it may be the **lift arm** [pseudo phonological ambiguity for 'left arm'] or the right arm, and the more **it lifts** the more your unconscious can signal to us that something wonderful is taking place for you. [If the arm doesn't lift] And other people find that their unconscious mind prefers to let those arms rest and relax there in order to show you and me that you are comfortable about making changes without having to do anything about it. And whether your unconscious chooses to let one of **those arms lift up now**...or whether it just wants those arms to rest and relax where they are as you make the changes the choice is yours – unconsciously of course.'

Arm Levitation (3) – Richard Bandler Style

Richard Bandler has a very useful way to facilitate arm levitation. It's like a combination of arm 'hovering' and arm catalepsy, but, in my observation, without the rigidity often associated with full arm catalepsy. He lifts the client's arm up for them (!) and then suggests it will remain there (for a while). He then creates resources for change using hypnotherapeutic principles and then suggests that the arm begin to move back towards the client's lap in proportion to the speed at which the changes are being made.

For instance, something like this:

'And in a moment I'm going to lift that left arm up. Here we go (lifts the arm). That's it. You've got it. Just let it rest up here. That's right – like that. Aaaaand – you're unconscious caaaan start to generate new and exquisite ways for you to be able to aaaalways do ABC in better and really...I mean reaaaally ... amazing ways. [At which moment some targeted therapeutic work could occur – followed by perhaps something like this...] And I waaant your unconscious noooow to only let that left arm begin to move back down into your lap at the rate at which IT IS making these change-is happening foooor you!' (Notice the way certain words are emphasised in order to enhance the client's therapeutic reaction to the process.)

Associated Language

[See Association]

Association

Association, as the word suggests, is the phenomenon of being highly involved (associated) in an event (real or imagined).

An example to demonstrate the impact that association has on our senses has been used by Anthony Robbins to good effect. He has a NLP training video which first shows some film of someone <u>observing</u> a group of people enjoying a ride at a roller coaster park, in the distance. Note: The film, then, is first shown from the **dissociated** vantage point of that of an observer watching other people on the ride which is taking place 'over there'. Then, in order to teach the viewer how powerful the same scenario can be when it's experienced from an associated position the observer's perspective is dramatically switched. Note: This time the viewer is placed, in effect, **in a front seat position**, looking at the ride from the vantage point of actually being **in the car** as it races up and down the tracks. And twist and turn it does; first making its way up to the top of the 'mountain' (which increases the sense of height) and then teetering on the summit (building anticipation of what's about to follow) just before it plunges down into the 'ravine' spinning, twisting and turning rapidly this way and that, as the 'other' people involved are screaming wildly. This naturally has the effect of powerfully associating the 'experiencer' to all of the twists and turns the car makes and to the view of the fair ground from '**in here**'. As you can imagine the two experiences are radically different. And very insightful. Often even just reading about it like this has the same sort of result – a switch in perspective.

I'm aware of an NLP Practitioner who once used this principle to explain the difference between Association and Dissociation to a Women's Institute meeting. He did such a good job (perhaps too good!) of building up the participants' involvement in the imaginary roller coaster ride that one of the delegates (an elderly lady) actually fell off of her chair and needed to be taken out of the room to recover from the experience of 'hurtling down the tracks at 90 miles an hour, with your hands tightly gripping the rails of the roller coaster...' (or words to that effect). It was a very powerful example of how association can enable a person to 'get inside' an experience in a very real way.

More often it's used therapeutically to assist clients to link to good, helpful feelings and resources of various kinds. For instance: take a moment to think of a time when you felt really optimistic about something. It can be anything that you felt really optimistic and positive about. Remember where you were, what it was about, what it was like to feel good like this. Now, imagine bringing that experience closer and closer so that you are actually stepping inside that moment right now...so that now you're in the moment, feeling what you're feeling again, seeing what you're seeing now in this moment again, hearing what you're hearing in this moment now again, sensing everything about reliving this optimistic positive moment right now. Being in yourself in your optimistic positivity, here right now. That's right. Really getting inside the experience.

You'll have noticed that the more you allowed yourself to fully enter into the experience – in direct proportion – the more associated you became. This is an example of how by enabling your clients (when necessary) to associate into helpful experiences (real or imagined) it can help them to be in much more conducive states to facilitate 'change work' (a term that we use in Indirect Hypnotherapy to signify the process of therapy to create generative change). You'll also have noticed that the language used in the above example itself switched from **dissociated language** to **associated language** from phrases like: '...what it was like...', to '...feeling what you are feeling'. From: 'remember where you were...', to '...now you are in the moment...'. And: 'what it was about...', to ' feel**ing**... see**ing**... hear**ing**... sens**ing**... reliv**ing**...', etc.

As You Do That...

The Pattern:

1) 'It can be nice to let yourself unwind and as you do that...that helps you do this... you can think about how nice it is to change for the better...'

2) 'Or you can think about how much better your future is now...and as you do that...that helps you do this...you can create better feelings inside...'

3) 'Better feelings that help you to be true to yourself... and as you do that...you can do this... you can relax and just let it all happen...'

4) 'Because it can be nice to just relax and let it all happen...and as you do that...that helps you do this... you can trust your inner self to do what is most helpful, healthful and appropriate to help you in all the best ways...'

5) 'Because changes like this which happen in normal, balanced and harmonious ways are always the best to experience this now...and as you do that...that helps you do this... you can just let it all work for you starting again right now...'

The Structure:

The 'And as you do that...that helps you do this...' pattern can be employed to generate a link (much like a traditional Contingent Suggestion) in which the phrase 'and as you do that...that helps you do this...' is said <u>after the first suggestion</u> has been made and as a result provides the aforementioned link to the follow up suggestion. The fact that the suggestion says '...that helps you do this...' is likely to be more acceptable than, for instance: 'And as you do that...you are compelled to do this...', which will have limited acceptability in clients. Whereas the more liberal phrase '...helps you do this...' is less open to resistance and more readily lends itself to appropriate interpretation and actioning by the client, in ways that suit his or her life circumstances.

1) 'It can be nice to let yourself unwind **and as you do that...that helps you do this**... you can think about how nice it is to change for the better...'

2) 'Or you can think about how much better your future is now...**and as you do that...that helps you do this**...you can create better feelings inside...'

3) 'Better feelings that help you to be true to yourself... **and as you do that...you can do this**... you can relax and just let it all happen...'

4) 'Because it can be nice to just relax and let it all happen...**and as you do that...that helps you do this**... you can trust your inner self to do what is most helpful, healthful and appropriate to help you in all the best ways...'

5) 'Because changes like this which happen in normal, balanced and harmonious ways are always the best to experience this now...**and as you do that...that helps you do this**... you can just let it all work for you starting again right now...'

Attribution Of Emotions (1)

The Pattern:

1) 'Now I know that sometimes you feel restless about this situation and that you want to change it now...'

2) 'I know and you know that you are fed up with being in this rut so now is the time to do something about it...'

3) 'You're getting enthusiastic about this aren't you? And that's really good...'

4) 'You're much happier now...'

5) 'And because you are a calm person you will handle this with ease...'

The Structure:

A simple yet very therapeutic language pattern in which an (to quote Bruce Lee) 'emotional content' is attributed to the client. Generally, to do so, the hypnotherapist would take a noticed emotion and then use that as a point of leverage. There are times when a therapist can elicit emotional states which have not been observed, as demonstrated in example (3) below.

Attribution Of Emotions (2): Observed Emotions Attributed To The Client (To Create Leverage)

1) 'Now I know that sometimes you feel <u>restless</u> about this situation and that you want to change it now...'

2) 'I know and you know that you are <u>fed up</u> with being in this rut so now is the time to do something about it...'

3) 'You're getting <u>enthusiastic</u> about this aren't you? And that's really good...'

4) 'You're much <u>happier</u> now...'

5) 'And because you are a <u>calm</u> person you will handle this with ease...'

Attribution Of Emotions (3): Unobserved Emotions Attributed To The Client (In Order To Help Elicit Them For The Client)

'And, you know, you are an amazing person. If I were to mention the emotion of happiness you'd understand what I meant by it. If I were to mention joy, which is very similar to happiness, you'd understand what I mean. And this means that at some level within, you already understand what happiness and joy... and many other positive emotions are like... because in order to be able to understand what they mean you have to have an internal understanding of them. We need to understand <u>what</u> something is... in order to <u>know</u> what it is. Which means that you already have them within you. You know what they are <u>because</u>

you have an <u>inner</u> <u>representation</u> of them in order to let you know that you know what they are. And, if you thought about it for a few more moments you could probably even begin to notice how you know what the difference is for you between happiness and joy. You could think about - how does happiness feel? And also - how does joy feel? Because you already have them inside! And I'm going to ask your powerful unconscious mind to begin to let you experience more of these feelings which you already understand deeply in a profound way. After all, <u>they</u> <u>are</u> <u>already</u> inside so it seems to me that you may as well experience them consciously too. And I wonder, how many other positive emotions are there which you already unconsciously have within that you will start to notice more and more of at a conscious level too which your unconscious mind is even now starting to get ready for you to experience them?'

This example uses a layered approach to introduce, first of all, the concepts of happiness and joy. It then gains agreement by stating that 'you'd understand what I meant...' (by the terms 'joy and 'happiness'). This point of reference is then linked with a Complex Equivalence, using the words, 'which means that' in order to reinforce a Truism that follows, and that is, that at some level, the client already has some level of understanding of what those emotions are like (even if they don't experience them often). However, because they already have an inner understanding, and because with hypnotherapy much of the work takes place on an inner level too, the frame is set to ask the client's unconscious mind to let them begin to experience more of these feelings, which '<u>you</u> <u>already understand deeply</u> in a profound way.' By working at this level it side-steps any conscious resistance as to whether or not the client can feel happy or joyous. The phrase: 'After all, they are already inside so it seems to me that you may as well experience them consciously too', is the kind of approach that Dr. Richard Bandler employs. It's very effective. The words 'after all' and 'they are already', changes the frame of reference for the client from one of (previously) trying to 'work up' (probably with difficulty) positive emotions into his/her life to one in which, even in a casual manner, they already have those emotions available and since they already do, then they 'may as well' experience them consciously 'too'. This implies that they already experience them within, even if purely at the level of having the natural range of human emotions that everyone else has available to them too. So, the emotions are 'already inside'. Then, from this reference point, things are expanded upon even more to include 'many other positive emotions' that the client will start to notice at a conscious level 'more and more'. The use of the words 'more and more' also allows for things to happen in their own good time. This helps to deal with any sense of failure that might occur in the client's reasoning if he/she doesn't immediately notice more of the positive emotions (although it's likely that they'll actually be feeling a change already).

So by utilising the Attribution of Emotions pattern in this way it's possible for the therapist to start to help the client to begin to therapeutically elicit the attributed emotions.

Auditory Coordinates

Developing an awareness of subjective Auditory Coordinates can support the client in the process of 'tuning into' helpful sounds and/or help to alter how the client relates to unwanted subjective auditory experiences.

Example: 'And when you say you hear a nice voice – where specifically is that nice voice?'

Avoidance Binds

The Pattern:

1) 'Would you like to do your homework now or after I've given you your pocket money (this example is also sometimes known as a bribe ☺).'

2) 'Are you going to make that presentation before or after you take your holiday in France?'

3) 'When do you think is the best time to go about asserting yourself and letting him know that that behaviour is unacceptable...before our second or third coaching session together?'

4) 'What do you think is the best way to do this? Before you become a non-smoker or afterwards when you're enjoying all of that extra money and good health?'

The Structure:

In the above examples choices are given, one of which may be less favourable (but required) while the other(s) is likely to be more desired (perhaps even considered to be something of a **reward**). Therefore, while there is likely to be a factor of avoidance in one of the presented choices, by introducing an element of 'reward' into the equation too, the client then more easily accepts the premise that the 'less desirable' task will take place (because it's 'wrapped up in' the desired aspect of the Bind). The 'Bind' [see Binds] occurs, for instance, in that by choosing to have the pocket money before or after completing the homework the person involved is, by implication, accepting to do his/her homework. Whichever choice he/she makes, it's in the direction of the required outcome.

B

Become

The Pattern:

1) 'And as you continue to become the fullest positive expression of yourself in every good and every wonderful way...'

2) 'While your unconscious mind helps you to become the vibrant and creative person that you really already are...'

3) 'It's a wonderful thing to start to become more relaxed about life...'

4) 'Some people find that they become non-smokers just by relaxing the changes to happen...I wonder how you will find that you are becoming a happy healthy non-smoker now?...'

The Structure:

Become is a useful word. It implies progressive action, forward movement, a change of direction towards a desired outcome.

1) 'And as you continue to **become** the fullest positive expression of yourself in every good and every wonderful way...'

2) 'While your unconscious mind helps you to **become** the vibrant and creative person that you really already are...'

3) 'It's a wonderful thing to start to **become** more relaxed about life...'

4) 'Some people find that they **become** non-smokers just by **relaxing the changes to happen**... I wonder how you will find that you are **becoming** a happy healthy non-smoker now?...'

[see also: Relaxing the Changes to Happen]

Best Guess

This is a very useful technique that I learnt from Ian Berry of NLP Northeast, when I was completing my NLP Master Practitioner training. He demonstrated how to help a person move from a position of limited resourcefulness to solution-focussed thinking with the use of the words Best Guess. Here's an example:

Client: 'This is a really difficult decision.'

Therapist: 'What do you think you should do first?'

Client: 'I don't know?'

Therapist: 'Do you have any idea?'

Client: 'No.'

Therapist: 'Well okay – what's your best guess instead then?'

Since first learning this method I've found that it can be really useful (and very subtle) to employ to gently encourage clients to change perspective from narrow thinking to more resourceful frames of reference. The client doesn't feel like he/she is having to commit to a specific course of action, after all, he/she is only offering a 'best guess'. Nevertheless, once they've moved out of their self-imposed limitation what naturally follows is more progressive thinking. And the 'best guess' often turns into a good idea.

A couple of variations which work on the same principle are in the form of the examples given immediately below, which are of the type that I saw Anthony Robbins use during one of his seminars. The moment went something like this:

Participant: 'I can't think of a better way to do it.'

Anthony Robbins: 'I know you can't – but if you could what would it be?'

Participant: 'I expect it would be like…'

Rather than create resistance and challenge the seminar participant's perceptions about what could take place Anthony instead met her at 'her level' and then helped her to side step her own 'resistance' and move directly to a solution. Another similar approach could be to respond by saying: 'I know you don't but if you did…'.

Better Ways Than That / Comparative Pattern

The Pattern:

1) '...And you used to do ABC while feeling XYZ but now that your unconscious mind is helping you can generate better ways than that...'

2) 'It's not important what used to happen because now you have better ways than that to do it...'

3) 'Why bother wasting time thinking those same old thoughts again? You've spent enough time going over them already. Since things are changing and you now know that there are better ways than that to spend your time...how about doing more of the things that make you feel good about yourself more often...'

The Structure:

1) '...And you used to do ABC while feeling XYZ but now that your unconscious mind is helping you can generate **better ways than that**...'

2) 'It's not important what used to happen because now you have **better ways than that** to do it...'

3) 'Why bother wasting time thinking those same old thoughts again? You've spent enough time going over them already. Since things are changing and you now know that there are **better ways than that** to spend your time...how about doing more of the things that make you feel good about yourself more often...'

This pattern is known as a Comparative Pattern in which a less empowering response is measured against a preferred choice (which may or may not be known consciously to the client). And the preferred response is, by intonation as well as implication, the Desired Direction that the client wants to move towards and which the therapist is helping them move toward, by utilising the Better Ways Than That pattern. The old response, by comparison becomes less desirable.

Variations include: 1) Other ways than that, 2) Different ways than those, etc.

Bind / Simple Bind

The Pattern:

1) 'Would you like to sit in this chair or that chair to go into a trance?'

2) 'Would you like to go into a trance now or in a moment?'

3) 'Would you like to go into trance with your eyes open or closed?'

4) 'How do you prefer to go into a trance now, while sitting down or lying down?'

The Structure:

Milton often employed the Bind technique (also known as a Simple Bind). In these examples each of the above suggestions implies that the client has some choice in the matter (and they do – albeit very limited).　While the presupposition inherent within all of the suggestions is that the client will **go into a trance** (Which is the desired outcome. It doesn't really matter whether they go into trance, sitting or lying down, for instance.　The 'choice' element, in a sense, is something of a 'smoke screen' which is used to help offer the suggestion in an indirect manner.).　A distinguishing factor of a Bind, which is to be differentiated from other forms of Binds, is that the choice can be made by the client at a conscious level.　This means that the client can choose to go into trance with their eyes open **or** eyes closed for instance (it's the going into trance – not so much how they go there – which is the Bind part of the pattern). Sales people often use Binds when seeking to persuade others to buy from them.

Here are the same examples – with the desired outcome highlighted:

1) 'Would you like to sit in this chair or that chair to **go into a trance**?'

2) 'Would you like to **go into a trance** now or in a moment?'

3) 'Would you like to **go into trance** with your eyes open or closed?'

4) 'How do you prefer to **go into a trance** now, while sitting down or lying down?'

<u>Binding A Suggestion</u>

To further identify the pattern and structure of binds here below are some non-bound phrases, which are then turned into binds for your reference.

Non-bound phrase:

'What will you do next about the dog and the car?'

Bound phrase:

'Will you wash the car next or walk the dog first?'

The difference is that in the first example the person concerned could more easily just respond by saying 'nothing'. However, in the second example they are, in effect, given a 'choice' between two desired courses of action. They could of course still say 'neither', but it's less likely to happen because of the way the situation's been presented.

Biofeedback Strategy

The Biofeedback strategy is employed by commenting on a client's ongoing experience in order to reinforce the experience.

<u>The Pattern</u>:

1) 'And as you listen to my voice your eyelids are beginning to close.'

2) 'As you're sitting here your breathing is becoming more relaxed.'

3) 'The muscles in your forehead are beginning to loosen up quite nicely...I wonder where that relaxation will spread to next?'

The Structure:

The golden rule of the Biofeedback Strategy is that 'you should never refer to an event unless it's actually happening'. For instance, it wouldn't be a good idea, in most cases, to say 'your eyes are starting to close' unless you actually observed that happening. If you said they were when they weren't it could break rapport with your client and be counter-productive. However, as you comment on the trance phenomena that you observe developing, by feeding your observations back to your client, it creates a biofeedback loop which most likely results in the client generating more hypnotic phenomena.

1) 'And as you listen to my voice **your eyelids are beginning to close**.'

2) 'As you're sitting here **your breathing is becoming more relaxed**.'

3) 'The **muscles in your forehead are beginning to loosen up** quite nicely...I wonder where **that sensation will spread** to next?' (This example includes an indirect suggestion that more of the same will follow.)

'Brooks Rule'

I remember hearing Stephen Brooks suggest that 'you should never ask a question to which you don't already know the answer', or words to that effect. While, in real life, in all circumstances, this may prove to be impossible to accomplish, as a heuristic 'rule', which is no doubt what he meant, it's a useful principle to remember during therapy and coaching sessions.

Building Excitement And Expectations

The Pattern:

1) 'In a moment I'm going to tell you something really exciting.'

2) 'Soon you'll discover a whole new way of using language which will be really useful for you.'

3) 'By this time tomorrow you'll be surprised by how many new things you've learned.'

4) 'People say it's the best seminar ever. Just you wait and see.'

The Structure:

In essence this pattern is probably one that everyone's used at sometime or other, just, perhaps, without knowing the 'label' that goes with it. However, by having knowledge of the label/pattern it provides us with the potential for strategic choice of when and how to utilise it. And I expect you'll be really impressed by the good things that happen as you start to choose to use it more often (☺).

This pattern is also known as…

Building Response Potential

It's useful to remember that it can often be therapeutically apt to Build Response Potential in your clients before utilising a particular strategy. For instance, before utilising anchors with them it may be helpful to build their response potential by sharing examples of other clients that you've helped with anchoring techniques; including, perhaps, <u>what</u> you did together and specifically <u>why</u> it benefited them. This often helps to generate a positive expectancy towards the work you're doing together.

[See also Indirect Framing.]

But Don't

<u>The Pattern</u>:

1) Therapist: 'That's it...and you can enjoy this trance...but don't go all the way down...just go to the level that's most comfortable for you here today.'

2) Therapist: 'Okay. Now that you have all those new ideas you have a lot more scope about what to do next. But don't do everything all at once. Take each stage, one at a time.'

3) Therapist: '...well done! It's really good to discover...is it not...just how many resources you have created...but don't try to consciously force yourself to use them....just let your unconscious mind generate them in better ways than that for you now...'

<u>The Structure</u>:

The words 'but don't' seem to limit the receiver's choice. However, really, they actually suggest more choice. For instance, the suggestion: 'That's right, go into the deepest trance possible', actually itself implies limitation. Because when the client reaches 'the deepest level' that means that there is no 'deeper' place to go. Whereas: 'But don't go all the way down…' implies that however deeply they go into trance there will always be 'deeper' levels to explore.

1) Therapist: 'That's it…and you can enjoy this trance…**but don't** go all the way down…just go to the level that is most comfortable for you here today.'

2) Therapist: 'Okay. Now that you have all those new ideas you have a lot more scope about what to do next. **But don't** do everything all at once. Take each stage, one at a time.'

This example can be used to help encourage a client to start to take measurable (appropriate) action. If the idea of initiating action appears 'daunting' to the client, the suggestion of making major change could be counter productive. However, by suggesting that the client has all the ideas he/she needs, **but** that he/she is only to action them in a measured way it will make the proposition more likely to be accepted.

3) Therapist: '…well done! It's really good to discover…**is it not**…just how many resources you have created…**but don't** try to consciously force yourself to use them….just let your unconscious

mind generate them in **better ways than that for you now...'**

This example is one in which the therapist, in effect, is suggesting that the client needn't consciously try to force a solution into existence, but rather that he/she should let the more powerful unconscious mind do it for them (it also therefore contains elements of a Conscious Unconscious Double Bind within it – plus the Better Ways Than That pattern, along with a Tag Question).

C

Calibration / Dialling

Calibration is an expression that's been utilised from the engineering world in order to measure a client's affective response/reaction to a variety of situations. By introducing the concept of the ten-point calibration scale to a client (1 being a very low affective response – 10 being a very high one) this has the advantage of turning something that is 'beyond measurement' into something that's quantifiable. This in turn immediately gives the therapist a means of introducing change to the 'affective system.' In essence, what often happens is that the therapist will calibrate by asking: 'On a scale between 1 to 10, whereabouts is that feeling for you now?' Then based on the client's self-assessment, the therapist can enter into a course of changework with the client and at various points, have the client re-assess their 'level'. This itself implies that movement will occur. In so doing, by regularly referencing the client's affective response level, in relationship to the therapy taking place, incremental changes can be generated, which helps the client to reduce an unwanted response (or heighten a preferred affective response).

For instance:

Client: '...and every time I think of ABC I get a sick feeling in the pit of my stomach.'

Therapist: 'On a scale of 1 – 10 what level would you say that feeling is?'

Client: 'Oh – it's about an 8 or a 9.'

Therapist: 'About an 8 or a 9.'

The therapist then proceeds to utilise his or her skills to help the client alter his or her reactions. At appropriate moments the therapist may ask:

Therapist: 'Okay – well done. When you try and get that unwanted feeling that you used to have in the past, how little of it can you notice now?'

Client: 'Less than before. It's about a 3 or a 4.'

And so on. The act of calibration is an indirect means of introducing the concept of graduated change into a, hitherto, stuck system. The units of measurement imply change in a way that a client can accept. Sometimes the concept of making change can seem 'too big' for a client to contemplate; whereas, by transforming the affective response's relationship to a ten point scale - change can take place, in realistic and measurable ways.

Dialling, which is the same principle as above, in a slightly different form, is often used to help increase a client's desired response to a given situation. In effect, the therapist will introduce the concept of a dial (again with a 10 point scale on it) and <u>create a relationship</u> between the imagined dial and a desired (by the client) response.

For instance: in a situation in which a client feels confident socially but lacking in confidence at work the therapist could utilise Dialling in the following way:

Therapist: 'That's right. You do know how to feel confident when you're out with your friends. Which means that you already know what confidence feels like and that you find that you naturally experience it quite often. Which means that all we need to ask your unconscious mind to do for you now is turn your natural confidence up when you're at work too. It's that simple! Now – I know that you know that your unconscious knows what a dial looks like. In fact it knows so well that you don't even have to consciously recall one now. Maybe with the numbers 1 to 10 around this dial. And your unconscious knows already how easy it is to turn that dial up to a level that lets you feel good when you're out with your friends. It just happens all by itself. Does it not? That confidence just gets turned up to a good level without you having to think about it. And I'd like to thank your unconscious for being so helpful and reliable for doing this for you so often already. And, because you're unconscious is so resourceful like this I'd like to invite your unconscious mind to turn that confidence dial up in the same kind of way, when you're at work, now and in the future. So that you can experience the same kind of helpful confidence just as easily as you already know that you know how to do this. You don't even have to consciously notice what changes your unconscious self is making right now and to what good level that confidence dial is being set, for you, at work, now. Your inner self knows and that's a nice way to change...for the best...work is yet to come...on and feel good...'

And so forth, with the theme being followed throughout the trance, interspersed with other examples of how change can take place and suggestions aimed to help the client develop more self-esteem, for instance.

You can, of course, depending on your client, be more **direct**: 'Okay, so that confidence dial is already at a 5. That's good. And I'm going to ask you inner self now to turn it up a bit further. First to a 6. Not too fast, do it in your own time. Just nod to me when it's starting to happen. [Nod.] Great! You've got it. Now...of course...we're not going to turn it all the way up today...but let's turn it up to an 8, if <u>that is okay</u>. Is that okay too? [Nod.] Good, okay, just let your inner self turn it up, turn it up to an 8. And notice even more of those good feelings. And let me know again when you sense that this is starting to happen. [Nod.] Thanks. And as you do that...'

Cartesian Logic

<u>Client statement</u>:

'I really fancy Sally but I don't know if she'll go out with me. So I'm afraid to ask her out.'

1)

Theorem: 'What would happen if you did?'

Client: 'I would know if she'd go out with me.'

2)

Inverse: 'What would happen if you didn't?'

Client: 'I would still be unsure.'

3)

Converse: 'What won't happen if you did?'

Client: 'I won't be unsure any more.'

4)

Non mirror image reverse: 'What won't happen if you didn't?'

Client: 'I won't know whether she will or won't if I don't.'

The Cartesian Logic questions are useful for helping clients to consider all of the possible ramifications to a course of action. If the client's decisions to each response all lead to the same overall conclusion, then the 'logic' of the response the model says can be held to be reliable.

Cause And Effect

The Cause and Effect language pattern is derived from Bandler and Grinder's Milton Model, which is itself based on the Indirect Hypnosis Language patterns developed and utilised by Dr. Milton Erickson.

The Pattern:

1) 'Listening to me will make you relax more...'

2) 'Breathing slowly can help you make changes...'

3) 'Being curious can activate your unconscious...'

4) 'When I click my fingers you will relax more into trance...'

The Structure:

You'll notice in the above examples that listening, breathing, being curious and the clicking of fingers are the 'cause', which can generate the effects of, relaxation, changes, activation of unconscious resources and more...trance. [See also Compound Suggestion].

Here's an example of some multiple Cause and Effect suggestions delivered in the kind of way they could easily be utilised in a therapy session:

'That's right. And as your eyes are closing [cause] you can [effect] begin to start to experience more of your experience. So that with each sound of the gentle music you hear [cause] you will continue to [effect] enjoy relaxing. Now, in a moment, when I click my fingers [cause] your unconscious mind can [effect] consider a new alternative that works for you ecologically, in your personal and private life.'

Another useful cause and effect phrase to remember is: '...will make...'.

...and so on.

Certain

The Pattern:

There is a certain word that indirect hypnotherapists often employ which can allude to a wide variety of possible meanings. Here are some examples of how the word 'certain' can be utilised in therapy:

The Structure:

1) 'There is a **certain** helpful skill that you have which you may not have used for a while, or perhaps even never, **yet**, but which can begin to become available to you. I wonder if you even consciously know what it is **yet**?'

2) 'On a **certain** day, perhaps within a month or even sooner you will notice...'

3) 'There is a **certain** positive feeling which you can become aware of...'

4) 'It's not about taking years of consideration and being absolutely specific to the nth degree, sometimes it's just nice to get a **certain** overall new idea about how different things could be...'

Chaining Modal Operators

Chaining is a method whereby the Modal Operator language patterns are 'chained' together to create powerful suggestions. You can start with Modal Operators of Necessity and lead into Modal Operators of Possibility. Like this:

1) 'You said that you feel that you must [necessity] do this right away and since there is nothing to stop you, you know that you can [possibility] get on with it right now.'

2) 'If you should [necessity] happen to send that application in, what will you be able to [possibility] do when it is accepted?'

Or, conversely you can lead with possibility into necessity, like this:

1) 'You said that you thought you could [possibility] phone by tomorrow. Some people might say that you shouldn't [necessity] let an opportunity like that pass by. What do you think?'

2) 'I agree. Anything is possible [possibility] now that you have started to take responsibility for your own decisions. What do you think you ought [necessity] to take action on first?'

<u>Multiple chaining between Modal Operators</u>:

'You know that you have [necessity] to do something right away because things will deteriorate if you don't. Out of these options, which one must [necessity] you handle first, that is possible [possibility] to start with? And since you can [possibility] begin to deal with that and because there are only one or two others that must [necessity] follow, and because you have more time, which means you are able [possibility] to allow yourself to focus on this for a while, don't you think you ought [necessity] to do yourself a favour and sort the whole thing out bit by bit starting now?!'

Challenge (Sleight Of Mouth)

Sleight of Mouth principles were first delineated by Robert Dilts as he himself modelled Richard Bandler's language patterns. Additional contributions have been made by Steve and Connirae Andreas. A number of Sleight of Mouth patterns now exist, which are covered in this book. Sleight of Mouth patterns are utilised to unravel and in the process depotentiate adverse Complex Equivalence and/or Cause and Effect statements made by the client. [See: Analogy, Another Outcome, Apply To Self, Challenge, Change Of Reference Frame Size, Chunk Size, Consequences, Counter Example, Hierarchy Of Criteria, Intention, Meta Frame, Model Of The World, Reality Strategy, Redefine, Switch Referential Index.] In this example the principle of Challenge is employed.

<u>Cause and Effect Example</u>:

Client: 'Every time I go to that club it makes me get angry.'

'(A) Every time I go to that club (B) it makes me get angry'.

Therapist (A): 'Every time?'
Therapist (A): 'How can you be sure it's only that club?'
Therapist (B): 'Are you sure it's anger – could it be frustration?'
Therapist (A/B): 'Is it possible that it isn't really every time? After all why would you ever go there if that's all that ever happened? And if it isn't always anger that must mean that you sometimes also feel other feelings as well.'

Complex Equivalence Example:

'I didn't go to Eton that means I'll never succeed.'

'(A) I didn't go to Eton (B) that means I'll never succeed.'

Hypnotherapist (A): 'Maybe it's a good thing that you didn't go to Eton.'

Hypnotherapist (B): 'Oh – so you're psychic too. You've already seen your own future. If you're that psychic why haven't you won the lottery yet?'

Hypnotherapist (A/B): 'But you did go to Winchester, like Churchill and he succeeded'. Client: 'But I'm not a Sir Winston Churchill'. Therapist: 'Neither was he until after he'd gone to Winchester and then subsequently succeeded at many things. And they told him he would fail too. But he didn't!'

Challenging

Basic 'challenging' means that when you notice inconsistencies in what your client is saying, or how they're responding, it can be useful to challenge the inconsistencies. I remember once myself when I was on my first training course as a trainee counsellor, during a group work session (which took place with all of the students sitting in a circle, overseen by the tutors, and then, one by one, but in no particular order, we would each 'open up' to discuss personal issues, during which we would each receive counselling from the rest of the group, group-member by group-member, also in no fixed sequence, as the conversation flowed) how I (and others) experienced a very powerful example of the therapeutic benefits of appropriate and tactful challenging. I noticed that one group member, while explaining how her philandering father had brought lots of pain into the family home, incongruently smiled as she explained, in minutiae, all of the unpleasant details to the rest of the group. At that stage in my life I'd only read some NLP books and listened to some Anthony Robbins tape sets, but I noticed the obvious incongruity between what she was explaining and her facial expressions. So I chose my moment and then interjected, saying something along the lines of: 'Heather (not her real name) I just noticed that every time you mentioned how painful those experiences were for you and your family and how many problems your dad had caused, you actually smiled each time you told us about them. The smile just didn't seem to fit with what you were saying…'. 'Heather' stopped in her tracks and was quiet for quite a while, thinking about the state of affairs… and then she began to honestly deal with her feelings relating to the situation, which she said, after consideration, she felt the smile had been used to mask. Her demeanour altered rapidly as she really began to sort out the emotional content, which she had, hitherto, it seemed, been avoiding. It was a very powerful moment for her - and for us. My intention to help her really deal with the issue she was presenting rather than 'role play' her way around it was on the mark and she benefited a lot from that moment and during the rest of the session.

Change Of Place Verbs

<u>The Pattern</u>:

1) 'When you start to move forward some more you'll arrive at your outcome before you know it.'

2) 'Come on – you can do it – really notice how much better things will be...'

3) 'And as you enter into that agreement with your inner self that you will continue to be true to yourself...'

4) 'As you shift your expectations and reach a better way of thinking...'

5) 'That's it. You can leave all of that old stuff behind and step into a new and brighter future.'

6) 'When will you first go and talk to her about this?'

7) 'And as those old feelings finally depart for good...'

8) 'It's always a good thing to land up being successful like you are doing...'

<u>The Structure</u>:

Words are used which suggest a change of place:
1) 'When you start to <u>move</u> forward some more you'll <u>arrive</u> at your outcome before you know it.'

2) '<u>Come</u> on – you can do it – really notice how much better things will be...'

3) 'And as you <u>enter</u> into that agreement with your inner self that you will continue to be true to yourself...'

4) 'As you <u>shift</u> your expectations and <u>reach</u> a better way of thinking...'

5) 'That's it. You can <u>leave</u> all of that old stuff behind and <u>step into</u> a new and brighter future.'

6) 'When will you first <u>go</u> and talk to her about this?'

7) 'And as those old feelings finally <u>depart</u> for good...'

8) 'It's always a good thing to <u>land up</u> being successful like you are doing...'

Change Of Reference Frame Size (Sleight Of Mouth)

Sleight of Mouth principles were first delineated by Robert Dilts as he himself modelled Richard Bandler's language patterns. Additional contributions have been made by Steve and Connirae Andreas. A number of Sleight of Mouth patterns now exist, which are covered in this book. Sleight of Mouth patterns are utilised to unravel and in the process depotentiate adverse Complex Equivalence and/or Cause and Effect statements made by the client. [See: Analogy, Another Outcome, Apply To Self, Challenge, Change Of Reference Frame Size, Chunk Size, Consequences, Counter Example, Hierarchy Of Criteria, Intention, Meta Frame, Model Of The World, Reality Strategy,

Redefine, Switch Referential Index.] In this example the principle of Change Of Reference Frame Size is employed.

<u>The Pattern</u>:

1)

Client: 'And that's the way it's always been in my life. There's no hope.'

Therapist: 'Pardon me, I was just thinking about how expressive you are. Many people would love to be as expressive as you. It would open up so many other possibilities for them. I wonder how you can use your range of self-expression constructively like that?'

2)

Client: 'I'm always confused.'

Therapist: 'That must be confusing. I wonder have you ever thought that you'd prefer to feel more certain?'

Client: 'Yes…of course I would!'

3)

Client: 'I'm beyond help. I don't even know why I saw the other therapists or why I've come to see you today.'

Therapist: 'Well, if you don't know, I don't. However, what do you think the reason might have been?'

4)

Client: 'You can't trust anyone these days!'

Therapist: 'Can you really trust yourself when you say that? Or are you responding more emotionally and less accurately?'

5)

Question: 'Okay then, just what can my country do for me?'

President Kennedy: 'Don't ask, 'what can my country do for me?' but rather ask 'what can I do for my country?'!'

<u>The Structure</u>:

1)

Client: 'And that's the way <u>it's always been</u> in my life. There's <u>no hope</u>.'

Therapist: 'Pardon me, I was just thinking about how <u>expressive</u> you are. Many people would <u>love to be as expressive as you</u>. It would <u>open up</u> so many <u>other possibilities</u> for them. I wonder how <u>you can use</u> your range of <u>self-expression constructively</u> like that?'

A key to working with Change of Reference Frame Size: notice what the client isn't currently consciously aware of.

In this first example the client is expressing hopelessness. The therapist notices a Truism (the client's ability to be expressive, and mentions it, thereby changing the frame's reference size) and side-steps the defeatist attitude and instead draws upon the Truism of expressiveness. The therapist then mentions how other people would love to be more expressive (a Truism for many people – which also changes the frame again from the focus being on the client to other people's desire for more of what the client already has) and then the therapist rhetorically asks how the client could use their self-expression (which itself is like self-esteem – and is itself a change of frame again) constructively (which is a total turn around from the original 'no hope' statement).

2)

Client: 'I'm <u>always confused</u>.'

Therapist: 'That must be confusing. I wonder have you ever thought that you'd prefer to <u>feel more certain</u>?'

Client: 'Yes...of course I would!'

The client expresses confusion. The therapist, in this example, uses the same measurement criteria (confusion) back on the client's statement to loosen things up a bit (while paradoxically meeting the client in their model of the world – confusion – albeit from a different vantage point). The therapist then asks a question, the answer of which was implied in the client's opening statement: '...have you ever thought that you'd prefer to feel more certain?'. The answer is, as in this example, likely to be in the affirmative (which also amounts to a change of reference frame size).

3)

Client: 'I'm beyond help. I don't even know why I saw the other therapists or why I've come to see you today.'

Therapist: 'Well, if you don't know, I don't. However, what do you think the reason might have been?'

In this example the therapist meets the client in his/her second stated reference frame 'I don't even know why...' and then helps the client to change perspective by asking: '...what do you think the answer might have been?'. This in turn, indirectly, also assists the client to stop thinking about being 'beyond help' and about solutions instead, without the client's statement ever having been directly challenged or addressed by the therapist.

4)

Client: 'You can't trust anyone these days!'

Therapist: 'Can you really trust yourself when you say that? Or are you responding more emotionally and less accurately?'

Again, in this example the therapist utilises the client's own measurement criteria (distrust) and applies it to the client's own statement. The therapist then offers a likely alternative interpretation to why the client is responding so globally in attributing untrustworthiness to everyone, and that alternative is to do with emotion (this changes the frame size from other people's trustworthiness to the client's emotionally pessimistic directed thinking). Implicitly a solution is suggested by the term 'less accurately'. That's because the term 'less accurately' suggests that if the client reduces his/her negative emotional content he/she will discover a more accurate interpretation about the situation (which also helps to shift the reference frame towards outcomes) and therein rests a key to a solution-focussed result.

5)

'Okay then, just what can my country <u>do for me</u>?'

'Don't ask 'what can my country do for me?' <u>but rather ask</u> 'what can I <u>do for my country?</u>'!'

A great John F. Kennedy example of changing the frame size, from one of 'get' to one of 'give'. From self (small Self) to others. Whether or not anyone ever actually asked him that question ('What can my country do for me?') is a moot point. The fact that he raised it himself in one frame and then changed the frame size as magically as he did – and a nation's perspective in the process - is a wonderful example of this approach.

Change Of State Verbs

<u>The Pattern</u>:

1) 'And as you discover yourself becoming more and more successful...'

2) 'Now and in the future as you start to change the way you feel...'

3) 'I really like it when you smile like that, a certain transformation happens and your energy rises in a really nice way.'

4) 'When you alter the way you feel...'

5) 'Feelings are just energy and your inner self can convert energy and use it in many ways. When will you first notice that that anger is being converted into determination?'

6) 'Adjust your thinking for just a moment or two and consider...'

7) 'And as you amend your responses to be the kind of responses and feelings that you choose to have instead of just letting them happen to you...'

8) 'It's not about a massive turn around in one 'giant leap'. You can modify things, a bit at a time, and see how soon you start to notice the difference...'

The Structure:

In all of these examples words are used which themselves convey the meaning of a change of state taking place:

1) 'And as you discover yourself <u>becoming</u> more and more successful...'

2) 'Now and in the future as you start to <u>change</u> the way you feel...'

3) 'I really like it when you smile like that, a certain <u>transformation</u> happens and your energy rises in a really nice way.'

4) 'When you <u>alter</u> the way you feel...'

5) 'Feelings are just energy and your inner self can <u>convert</u> energy and use it in many ways. When will you first notice that that anger is being <u>converted</u> into determination?'

6) '<u>Adjust</u> your thinking for just a moment or two and consider...'

7) 'And as you <u>amend</u> your responses to be the kind of responses and feelings that you choose to have instead of just letting them happen to you...'

8) 'It's not about a massive turn around in one 'giant leap'. You can <u>modify</u> things, a bit at a time, and see how soon you start to notice the difference...'

Change Of Time Verbs And Adverbs

<u>The Pattern</u>:

1) 'You'll be surprised by how you stop doing that and start doing this instead...'

2) 'When you begin to take some time for yourself...'

3) 'You already know at least two better ways of doing this. I wonder how many more you can begin to think about...'

4) 'Okay. So let's continue with this idea some more...'

5) 'So, this means that whereas previously you used to do ABC you will instead proceed to do XYZ even though you have yet to know how exactly you will do this...'

6) 'Making changes can be easy. We don't have to spend years trying to find a 'root cause' anymore. We can instead start to make changes in the present that can continue right into the future. The past is the past and it no longer exists. If a person drove a car while continuously looking in the rear view mirror they'd soon crash. It's better to glance back now and again, while keeping your eyes focussed on what's taking place in front of you. That way you can proceed safely in the right direction.'

The Structure:

Temporal words are used to suggest a change of reference in relation to time:

1) 'You'll be surprised by how you <u>stop</u> doing that and <u>start</u> doing this instead...'

2) 'When you <u>begin</u> to take some time for yourself...'

3) 'You <u>already</u> know at least two better ways of doing this. I wonder how many more you can <u>begin</u> to think about...'

4) 'Okay. So let's <u>continue</u> with this idea some more...'

5) 'So, this means that whereas <u>previously</u> you used to do ABC you will instead <u>proceed</u> to do XYZ even though you have <u>yet</u> to know how exactly you will do this...'

6) 'Making changes can be easy. We don't have to spend years trying to find a 'root cause' <u>anymore</u>. We can instead <u>start</u> to make changes in the present that can <u>continue</u> right into the future. The past is the past and it no longer exists. If a person drove a car while continuously looking in the rear view mirror they'd soon crash. It's better to glance back now and again to learn from what's behind, while keeping your eyes focussed on what's taking place in front of you. That way you can <u>proceed</u> safely and in the right direction.'

Change Work

A generic expression that Indirect Hypnotherapists and NLP exponents apply to the work that we do.

Characterisations

<u>The Pattern</u>:

1) 'And as you are dynamic and creative you'll notice more and more...'

2) 'Now that you are an energised person you'll feel more and more...'

3) 'Your natural assertiveness means that you will be able to...'

4) 'Because you are tough by nature you can crack through this challenge with ease...'

5) 'It's because you are compassionate that you want to do something to help...'

6) 'Your natural empathy will help make the difference.'

7) 'Wouldn't it be great if everyone was as humorous as you?'

8) 'That's good. You're curious by nature.'

9) 'He's just a greedy so and so...'

10) 'He's so kind and so caring...'

The Structure:

The Characterisations pattern attributes characteristics that are assumed to be identified with the object (or client) in an enduring way. It's as if the attributed aspects are equated to being a factor of the object (or client). In fact, the aspects could even be deemed (in this context) to be a part of the object's (or client's) identity.

1) 'And as you are <u>dynamic</u> and <u>creative</u> you'll notice more and more...'

The 'dynamic' and 'creative' elements are mentioned in a way that helps to reinforce the client's positive beliefs about him/herself.

2) 'Now that you are an <u>energised</u> person you'll feel more and more...'

This implies that the person is 'now' an 'energised' person, and that this energised element of their personality, in the right contexts, is an intrinsic part of their nature. It's important to frame suggestions well in order to make them context specific. The above suggestion, and others like it would best be set in a framework that is clear regarding what type of specific situations the client will find himself/herself 'energised' in (or whatever the characteristic is that's being attributed).

3) 'Your natural <u>assertiveness</u> means that you will be able to...'

This presupposes that the client is naturally assertive and that this assertiveness is an enduring facet of 'who they are' and can be called upon.
4) 'Because you are <u>tough</u> by nature you can crack through this challenge with ease...'

Suggestions are offered which are designed to elicit the client's 'tough' nature to help them handle a challenge.

5) 'It's because you are <u>compassionate</u> that you want to do something to help...'

Here a reason is being offered for why a client wants 'to do something to help', and that is because they are 'compassionate'.

6) 'Your natural <u>empathy</u> will help make the difference.'

The client is empathic.

7) 'Wouldn't it be great if everyone was as <u>humorous</u> as you?'

The client is humorous.

8) 'That's good. You're <u>curious</u> by nature.'

The client is curious.

9) 'He's just a <u>greedy</u> so and so…'

The person has greed attributed to him as an identifying characteristic (this example would more likely be used, in a therapy context, with a friendly smile and a Provocative Therapy 'twinkle in your eye').

10) 'He's so <u>kind</u> and so <u>caring</u>…'

The person has kindness and a caring nature attributed to him in a permanent way.

Chunk Size (Sleight Of Mouth)

Sleight of Mouth principles were first delineated by Robert Dilts as he himself modelled Richard Bandler's language patterns. Additional contributions have been made by Steve and Connirae Andreas. A number of Sleight of Mouth patterns now exist, which are covered in this book. Sleight of Mouth patterns are utilised to unravel and in the process depotentiate adverse Complex Equivalence and/or Cause and Effect statements made by the client. [See: Analogy, Another Outcome, Apply To Self, Challenge, Change Of Reference Frame Size, Chunk Size, Consequences,

Counter Example, Hierarchy Of Criteria, Intention, Meta Frame, Model Of The World, Reality Strategy, Redefine, Switch Referential Index.] In this example the principle of Chunk Size is employed.

The term 'chunk size' relates to terminology used in NLP to denote scale. 'Chunking up' basically means going up in scale (big picture/abstract) whereas 'chunking down' means going down in scale (detail/specificity). Bandler and Grinder's 'Milton Model' is placed at the 'chunking up' end of the scale, whereas their 'Meta Model' is placed at the 'chunking down' end of the spectrum.

Chunking Down (focussing on specifics)

The Pattern:

1)

Client: 'Things would be better if I had a different job.'

Hypnotherapist: 'What kind of job are you talking about?'

Client: 'Something that involved working outdoors.'
Hypnotherapist: 'I see. Doing what?'

Client: 'Working for the Forestry Commission.'

2)

Client: 'They are just unthinking when they do that.'

Hypnotherapist: 'When you say 'they are just unthinking...', who specifically are you talking about?'

Client: 'The ABC group.'

Hypnotherapist: 'Which members of the ABC group are you specifically referring to?'

Client: 'Well – it's actually Jack and Phoebe.'

The Structure:

In this example you'll notice that the word 'what' is used to help the client focus in on specifics.

1)

Client: 'Things would be better if I had a different job.'

Hypnotherapist: '**What** kind of job are you talking about?'

Client: 'Something that involved working outdoors.'

Hypnotherapist: 'I see. Doing **what**?'

Client: 'Working for the Forestry Commission.'

The Structure:

In this example you'll notice that the word used to help the client 'chunk down' to the most relevant detail is 'specifically'.

2)

Client: 'They are just unthinking when they do that.'

Hypnotherapist: 'When you say 'they are just unthinking...', **who specifically** are you talking about?'

Client: 'The ABC group.'

Hypnotherapist: 'Which members of the ABC group are you **specifically** referring to?'

Client: 'Well – it's actually Jack and Phoebe.'

Chunking Up (the 'big picture')

The Pattern:

1)

Client: 'I'd like to be a therapist of some kind.'

Hypnotherapist: 'What would that do for you?'

Client: 'I'd get job satisfaction out of helping people.'

2)

Client: 'I'd like to drive.'

Hypnotherapist: 'For what reason or purpose?'

Client: 'It would open up so many more career choices.'

<u>The Structure</u>:

In this example the hypnotherapist's question 'what would that do for you?' encourages the client to consider what is important to them in relation to being a therapist.

1)

Client: 'I'd like to be a therapist of some kind.'

Hypnotherapist: '**What would that do for you**?'

Client: 'I'd get job satisfaction out of helping people.'

2)

In this example the hypnotherapist's question 'for what reason or purpose' causes the client to consider the wider implications of their reason for wanting to drive.

Client: 'I'd like to drive.'

Hypnotherapist: '**For what reason or purpose**?'

Client: 'It would open up so many more career choices.'

<u>Chunking: an example based on Anthony Robbins</u>

I remember listening to an audio tape of Anthony Robbins at a 'guest event' presentation in which he was working with a member of the audience. The audience member told Anthony that he wanted to buy his mother a house (or something like that).

Anthony used a similar principle to the above, by repeatedly asking the client a question like: 'and what would that do for you?'. The session went something like this:

Client: 'I'd like to buy my mom a house.'

AR: 'And what would that do for you?'

Client: 'I would know that my mom has a better standard of living.'

AR: 'And what would that do for you?'

Client: 'I could visit her more often because I'd buy one close to my home.'

AR: 'And what would that do for you?'

Client: 'I'd know that my mom is more secure.'
AR: 'And what would that do for you?'

Client: 'Umm. It would make me feel good.'

AR: 'Aha! It would make you feel good! So the bottom line is that you want to buy your mom a house because it would make you feel good.'

Anthony helped the client to discover the detail which provided him with the impetus to consider buying his mum a house. In-so-doing the client was able to learn something about what motivated him in such a way that he (and all those others who heard the session) could develop more clarity about why he did what he did in life. (This is not a verbatim representation of the situation in question, it's based on my recollection of the tape which I listened to a number of years ago, but it does, I believe, closely demonstrate the gist of what Anthony was so skilfully doing).

Clean Language

Clean Language is a model of communication which seeks to, as the name suggests, ensure that the therapist-client cycle of communication doesn't become deleted, distorted or generalised by the therapist using words which he or she may think mean the same thing as those the client is using, but which in actual fact don't, thereby unwittingly 'contaminating' the communication cycle.

Here is a non Clean Language example:

Client: 'And it makes me feel frustrated.'

Hypnotherapist: 'Oh I see. So your temper starts to boil.'

In this very obvious faux pas the therapist has attributed 'temper' to mean that 'same' thing as 'frustrated' does to the client. Now, it's possible that the words 'frustrated' and 'temper' are synonymous in meaning for the therapist, but it's quite possible also that they have very different meanings for the client. If the therapist pursued the cycle of communication in this manner things could become muddled.

Here are some examples utilising the basic Clean Language model:

Client: 'And it makes me feel frustrated.'

1) Hypnotherapist: 'And is there anything else about [frustrated]?'

2) Hypnotherapist: 'Frustrated. And then what happens?'

3) Hypnotherapist: 'Frustrated. And what happens next?'

4) Hypnotherapist: 'Frustrated. And what happens just before ['...it makes me feel frustrated...']?'

5) Hypnotherapist: 'And where could (that) [frustrated] come from?'

6) Hypnotherapist: 'And what kind of [frustrated] is that [frustrated]?'

In the above examples, rather than interpret what the word frustrated might mean to the client, the therapist keeps the communication 'clean' and utilises the client's own words, thereby, reducing the chances of a miscommunication occurring.

Basic Clean Language Questions

Here, below are the basic Clean Language Questions.

Developing Questions

'And is there anything else about [what the client described]?'

'And where is (that) [what the client described]?'

'And whereabouts is (that) [what the client described]?'

'And then what happens?'

'And what happens next?'

'And what happens just before [what the client described]?'

'And where could (that) [what the client described] come from?'

Shifting to Metaphor

'And what kind of [what the client described] is that [what the client described]?'

'And that's (a) [what the client described] like what?'

My own training in Clean Language was with Caitlin Walker of NLP Northeast. Caitlin has worked closely with James Lawley and Penny Tompkins who are the authors of 'Metaphors in Mind'. Clean Language, as a model, has been developed by David Grove. Space in this volume does not permit a further, more detailed, exposition of the principles of Clean Language, therefore, I suggest that the interested reader purchase a copy of Metaphors in Mind, to learn more.

Basic Theme Development

Here is an example of how a theme could be developed based on the client's statement: 'I'm unhappy'.

Developing Questions

'Unhappy. And is there anything else about [unhappy]?'

'And where is (that) [unhappy]?'

'And whereabouts is (that)[unhappy]?'

'Unhappy. And then what happens?'

'Unhappy. And what happens next?'

'And what happens just before [unhappy]?'

'And where could (that) [unhappy] come from?'

Shifting to Metaphor

'And what kind of [unhappy] is that [unhappy]?'

'And that's (an)[unhappy] like what?'

Further Theme Development

Staying with the client's statement: 'I'm unhappy', using Clean Language, the theme could be further developed thus:

Developing Questions

Hypnotherapist: 'Unhappy. And is there anything else about [unhappy]?'

Client: 'Yes, it makes me feel weak.'

Hypnotherapist: And where is (that) [weak]?

Client: 'It's in the pit of my stomach.'

Hypnotherapist: 'And then what happens?'

Client: 'I feel like I'm worthless.'

Hypnotherapist: 'Worthless. And what happens next?'

Client: 'I see pictures in my mind of me getting everything wrong.'

Hypnotherapist: 'And whereabouts is (that)[getting everything wrong]?'

Client: 'Right in front of me.'
Hypnotherapist: 'And where could (that) [right in front of me] come from?'

Client: 'From within me. I always see myself making mistakes like this.'

Hypnotherapist: 'And what happens just before [making mistakes like this]?'

Client: 'I hear my uncle's voice telling me I'll never get anywhere in life. And it really upsets me. It makes me feel low.'

Shifting to Metaphor

Hypnotherapist: 'And what kind of [low] is that [low]?'

Client: 'Like someone has put heavy weights on me making it difficult to move forward in life. A really low feeling.'

Hypnotherapist: 'And that's [a really low feeling] like what?'

Client: 'Like I'm being held down by other people's negativity.'

In this example you'll notice how, by staying with the client's own words the hypnotherapist is able to help the client move from a position of 'unhappy' to a metaphor which the client feels represents his/her current life situation. At this point the hypnotherapist could help the client to explore the metaphor in ways that help him/her to move towards solution-focussed metaphor(s) and in the process workable approaches in order to feel a wider range of positive emotions more often. For instance:

Hypnotherapist: 'And when 'held down by other people's negativity' what would you rather feel?'

Client: 'Freer!'

Hypnotherapist: 'Freer! And what kind of freer is that freer?'

Client: 'Like life is bright and vibrant again.'

Hypnotherapist: 'Bright and vibrant again (which is also an Embedded Suggestion back to the client) ...and then what?'

Client: 'Then I'd feel like I have more energy.'

Hypnotherapist: 'And when 'more energy' what happens next?'

Client: 'I feel like I can accomplish more. That I can face the challenges and beat them. Even enjoy them!' (In these three sentences the client has shifted to the present tense which indicates that the therapy is helping the client to make changes.)

...and so on.

Cleft Sentence

The Pattern:

1) 'It's probably your creativity that will enable you to think of some more solutions.'
2) 'It was your compassion that no doubt will have enabled you to become more tolerant of people.'

3) 'Is it your sense of humour or your relaxed attitude that will be most useful when you make that presentation?'

The Structure:

1) '<u>It's</u> probably your creativity <u>that</u> will enable you to think of some more solutions.'

The words following 'it's' are used to generate a receptive frame for the presupposition-suggestion which follows the word 'that', which, in this case is: '...will enable you to think of more solutions.' They act as both a 'primer' and as a source of distraction. The client, in effect, is distracted by the opening remark about creativity, while the follow up remark about new solutions is designed to 'slip under the threshold' without being challenged.

2) 'It was your compassion that no doubt will have enabled you to become more tolerant of people.'

In this example the opening phrase about compassion is employed to both prime and distract the client from the following presupposition element located after the word 'that', which is designed to 'slip under the threshold' to elicit tolerance.

3) 'Is it your sense of humour or your relaxed attitude that will be most useful when you make that presentation?'

In this example the presupposition suggestion which 'slips under the threshold' about the client being able to make a certain presentation after the use of the word 'that' is double front-loaded with primers/distracters, in this case being a 'sense of humour' and a 'relaxed attitude'. This is achieved with the combined use of the question 'Is it?' and the word that invites a cross referencing of the situation 'or', which distracts and primes the client to be more open to the idea that they already have the resources they need to make the presentation (which invariably they do, they often just don't believe they do, which is a different situation entirely).

I remember reading some work by Dale Carnegie a long time ago in which he said something about giving a person a high ideal/reputation to live up to, because it will act as a motivating influence upon them. It's a similar principle to that being employed in these examples.

Client's World

Indirect Hypnotherapists seek to understand the client's 'world model'. This means that, rather than looking at the client through a range of generic theories and classifications, which may or may not snugly fit the specific individual presenting for therapy, the hypnotherapist, instead, seeks to understand the unique circumstances of the client's outlook and relationship to their problem(s)/challenge(s). It could be viewed as the difference between a one-size-fits-all garment and a carefully tailored suit. The one-size-fits-all may bear some resemblance to a person's overall physique, whereas the tailored suit will fit much more closely and look a lot better. Indirect Hypnotherapists then have an understanding of theory and classifications, but place emphasis on individuals, their circumstances and responses.

Clustered Suggestions

Clustered suggestions are suggestions, with a specific theme, clustered together. They're usually followed by another constellation of related, but different, suggestions during the trancework. While similar to Milton's interspersal techniques, rather than the suggestions being interspersed throughout a hypnotherapy session, they are instead clustered at specific points, or intervals, in the change work. For instance, during a therapy session in which an unwanted behaviour is being replaced with a more desired response, at the point at which the emphasis is on leaving behind the old, unwanted, behaviour pattern, suggestions would be clustered which denote 'change', 'moving on', 'getting rid of'..., etc, whereas when the emphasis is on installing the desired new response they would be clustered around incorporating 'better feelings', 'looking good', 'feeling good', etc.

<u>Here's an example</u>:

'...because you know it's a good thing down deep inside to <u>change</u> and <u>let go</u> of that old fashioned way of doing things. You know you want to, so now you can. <u>You're moving on</u>, and getting rid of those <u>outdated feelings</u> which <u>you have now left behind</u>...so that now, <u>instead</u>, you <u>begin to sense how much better things are</u> as you let yourself start to <u>feel even better</u> from somewhere special inside. And as <u>you experience more of these better feelings</u>, and <u>notice that you're looking good</u> and <u>feeling good</u> things can <u>begin to improve</u> even more quickly than you may have expected...' (the word 'instead' is the pivotal point at which the emphasis shifts from leaving behind the unwanted behaviour and towards choosing more life-enhancing responses.)

Commentary Adjectives And Adverbs

<u>The Pattern</u>:

1) 'And it's wonderful to know that you can learn this'.

2) 'You don't necessarily have to say it like that.'

3) 'He hesitantly replied.'

4) 'She uncharacteristically said no.'

5) 'She fortunately agreed with us.'

6) 'I think it's great that he is so lucky.'

<u>The Structure</u>:

1) 'And it's <u>wonderful</u> to know that you can learn this.'

2) 'You don't <u>necessarily</u> have to say it like that.'

3) 'He <u>hesitantly</u> replied.'

4) 'She <u>uncharacteristically</u> said no.'

5) 'She <u>fortunately</u> agreed with us.'

6) 'I think it's <u>great</u> that he is so <u>lucky</u>.'

Certain words are used which are designed to add enhanced meaning to what's being said. The inclusion of the Commentary Adjectives and Adverbs word(s) gives greater meaning to the communication. For instance the phrase: 'And it's <u>wonderful</u> to know that you can learn this' has a very different sense to it than saying only '...you can learn this'. And 'He <u>hesitantly</u> replied' sends a very different message from 'He replied'.

Some other useful words: outstanding, great, lucky, happily, good, excellent, fortunate, remarkable, innocently, enjoyable, wryly, curiously, different, arguably, stunning, formidable, lazy, industrious.

Comparative – As

<u>The Pattern</u>:

1) 'You will find that you learn this pattern as easily as that.'

2) 'A wonderful thing about learning like this is that as much as you already know now you can be sure there are always more good things to learn ahead.'

3) 'While your protective unconscious mind is generating as many resources as you need, you may allow yourself to sense a sense of developing curiosity about how you will positively notice them occurring for you.'

4) 'Well done! As you connect with your inner self as much as you like to now you can make some more changes which help you. That's right and you can sense it's as simple as allowing yourself to relax the changes to happen.'

5) 'That's right. And going into trance like this can be as nice as you like it to be.'

<u>The Structure</u>:

1) 'You will find that you learn this pattern <u>as</u> easily <u>as</u> that.'

The Comparative As pattern manifests in the use of the word 'as', which is repeated in close succession. This has the effect of amplifying the meaning of the context in which it's used. For instance, the phrase 'as easily as that', implies more than the simple alternative 'easily' does, when used alone. It is also presupposed that the reader will learn this language pattern. The client is most likely to take conscious notice of the 'as easily as that' element of the message while indirectly absorbing the presupposition element without conscious resistance.

2) 'A wonderful thing about learning like this is that as much as you already know now you can be sure there are always more good things to learn ahead.'

The same Comparative As principle is applied here, with a presupposition that learning is taking place. As in the above example the presupposition element 'learning like this' is 'slipped under the threshold' of awareness through the rest of the language pattern's content.

3) 'While your protective unconscious mind is generating as many resources as you need, you may allow yourself to sense a sense of developing curiosity about how you will positively notice them occurring for you.'

The presupposition here is that the client has a protective unconscious mind. This is followed by the Comparative As principle. Positive suggestions follow about a 'developing sense of curiosity', and how the client will 'positively notice them occurring'.

4) 'Well done! As you connect with your inner self as much as you like to now you can make some more changes which help you. That's right and you can sense it's as simple as allowing yourself to relax the changes to happen.'

The presupposition here is that the client is connecting with their inner self. The Comparative As, used twice here, conveys the sense of 'as much as you like', and 'it's as simple as...'.

5) 'That's right. And going into trance like this can be <u>as</u> nice <u>as</u> you like it to be.'

Going into trance is presupposed. The Comparative As suggests that it's going to be a nice experience.

Useful phrases:

'As well as...'

'As much as...'

Comparative Deletion

<u>The Pattern</u>:

'And as your unconscious helps things to get better and better...'

<u>The Structure</u>:

Getting better is presupposed. However the word better, by its very nature implies that something is being measured against something else in order to arrive at the conclusion that it has, indeed, become better than the other unit of measurement. This means that, when said like this, the element against which it's being compared has been 'deleted'.

Another example:

The phrase 'You are going deeper', implies that a comparison of some sort has been made, the detail of which has also been deleted. We could ask ourselves the question: 'deeper than what?'. However, in the context of indirect hypnotherapy, employing comparative deletions can have excellent therapeutic results. Here are some examples of phrases which you could employ as a therapist to help your clients:

1) 'The positive changes can happen <u>quicker</u> / <u>more quickly</u>.'

2) 'As things get <u>better</u>.'

3) 'You can access <u>higher</u> levels of awareness which can help you make <u>better</u> choices.'

4) 'You can develop <u>more</u> ideas / <u>even more</u> ideas.'

5) 'Things can seem to happen <u>more</u> <u>slowly</u>.'

6) 'It's like you have a <u>greater</u> insight now.'

7) 'You notice that your response has <u>lessened</u>.'

Another useful comparative deletion phrase to remember is: 'Do things better more easily...'

Comparatives

<u>The Pattern</u>:

1) 'It doesn't matter whether your developing indirect hypnotherapy skills are currently lesser or greater than were Milton's, what is important is that you enjoy using them.'

2) 'As you discover more about the language of trance than you used to know you will find that you naturally develop more fluency with it.'

3) 'As you spend less time thinking about this situation the more time you will have available to think about the nice things in life.'

4) 'While you are developing a greater range of indirect hypnotherapy skills than you used to have, the more varied are the opportunities which are coming your way.'

<u>The Structure</u>:

Unlike the Comparative Deletion, in which the unit of measurement is deleted, the Comparative pattern retains the element against which the operative 'measuring' word is being measured. It also contains a presupposition in its structure.

1) 'It doesn't matter whether your developing indirect hypnotherapy skills are currently <u>lesser</u> or <u>greater</u> **than were Milton's**, what is important is that you enjoy using them.'

In this example the Comparatives used are the words 'lesser' and 'greater' and the element against which they are being measured are the words 'than were Milton's'. It is presupposed the person is developing indirect hypnotherapy skills.

2) 'As you discover <u>more</u> about the language of trance **than you used to know** you will find that you naturally develop more fluency with it.'

Here, the Comparative appears with the use of the word 'more' which is being measured in relation to the phrase 'than you used to know'. It's presupposed that the person will discover more about the language of trance.

3) 'As you spend <u>less time</u> **thinking about this situation** the <u>more time</u> you will have available to **think about the nice things** in life.'

Here 'less time' and 'more time' are being compared in relation to the words 'think about the nice things...' It's presupposed that the client will spend less time thinking about the situation in question.

4) 'While you are developing a <u>greater range</u> of indirect hypnotherapy skills **than you used to have**, the <u>more varied</u> are the opportunities which are coming your way **compared to before now**.'

The words 'greater range' and 'more varied' are the Comparatives which are being measured against the phrases 'than you used to have', and 'compared to before now'. A developing range of hypnotherapy skills is presupposed.

Comparison Of Opposites

The Pattern (direct form):

'So...you will have this [problem] or this [solution] based on the choice that you make now...So now's never been a better time to make a good decision and choose the better course of action...the solution...'

The Structure (direct form):

This example helps to act as a catalyst that will assist the client to become very clear about the repercussions of his/her choices and ('in the spirit of Anthony Robbins') aid him/her to accept personal responsibility for decisions and the results obtained due to whichever course of action he/she takes. This implicitly teaches the client that he/she does have a significant degree of influence over the course of his/her life.

The Pattern (as a metaphor):

'Happiness and sadness are like a coin. There's always a bit of happiness in sadness and sadness in happiness. That helps us to know the difference – you have to feel hungry before you can enjoy a good meal.' (Stephen Brooks used this method in one of our seminars.)

The Structure (as a metaphor):

As a follow on to the above you could continue perhaps like this: 'So, what does this tell you? Let me tell you...it tells us that while things have been difficult they have within them the potential for a solution...all we need to do is look at the other side of the coin so to speak. Let's do that...let's consider what we can do to start to change things now...'

Complex Equivalence

The Pattern:

'As you relax in trance **this means that** your unconscious is beginning to open up more.'

The Structure:

A connection is made between relaxing in trance and the unconscious mind opening up. A Complex Equivalence is a linguistic structure which implies an equivalent connection between one thing and another, which in reality may not have existed, before it was suggested. It's like a mathematical sum. You can look at it like this: As you relax in trance = your unconscious is beginning to open up more.

Other examples:

1) 'Sitting quietly **means that** you are going inside.'

Here you will notice that an equivalent connection is made between the act of sitting quietly and (=) 'going inside'. We could ask ourselves the question 'How does sitting quietly **equal** that I am going inside?', however, the Complex Equivalence is an excellent linguistic tool for use in therapy. Here are some examples of phrases which you could employ as a therapist to help your clients:

2) 'And as you enter into trance <u>this means that</u> (=) you are ready to make some changes.'

3) 'So while you are thinking about this consciously this <u>indicates that</u> (=) you are searching for a positive outcome unconsciously.'

4) 'You are wondering about things <u>which tells us</u> (=) that you are conscientious.'

5) 'You don't even have to think about this right now. Because whether you do or whether you don't <u>it just means that</u> (=) you can let your inner self get on with helping you either way.'

6) 'Asking your unconscious to help you change <u>is the same</u> (=) as making the changes happen.'

7) 'Knowing that you've started to take action <u>is equal to</u> finding a solution. Now all you need to do is realise that you already know that you know what to do, when you sense the time is right.'

Another useful complex equivalence phrase to remember is: 'Which means that...'.

Compound Suggestion (1)

Version One

<u>The Pattern</u>:

1) 'You're now sitting in this chair, breathing in a certain way and you can begin to wonder how your unconscious will help you.'

2) 'You're sitting in this chair, breathing in a certain way and I wonder if you've begun to wonder how your unconscious will help you?'

3) 'You're hearing the sound of the music and you may sense that you're already starting to change...you're breathing in that certain way now and I wonder when you will first notice more resourceful ideas coming to you. So, this means that you are consciously listening to me right now and learning things at deeper levels as you do.'

The Structure:

This Compound Suggestion is a Truism – followed by a leading statement or a question - linked by the word 'and' or a pause.

1) 'You're now sitting in this chair, breathing in a certain way [Truism] <u>and</u> you can begin to wonder how your unconscious will help you [Leading Statement].'

2) 'You're sitting in this chair, breathing in a certain way [Truism] <u>and</u> I wonder if you've begun to wonder how your unconscious will help you [Leading Question]?'

3) 'You're hearing the sound of the music [Truism] <u>and</u> you may sense that you're already starting to change [Leading Statement]...you're breathing in that certain way now [Truism] <u>and</u> I wonder when you will first notice more resourceful ideas coming to you [Leading Question]? So, this means that you are consciously listening to me right now [Truism] <u>and</u> learning things at deeper levels as you do [Leading Statement].'

Compound Suggestions (2)

Version Two

The Pattern:

1) 'And when I click my fingers you will awaken feeling relaxed and at ease in every way.'

2) 'And when I say the word 'now' your trance will develop some more.'

3) 'And when I let your hand back down and as it touches your leg that will be a signal to you to let yourself feel good.'

The Structure:

The implication is that the desired result is 'triggered' by the hypnotherapist's actions. The result is therefore compounded by the hypnotherapist's actions.

1) 'And when I <u>click my fingers</u> **you will awaken feeling relaxed and at ease** in every way.'

2) 'And <u>when I say the word 'now'</u> **your trance will develop** some more.'

3) 'And <u>when I let your hand back down and as it touches your leg</u> **that will be a signal to you to let yourself feel good**.'

Compound Suggestions (3)

Version Three

<u>The Pattern</u>:

1) 'You're going to notice some positive changes. Positive changes are nice. Aren't they?'

2) 'Now you're feeling relaxed. It's nice to feel relaxed.'

3) 'Now you're discovering how to feel happier. It's good to know that things can improve.'

<u>The Structure</u>:

A statement is made which includes a suggestion, which is then 'cloaked' by a follow up statement. The follow up statement distracts the conscious attention and allows for the opening suggestion to be more readily absorbed.

1) 'You're going to <u>notice some positive changes</u>. Positive changes are nice. Aren't they?'

2) 'Now <u>you're feeling relaxed</u>. It's nice to feel relaxed.'

3) 'Now <u>you're discovering how to feel happier</u>. It's good to know that things can improve.'

Confusion Technique

<u>The Pattern</u>:

'And as you think about what you're noticing or noticing what you're thinking about you don't have to listen to what you consciously haven't heard...but when you do unconsciously listen to everything that you hear you know... you can relax.'

<u>The Structure</u>:

This technique is used to confuse the conscious mind – for therapeutic purposes. When the mind is confused it searches for an answer, for something that it understands, in order to end the confusion. This means that when a therapist uses the confusion technique to generate uncertainty the client will more <u>readily accept the next direct suggestion</u> which follows in order to end their state of confusion. Notice the difference as you read this example:

'And as you think about what you're noticing or noticing what you're thinking about you don't have to listen to what you consciously haven't heard...but when you do unconsciously listen to everything that you hear you know... **you can relax**.'

<u>Here's another example</u>:

'That's right and you don't have to not know how you know what isn't happening inside outside of your awareness but when you... **feel better now**.... you can remember what you didn't know you knew... don't get confused now will you...**feel better**...'

Conjectures And Conclusions

<u>The Pattern</u>:

Type One (those generated by the client):

1)

Client: 'Me! No one will ever love me!'

Hypnotherapist: 'How can you be sure, I mean really sure, that you're correct about that? Have you ever been wrong about anything before?'

Client: 'I suppose so.'

Hypnotherapist: 'There you are!'

2)

Client: 'I don't know why I even decided to come and see you about this. I'll never get over it.'

Hypnotherapist: 'I'm not going to disagree with you. You know you better than anyone else. But how can you be sure that you of all the millions of people who have been in this situation won't be able to improve things in your life? Even if you don't think so, I think you're more resourceful than that. But I'm not going to argue with you about this. If you want to sell yourself short that's up to you. Did you know by the way; someone with much fewer resources than you came to see me about this kind of thing once? And they didn't think they'd be able to deal with it either. But they did. You know how? They started to ...'

Type Two (those generated by the hypnotherapist):

1)

'So you know you have to take a different approach to this. That's the way to sort it out.'

2)

'Well – if you don't do it, someone else will.'

<u>The Structure</u>:

<u>Type One (those generated by the client)</u>:

The client makes a statement based on conjecture and draws a conclusion from it from which they then operate. The therapist, having spotted this, untangles the client from their ravelled thinking by challenging the client's statement.

1)

Client: 'Me! No one will ever love me!'

Hypnotherapist: 'How can you be sure, I mean <u>really</u> sure, that you're correct about that? Have you ever been wrong about anything before?'

Client: 'I suppose so.'

Hypnotherapist: 'There you are!'

The client makes a statement which is (in effect) based on conjecture. It's speculation. They have also reached a state of affairs based on a worst case scenario. The hypnotherapist challenges it by asking the question: 'How can you be sure, I mean <u>really</u> sure...' the word 'really' is emphasised to implant further doubt in the client's conjectured 'belief' (they may of course not really believe it, they may be 'playing victim', or some other role). Everyone has made a mistake or two in their lives. This introduces the possibility that this conjecture/conclusion of the client's is also likely erroneous. The hypnotherapist replies with: 'There you are!', as if it's a self evident conclusion that the client is, in all likelihood, equally wrong about the statement they made.

2)

Client: 'I don't know why I even decided to come and see you about this. I'll never get over it.'

Hypnotherapist: 'I'm not going to disagree with you. You know you better than anyone else. But how can you be sure that you of all the millions of people who have been in this situation won't be able to improve things in your life. Even if you don't think so, I think you're more resourceful than that. But I'm not going to argue with you about this. If you want to sell yourself short that's up to you. Did you know by the way; someone with much fewer resources than you came to see me about this kind of thing once? And they didn't think they'd be able to deal with it either. But they did. You know how? They started to ...'

In this example rather than be perceived by the client as disagreeing which (curiously) may result in the client retreating further into their self-limiting frame of reference (note: I believe it was either in the book Psycho-cybernetics by Maxwell Maltz, or in a Psycho-cybernetics audio set by Maxwell Maltz and Dan Kennedy that it was explained that sometimes a client will seek to protect their negative self-image vehemently; which, my experience indicates can sometimes, sadly, be very true. So it can be, on occasion, the therapist's job to help the client move out of such a limited frame), instead the hypnotherapist builds rapport by stating that he or she isn't going to disagree. He/she even seems to reinforce the client's belief by stating 'you know you better than anyone else'. It's then at this point (having gained two unspoken 'yeses', by implication, from the client) that the hypnotherapist begins to introduce the possibility of doubt. And he or she does so in such a way as to provoke the client (in the manner of Frank Farrelly's excellent Provocative Therapy approach) to imply that if the client carries on in this self-defeatist attitude he/she will be the 'one in a million' who did. This, in a subtle way, will likely cause the so-provoked client to begin to resist his/her own defeatist pattern. As Frank Farrelly's Provocative Therapy shows, it's often okay for us to say something negative about ourselves, but when someone else starts to agree, or, by comparison, imply that we are less able than others, we will become provoked at some level and actually begin to assert ourselves, while in the process disengaging ourselves from our stated 'belief'. Then, in the style of Dale Carnegie the hypnotherapist gives the client a high ideal to 'live up to', based on the hypnotherapist's true perception of the client's real abilities. Before the client can negatively counter the statement, the therapist, in order to embed the suggestion at an unconscious level, says: 'But I'm not going to argue with you about this...', which again, seems to indicate that the therapist isn't going to challenge the client's negative thinking pattern (at least not totally overtly). The therapist then places the responsibility for the situation onto the client, due to his/her attitude by adding: 'If you want to sell yourself short that's up to you'. This statement is also designed to therapeutically provoke the client more and begin to challenge his or her own negative reference point. The hypnotherapist then introduces an example from his or her previous client work in such a way that it too is designed to provoke the client some more, in the direction of therapeutic balance, by comparing him/her with another client who had 'fewer resources' in a similar situation: 'Did you know by the way; someone with much fewer resources than you came to see me about this kind of thing once? And they didn't think they'd be able to deal with it either.' The hypnotherapist then states that the previous client did manage to deal with the situation (with fewer resources remember, which implies that the current client can too). And is he/she going to let someone with fewer resources 'beat' him/her? Not likely. The therapist then appeals to the client's curiosity in a tantalising way with the words: 'But they did. You know how? They started to...', and then proceeds, by example to explain to the client what they could also do, based on what the previous 'less able' client did.

Type Two (those generated by the hypnotherapist):

In these two examples, the client could, at least in effect, challenge the hypnotherapist's statement being that there are elements of conjecture and conclusion in them. The difference is, that the hypnotherapist can offer more evidence to assert them than the client's previous two 'fluffy' statements. So, technically, it could be argued that there are elements of conjecture in what the therapist is saying, but on a point-by-point scoring system they're based more in the realm of reality and less in the realm of error.

1)

'So you know you have to take a different approach to this. ['Conjecture'] That's the way to sort it out. ['Conjecture'/Conclusion]'

Short and to the point. In reality the client could challenge this by saying: 'How do you know that?'. But it's unlikely that they will if they understand that a) it's true and b) the therapist has their best interests at heart.

2)

'Well – if you don't do it, someone else will. ['Conjecture'/Conclusion]'

A phrase that millions of people have used. In reality the client could challenge it, but, as above, in essence what's being said is a fact, that given the right kind of circumstances and time, it's likely that someone else will do 'it' and the client will have missed his/her opportunity.

Conjunctions

The Pattern:

1) 'You can sense your relaxation and make changes to the way you feel.'

2) 'While you experience this happening also you can feel differently about things.'

3) 'You can sense some of that old emotion again but don't become aware of your new inner happiness instantly. Just let it happen gently.'

4) 'You can feel how it feels and start to notice something different.'

5) 'As your experience develops you can also notice new sensations starting to occur.'

6) 'You can experience levels of relaxation but don't become fully comfortable until you want to.'

7) 'You can feel the pleasant temperature and feel different about your future too.'

8) 'You can explore the sensations of your eyelids closed while also feeling your trance developing.'

9) 'You are relaxing in a certain way and noticing certain sensations but don't change them for even more comfortable ones right away.'

The Structure:

1) 'You can sense your relaxation <u>and</u> make changes to the way you feel.'

2) 'While you experience this happening <u>also</u> you can feel differently about things.'

3) 'You can sense some of that old emotion again <u>but</u> don't become aware of your new inner happiness instantly. Just let it happen gently.'

4) 'You can feel how it feels <u>and</u> start to notice something different.'

5) 'As your experience develops you can <u>also</u> notice new sensations starting to occur.'

6) 'You can experience levels of relaxation <u>but</u> don't become fully comfortable until you want to.'

7) 'You can feel the pleasant temperature <u>and</u> feel different about your future too.'

8) 'You can explore the sensations of your eyelids closed while <u>also</u> feeling your trance developing.'

9) 'You are relaxing in a certain way <u>and</u> noticing certain sensations <u>but</u> don't change them for even more comfortable ones right away.'

Conjunctions are used to link one experience with another. It's done in a manner which implies or presupposes a connection between each element of the linked experience, even when one may not exist in reality. The words used to achieve this linking are: 'and', 'also' and 'but'. For instance, the phrase: 'You can sense your relaxation <u>and</u> make changes to the way you feel', implies a connection between the client sensing their relaxation AND making changes to the way they feel. In the following example: 'While you experience this happening also you can feel differently about things' the word 'also' links the client's ongoing experience with him/her feeling differently about things. While: 'You can sense some of that old emotion again but don't become aware of your new inner happiness instantly. Just let it happen gently' makes a therapeutic link from that 'old emotion' to new inner happiness with the word 'but'.

Conscious Association   Unconscious   Dissociation

The Pattern:

1) 'And I wonder what resource you already have which you are not yet consciously aware of which your unconscious can choose to let you remember and experience now in order to let this change happen for you might be?'

2) 'I'm curious to know which useful feeling that you've already felt before that your unconscious can let you remember consciously and begin to re-experience again when the time is right that will help you do this might be?'

The Structure:

This pattern is helpful in order to elicit a useful behaviour or resource from within the client in a way that is outside of their conscious awareness but which brings the idea of the resource into their conscious awareness. It does so in a way that does not invite challenge or 'resistance' but rather is so subtle that the client is considering the possible resources that they have without thinking about whether or not they actually have them. Consciously clients will sometimes protect a negative self-image, which is why it can be useful to help them draw upon other senses of self without critical conscious evaluation. This pattern can be used to do this.

1) 'And I wonder what <u>resource you already have which you are not yet consciously aware of</u> which your unconscious can choose to let you <u>remember</u>

<u>and experience now</u> in order to let this change happen for you might be?'

In this example it's presupposed that the client already has access to resources, but (as is often the case) they don't know what they are or how to reach them. However, as you follow the structure of the pattern the unconscious mind is prompted to choose to let them 'remember and experience now', which helps to shift the client to a better, therapeutic, position.

2) 'I'm curious to know <u>which useful feeling that you've already felt before</u> that your unconscious can let <u>you remember consciously and begin to re-experience again</u> when the time is right that will help you do this might be?'

Here the client is encouraged to consider the concept of a useful feeling that they already have experience of (which they may or may not have felt recently) that (again) their unconscious mind can help them to remember (elicit) and re-experience (revivify). This too side-steps conscious critical evaluation and appeals directly to unconscious intervention in a way that is rapidly consciously apparent as well.

Conscious Unconscious Double Bind

<u>The Pattern</u>:

1) 'Your conscious mind can wonder what solutions will happen while your unconscious is generating them for you.'

2) 'While your unconscious mind is creating solutions and your conscious mind is curious about how they will occur.'

3) 'I wonder what unconscious changes you will make and which will be the first one that you consciously notice happening?'

4) 'Your conscious mind can wonder how many new ideas your unconscious mind will create for you while your unconscious is already creating them.'

5) 'Your unconscious mind can change the way you feel quickly while your conscious mind is wondering just how quick that change will be.'

The Structure:

The Conscious Unconscious Double Bind is created in such a way that the conscious mind is, a) 'played down', that is to say it's implied that it has less influence in the way things are working out than the unconscious mind and, b) the person can't consciously decide how the suggested outcome will occur, they literally have to 'wait and see' what the unconscious mind will do to bring the therapeutic event to fruition. Neatly woven into the Bind is a therapeutic suggestion. For example:

1) 'Your conscious mind can wonder what solutions will happen while your unconscious is generating them for you.'

The suggestion is that solutions will happen. However, the conscious mind can only wonder how they will happen – while the (more resourceful) unconscious mind is generating them. This means that the client will consciously have to wait and see how the unconscious will go about introducing the new solutions into their life.

2) 'While your unconscious mind is creating solutions and your conscious mind is curious about how they will occur.'

Similarly, solutions are again suggested, which are being created unconsciously while the conscious mind is curious about how they will occur (which means that consciously <u>they don't know</u> how they will occur. They have to wait and see.).

3) 'I wonder what unconscious changes you will make and which will be the first one that you consciously notice happening?'

Unconscious changes are suggested – but there is a question mark over which one of those changes will be the first one that the client consciously notices. This itself implies that they may begin to experience the changes but not notice them consciously until after <u>they have already taken place a number of times</u>. This can be a powerful therapeutic suggestion.

4) 'Your conscious mind can wonder how many new ideas your unconscious mind will create for you while your unconscious is already creating them.'

New ideas are suggested, which the conscious mind can only wonder about while the unconscious mind is already creating them (which means that the conscious mind doesn't know what they are – it can only wonder, while the unconscious mind obviously knows what they are because it is the part that is creating them).

5) 'Your unconscious mind can change the way you feel quickly while your conscious mind is wondering just how quick that change will be.'

In this case a change of affect ('the way you feel') is suggested, which the unconscious mind is both creating and responsible for the speed of the change, while the conscious mind can only wonder just how quick it will turn out to be. This is another example of the unconscious mind knowing how an outcome will occur while the conscious mind can only 'wait and see'.

The Detailed Structure Of A Conscious Unconscious Double Bind:

1) Overt:

'I wonder how your conscious mind will notice those new resources as your unconscious mind creates them for you?'

'I wonder how your conscious mind [this is the conscious part of the Bind]'

'...will notice those new resources [this is what the Bind is focussed on generating, 'new resources']'

'...as your unconscious mind [this is the unconscious part of the Bind]'

'...creates them for you [referring again to the 'new resources' by implication 'ties the bind' tighter]'

Consciously the client can only wait and see how the new resources will manifest as the unconscious mind (which knows and is responsible for this) creates them.

2) Covert:

'And you can create resources while you don't have to think about them.'

'And you can create [this part is aimed at the unconscious mind]'
'...resources [this is the focus of the Bind]'

'...while you don't have to [this part is aimed at the conscious mind]'

'...think about them [by implication this is referring again to the resources, and it 'ties the bind']'.

In this covert example the words conscious and unconscious are not even used, they're implied.

Here are some more Covert Conscious Unconscious Double Binds:

1) 'And you can change while you wonder how it's happening.'

Change is the element on which the Bind is focussed. The first 'you' referred to is the unconscious while the second 'you' is the conscious mind.

2) 'And you don't have to listen because you can listen to me instead.'

It's suggested that the client will listen. However, the first time this is mentioned it's aimed at the conscious mind (the first 'you') by saying that they don't consciously have to listen because 'you' (the second you – the unconscious) can listen instead.

3) 'Don't think about this now because you can think about this now.'

Thinking about the hypnotic suggestions is further suggested in a way that removes responsibility for doing this from the conscious mind, to the unconscious mind. In this example the conscious 'you' is totally implied whereas a 'you' is included to focus the attention on the unconscious mind.

4) 'You don't have to make any changes at all, because you can make them.'

And the same type of covert theme is employed here.

5) A couple I learned from Stephen Brooks that I like are: 'I can talk to you – and I can talk to you' (followed by an appropriate comment or suggestion, such as, perhaps: 'as you make the changes...'); and: 'I can talk to you and your unconscious mind can listen' (followed by an appropriate comment or suggestion, such as, perhaps: '...as you learn what you need to know').

Conscious Unconscious Double Dissociated Double Bind

<u>The Pattern</u>:

1) 'And you can consciously explore a thought without knowing where it comes from or unconsciously know where it comes from without exploring how you're thinking it.'

2) 'And you can consciously consider an idea without knowing how you're doing so or unconsciously know how you're doing so without considering how you are.'

3) 'As you consciously ponder a new alternative without knowing how it's happening or unconsciously know how it's happening without pondering where it is.'

4) 'While you consciously sense a new sensation without knowing where it's coming from or unconsciously know where it's coming from without wondering what it is.'

5) 'You can consciously think of new solutions without knowing how you're doing it or you can unconsciously know how you're doing it without thinking of where they're coming from.'

6) 'You can consciously sense a better emotion without understanding how or you can unconsciously understand how without sensing how you do.'

7) 'You consciously can think of new ideas without realising how you're doing it or you can

unconsciously realise how you do it without thinking about where they're from.'

8) 'Even if you consciously consider changing without knowing how you'll do it you can unconsciously know how you'll do it without thinking about how it's done.'

9) 'As you become a healthy non-smoker without consciously sensing when or you may unconsciously sense when without having to think about how.'

10) 'Special changes can occur without you consciously thinking about them or you can unconsciously think about them without considering what they are.'

11) 'You can learn conscious unconscious double dissociated double binds easily and not consciously think about how you're doing it, or you can unconsciously think about how you're doing it without thinking about what this means.'

12) 'You can consciously think about how you're learning without unconsciously considering why you are or you can unconsciously consider why you are without consciously thinking about what that learning is.'

The Structure:

Just as in the above examples of the Conscious Unconscious Double Bind, the Conscious Unconscious Double Dissociated Double Bind, employs the same effect of developing the phraseology in such a way that it's not possible for the conscious mind to choose when, or how, the suggested result will manifest. It's left up to the unconscious mind to do that. However, in this pattern some further elements are introduced which help to present the message in an even more embedded way to the unconscious mind. This takes place by double dissociating the focus of the suggestion, so that it is further removed from conscious processing.

1) 'And you can <u>consciously</u> explore a thought (the focus of the suggestion) without knowing where it comes from (dissociated) or <u>unconsciously</u> know where it comes from without exploring (dissociated) how you're thinking it.'

In this example the focus of the suggestion is on the receiver exploring a thought (the content of which could have previously been suggested in the trancework session). However it's suggested that while they may be able to consciously explore 'a thought', they also won't know where it's coming from (this dissociates it once). Then it's suggested that they may unconsciously know where it comes from 'without knowing how you're thinking it' (this dissociates it for the second time, resulting in the double dissociation effect). So, the person's conscious mind will have become lost in the sentence structure, while the overall message, of exploring a thought can be picked up and acted upon at deeper levels.

2) 'And you can <u>consciously</u> consider an idea (the focus of the suggestion) without knowing how you're doing so (dissociated) or <u>unconsciously</u> know how your doing so without considering how (dissociated) you are.'

3) 'As you <u>consciously</u> ponder a new alternative (the focus of the suggestion) without knowing how (dissociated) it's happening or <u>unconsciously</u> know how it's happening without pondering where (dissociated) it is.'

4) 'While you <u>consciously</u> sense a new sensation (the focus of the suggestion) without knowing where it's coming from (dissociated) or <u>unconsciously</u> know where it's coming from without wondering what (dissociated) it is.'

5) 'You can <u>consciously</u> think of new solutions (the focus of the suggestion) without knowing how you're doing it (dissociated) or you can <u>unconsciously</u> know how you're doing it without thinking of where they're coming from (dissociated).'

6) 'You can <u>consciously</u> sense a better emotion (the focus of the suggestion) without understanding how (dissociated) or you can <u>unconsciously</u> understand how without sensing how you do (dissociated).'

7) 'You <u>consciously</u> can think of new ideas (the focus of the suggestion) without realising how you're doing it (dissociated) or you can <u>unconsciously</u> realise how you do it without thinking about where they're from (dissociated).'

8) 'Even if you <u>consciously</u> consider changing (the focus of the suggestion) without knowing how you'll do it (dissociated) you can <u>unconsciously</u> know how you'll do it without thinking about how it's done (dissociated).'

9) 'As you become a healthy non-smoker (the focus of the suggestion) without <u>consciously</u> sensing when (dissociated) or you may <u>unconsciously</u> sense when without having to think about how (dissociated).'

10) 'Special changes can occur (the focus of the suggestion) without you <u>consciously</u> thinking about them (dissociated) or you can <u>unconsciously</u> think about them without considering what they are (dissociated).'

11) 'You can learn conscious unconscious double dissociated double binds easily (the focus of the suggestion) and not <u>consciously</u> think about how you're doing it (dissociated), or you can <u>unconsciously</u> think about how you're doing it without thinking about what this means (dissociated).'

12) 'You can <u>consciously</u> think about how you're learning (the focus of the suggestion) without <u>unconsciously</u> considering why you are (dissociated) or you can <u>unconsciously</u> consider why you are without <u>consciously</u> thinking about what that learning is (dissociated).'

This example was slightly more complex in that it twice includes the conscious/unconscious pivot elements.

The Detailed Structure of a Conscious Unconscious Double Dissociated Double Bind (using a Nominalisation - the word 'changes'):

'And you may consciously be sensing changes beginning to happen without wondering how

they are or unconsciously knowing how they are without wondering how you're doing it.'

'And you may consciously be sensing [this part is aimed at the conscious mind and it's associated]'

'...changes beginning to happen [this is the focus of the Bind]'

'...without wondering how they are [this is dissociated]'

'...or unconsciously knowing how they are [this part is aimed at the unconscious mind and it's associated]'

'...without wondering [this dissociates it]'
'...how you're doing it [this 'ties the bind'].'

The Detailed Structure of a Conscious Unconscious Double Dissociated Double Bind (using an emotional process):

'And you can consciously feel a new and better emotion occurring without knowing how it's happening or unconsciously you can know how it's happening without deciding how it will start.'

'And you can consciously feel a new and better emotion [this part is aimed at the conscious mind and it's associated]'

'... occurring [this is the focus of the Bind]'

'... without knowing how it's happening [this is dissociated]'

'... or unconsciously you can know how it's happening [this part is aimed at the unconscious mind and it's associated]'

'... without deciding [this dissociates it]'

'... how it will start. [this 'ties the bind'].'

Consequences (Sleight Of Mouth)

Sleight of Mouth principles were first delineated by Robert Dilts as he himself modelled Richard Bandler's language patterns. Additional contributions have been made by Steve and Connirae Andreas. A number of Sleight of Mouth patterns now exist, which are covered in this book. Sleight of Mouth patterns are utilised to unravel and in the process depotentiate adverse Complex Equivalence and/or Cause and Effect statements made by the client. [See: Analogy, Another Outcome, Apply To Self, Challenge, Change Of Reference Frame Size, Chunk Size, Consequences, Counter Example, Hierarchy Of Criteria, Intention, Meta Frame, Model Of The World, Reality Strategy, Redefine, Switch Referential Index.] In this example the principle of Consequences is employed.

The Pattern:

1)

Client: 'I don't have a solution and as a result I feel anxious.'

A)

Hypnotherapist: 'I understand what you're saying. However not having a solution means that you still have the pleasure of creating one.'

B)

Hypnotherapist: 'Okay. And not having a solution can make you feel more determined.'

C)

Hypnotherapist: 'Feeling anxious can encourage you to do something about it.'

D)

Hypnotherapist: 'Not having a solution could mean that you start to network with others to create one and in the process not only will your anxiety have no more reason to exist but it's likely that you'll be helping others in similar ways too.'

2)

Client: 'I don't understand what she means and it makes me angry.'

A)

Hypnotherapist: 'Because you don't understand that will give you the opportunity to learn more about her.'

B)

Hypnotherapist: 'However, not understanding can make you want to find out more about where she is coming from.'

C)

Hypnotherapist: 'Feeling angry is a signal that something isn't right and it's telling you that you need to take some positive action.'

D)

Hypnotherapist: 'Not understanding can make you determined to learn more about her, while in the process, learning how to become more calm also as you understand more.'

The Structure:

The Consequences pattern takes the stated issue(s) and attributes certain (in this case therapeutic) consequences to it/them.

1)

Client: 'I don't have a solution and as a result I feel anxious.'

A)

Hypnotherapist: 'I understand what you're saying. However not having a solution <u>means that you still have the pleasure of creating one</u>.'

This example is of using the Consequences pattern on the first part of the client's statement. In this case: 'I don't have a solution'. By using this element as the starting point the hypnotherapist is afforded the natural opportunity to apply the Consequences pattern to it, in order to create a therapeutic shift in the client's perceptions and cognition processes, moving in the direction of solution-focussed thinking. The Consequence of not having a solution is the pleasure of finding one.

B)

Hypnotherapist: 'Okay. And not having a solution can <u>make you feel more determined</u>.'

This example also applies the pattern to the first part of the client's statement, to create a therapeutic shift in awareness. The Consequence of not having a solution is that it can make the client feel more determined.

C)

Hypnotherapist: 'Feeling anxious can <u>encourage you to do something about it</u>.'

This example utilises the Consequences pattern on the second half of the client's statement: 'I feel more anxious'. In this case the results of the anxiety are transformed. No longer is anxiety the static end result, it is rather a catalyst in an ongoing process of encouraging the client to take some action to: 'do something about it'. The Consequence of the anxiety becomes doing something about it.

D)

'Not having a solution could mean that <u>you start to network with others</u> <u>to create one</u> and in the process not only will <u>your anxiety have no more reason to exist</u> but it's likely that you'll be helping others in similar ways too.'

In this example the Consequences pattern is applied to both elements of the client's statement. So that not having a solution becomes equal to or equals (=) being a catalyst to networking with others, which in turn will mean that the Consequence of such networking action is that the anxiety will have no more reason to exist. The Consequence of the lack of a solution is networking and the Consequence of networking is creating solutions and the Consequence of that is that the client will no longer 'need' to feel anxious, because the trigger for the anxiety will have vanished.

2)

Client: 'I don't understand what she means and it makes me angry.'

A)

Hypnotherapist: 'Because you don't understand <u>that will give you the opportunity to learn more about her</u>.'

The Consequence of not understanding is the opportunity to learn more.

B)

Hypnotherapist: 'However, not understanding can make you want to find out more about where she is coming from.'

The Consequence of not understanding is to make the client want to find out more about where she is coming from.

C)

Hypnotherapist: 'Feeling angry is a signal that something isn't right and it's telling you that you need to take some positive action.'

The Consequence of feeling angry is that it's a signal that they need to take some positive action.

D)

Hypnotherapist: 'Not understanding can make you determined to learn more about her, while in the process, instead of feeling angry you'll be learning how to feel more calm about things as you understand more.'

The Consequence of not understanding is determination to learn more about her and the Consequence of that is that the client will be learning to feel more calm about things.

Context Reframing:

<u>The Pattern</u>:

1) 'Client: I'm too shy to talk to her.'

2) 'Client: I've been wanting to change my career for years now. But I'm too mixed up and I just can't decide what I'd prefer to do.'

<u>The Structure</u>:

In essence a Context Reframe is a pattern that can be used to enable the therapist to help the client understand that his/her behaviour <u>is an appropriate response</u> – but in another context. This can be very helpful for the client, particularly if he/she has concluded that the behaviour in question is totally inappropriate.

This pattern can be applied in situations when a client says something like: 'I'm too ABC', or (he/she/it/they) is/are 'too XYZ'.
1) Client: 'I'm too shy to talk to her.'

Hypnotherapist Reframe: 'I'm glad that you aren't the kind who just 'blurts' things out. This tells me that you're giving thought and consideration to what you're going to say to her.'

2) Client: 'I've been wanting to change my career for years now. But I'm too mixed up and I just can't decide what I'd prefer to do.'

Hypnotherapist Reframe: 'Well maybe yes – maybe no. I think that you may simply be ensuring that you look at all your options rather than just rushing into something.'

Contingent Suggestions

(AKA Dependent Suggestion)

Version One:

A Contingent Suggestion 'hitch-hikes' a desired behaviour onto an ongoing behaviour: In effect the outcome of the suggested behaviour is contingent (or dependent) upon the first behaviour being in existence for the new, desired behaviour to be 'hitch-hiked' on to it.

Here's an example:

Suggestion: 'Turn the television on.'

Answer: 'No!'

Or:

Suggestion: 'As you're walking over to the bookcase, please turn the television on.'

Answer: 'Yes.'

Notice the difference. In the first (blunt) example of the suggestion (or in this case a command) to 'turn the television on', it's (not surprisingly) met with the answer 'No!'. However, for the purposes of demonstrating how a contingent suggestion 'hitch-hikes' onto an ongoing behaviour, in order to generate another desired outcome, the requester asks that the television is turned on <u>as</u> the other person is (already) walking over to the bookcase. This is much less confrontational, commanding, or overt. It is (as in the above example) much more likely to be met with an affirmative response. An important point to remember: the initial behaviour MUST already exist to some degree (or be perceived by the client to exist to some degree), in order for the secondary behaviour to be hitch-hiked on to it.

Here's an example that you're likely to use in a hypnotherapeutic context: '**As** you watch the clouds floating by, your eyelids **may** start to close'. The first statement (in this example) represents a Truism based on what the therapist can observe: that the client is starting to go into trance by observing some clouds through the view offered by the window in the treatment room. On this basis, onto this ongoing behaviour the therapist then 'hitch-hikes' the suggestion that the client's eyelids 'may start to close'.   Note also: the use of the word 'may', rather than will. At this stage of the trancework it's usually better to be very permissive and indirect regarding what the outcome will be, while, at the same time creating the right kind of environment for the therapeutic suggestions to generate a response.   If the therapist authoritatively stated that the client's eyes 'will' close, and they subsequently didn't do so, it would create a break in rapport.   However, later in the trancework, when the client is fully involved in the process, more direct Contingent Suggestions can be offered. Such as: 'So now, as you relax in the chair here and as you get ready to start to listen very carefully to what I say now...' In this example getting ready to listen carefully is hitch-hiked on to the ongoing behaviour of being relaxed in the chair. It's also more direct, in that the therapist says: '...as <u>you get ready</u> to start to listen very carefully...', rather than: 'As you <u>may</u> be getting ready to start to listen very carefully...'.

The words: 'as', 'when', 'will', 'probably', 'until', 'you can', 'can you', 'and as', 'I wonder', 'makes', 'during', 'before', 'after', 'while'... and the use of pauses can all be used to create Contingent/Dependent Suggestions. Here are some more examples:

1) '...And as you start to think about coming out of trance you can let the learnings integrate in exactly the right way. [The therapist observes the client beginning to return to the conscious state as a result of the suggestions to do so and follows with...] But don't come out of trance **until** your unconscious mind let's you know that the changes you've needed have occurred.'

The ongoing state of returning to conscious awareness has linked to it the suggestion that the client's return from trance is also a signal from the unconscious mind that the required changes have taken place.

2) **'While** you consciously notice the rhythm of your breathing your unconscious is making the necessary adjustments so that when you know you are ready you can begin to come out of trance.'

The ongoing state in this example is the client's breathing which has associated to it the suggestion that the unconscious mind is making 'necessary adjustments'.

3) 'That's right. And **while** you're thinking those thoughts that you're thinking you will **probably** start to notice that you can feel a certain sense of comfort starting to occur.'

The 'certain sense of comfort' is hitch-hiked onto the client's current thinking process.

4) 'Because now you've invited your unconscious mind to help you....**You Can** even remember at a conscious level now that you've invited your unconscious to help you. **And As** you think about this now your unconscious can start to make finer adjustments so that you do this more easily...so that **As** you continue to relax now **While** this happens changes can occur...**And As** you wonder what those changes may be...**I Wonder** what you will start to notice first...and when you notice whatever you're noticing now **You Can** use the idea that your unconscious is making available to you to help things get better...**When** you...'

Here is an example of some multiple-layered Contingent Suggestions. Remembering at a conscious level is linked by the words **'You Can'**, which themselves are 'hitch-hiked' on the back of the client having invited their unconscious to help them. This is followed by **'And As'** which hitch-hikes onto the back of the client thinking about what has just been mentioned, which in turn links to the suggested behaviour of the unconscious making 'finer adjustments', which is then linked by the word **'As'** to the client's continuing relaxation, while the word **'While'** is used to hitch-hike the suggestion that 'changes can occur', which is then itself followed by the words **'And As'**, these lead into the concept of wondering, followed by the words **'I Wonder',** which becomes the pivot for a suggestion that the client will 'start to notice changes', which in turn is soon followed by the words **'You Can'**, this leads into the suggestion that the client's unconscious is 'making available' an 'idea', to help things 'get better', and so on.

Version Two (Simple version):

Simple Contingent Suggestions are linked by **'And As'**, like this: 'So now you're completing your CV **and as** you do this you could decide which the best company is to approach with it first.'

1) **'And as** you breathe in that relaxed way your unconscious can begin to make changes...'

The fact that the client's breathing is an observable ongoing behaviour provides the opportunity to 'hitch-hike' the suggestion onto this behaviour so that the client's unconscious will begin to make changes.

2) **'And as** you think those conscious thoughts your unconscious can think unconscious thoughts to find a better way to do this now...'

The fact that the client is consciously thinking (a Truism) has provided the 'hitch-hiked' opportunity to link this truth onto the suggestion that their unconscious is thinking about how to find a 'better way.'

3) **'And as** you are sensing your experience developing your unconscious is listening. **And as** your unconscious listens it can think of new ways to

help you. **And as** it begins to do this you can start to consciously relax more...'

In this example the language is quite indirect in that after the words 'And As' are first employed, the expression 'you are sensing your experience developing' is added, which is quite vague. So, in actual fact, whatever the client is then sensing will fit this description. It therefore becomes a Truism based on whatever the client's current experience is. This is followed by the suggestion that their 'unconscious is listening'. Now, strictly speaking, this is not an observable phenomenon, but it can be a <u>perceived phenomenon</u> (either perceived by actual inner experience, belief, or, most likely, both). The words 'And as' are utilised again to suggest that (based on the unconscious listening) it (the unconscious) can think of new ways to help. This then becomes a perceived phenomenon, upon which, as a perceived Truism, the suggestion is made that 'you can consciously relax more'.

Contrary To Expectation

<u>The Pattern</u>:

1) 'If you should find that you don't know how to do it. I'll help you.'

2) 'If you should discover that you can't. Let me know.'

3) 'Oh! And if you should find that you **really** can't do it then I **suppose** we could consider something else.'

<u>The Structure</u>:

The use of the word 'should' implies that the speaker actually expects that the receiver of the communication can/will be able to do whatever is expected.   Comments   offered   like   this   can sometimes be less 'challenging' to the client than those conveyed in more direct ways.   In the third example the Contrary to Expectation implication is further enhanced by the hypnotherapist's emphasis of the word 'really'.   The addition of the phrase 'I suppose we could consider something else', with emphasis on the word 'suppose' also implies that the 'something else' isn't really an option and the expected outcome (that the client can and will 'do it') is what's really anticipated.

Conversational Hypnosis

This is another term that's used to describe Indirect/Ericksonian-style hypnotherapy.   As the name suggests the therapy is delivered in a conversational way, which characterises Milton's 'informal' approach.

Conversational Postulate

<u>The Pattern</u>:

1) 'Could you relax now and let me know when it's happening?'

2) 'Can you think of another option and share it with me?'

3) 'Will you work with me on this by taking a nice long deep breath in?'

4) 'Would you like to change the way you feel by telling me what you'd like to be different?'

The Structure:

A question is postulated, which, indirectly is designed to elicit a desired response.

1) 'Could you **relax now** and <u>let me know when it's happening</u>?'

This example is phrased as a question, but it's designed to act as a suggestion to reinforce relaxation and a communication cycle.

2) 'Can you **think of another option** and <u>share it with me</u>?'

This example is phrased as a question, but it's designed to act as a suggestion to generate solution-focussed thinking, in the form of 'another option'.

3) 'Will you **work with me on this** by <u>taking a nice long deep breath in</u>?'

This example is phrased as a question, but it's designed to generate rapport and a state of relaxation.

4) 'Would you like to **change the way you feel** by <u>telling me what you'd like to be different</u>?'

This example is phrased as a question, but it's designed to act as a suggestion to help the client start to change the way he/she feels.

Coué Bind

The Pattern:

1) 'That's right and if ever you try to think about that old problem you just try and stop a solution starting to appear as well. It will appear before you know it.'

2) '...Which means that if at sometime you try to think about that like you used to, you'll also discover, even if you try not to, that you'll begin to sense a better option becoming available to you.'

3) 'So this means if you try to start to think about that problem ever again and then not to think about it you'll begin to notice that without you having to do anything about it from somewhere inside better thoughts will happen and you won't be able to stop the better thoughts consciously even if you try. But then you wouldn't want to – after all it's better to let better things happen is it not? Which is why you will.'

4) 'And if you're ever faced with this challenge in the future your unconscious will help you immediately start to notice better ways of dealing with it. You just try and stop yourself – and you'll see how powerful this is.'

5) 'If you want to test this you can even try not to think of a better way of doing it when the time comes and you'll find that you will anyway.'

The Structure:

Emile Coué coined the phrase: 'What you resist persists'. It became known as Coués Law of Reversed Effect. Many clients are caught in what we call a Coué Bind, when they present with their problem(s). They will have tried hard to resist their habit, phobia, addiction, obsession or whatever else the problem may be centred around, but, paradoxically, very often, the harder they try to resist the more persistent the problem becomes. Think about it this way – try as hard as you can not to think about the actor Brad Pitt now. That's it, really try not to think about Brad Pitt. Don't think of his name. Certainly don't think of the movies Troy, Fight Club or Meet Joe Black. And don't think of any of the widely circulated images you may have seen of him on posters, cards and book covers. Please, go on, really try not to let even the merest glimmer of the thought of Brad Pitt enter into your mind right now.

I think you get the picture. This is an example of how 'trying' to resist something actually can have the opposite effect. Therefore, the therapeutic intention of a Coué Bind is to take this principle and transform it into a therapeutic Bind instead of the client's problematic one.

1) 'That's right and if ever you try to think about that old problem you just try and stop a solution starting to appear as well. It will appear before you know it.'

In this example, rather than suggesting that the client will 'never' think about their 'problem', instead, the hypnotherapist has taken an ongoing pattern and then reapplied the resistance pattern to the problem in the form of introducing a solution. So, should the client ever begin to get caught up again in the old loop of trying to resist the problem, because the habituated pattern has been altered by the introduction of a further suggestion of 'resistance' (that's not really encouraging resistance, but is rather an invitation) to a solution starting to appear, plus because an element of doubt has been introduced in the opening remarks with the words 'if ever', implying that the client might not ever think about the old issue, it's likely that the old habituated response will be interrupted to one degree or another. The phrase: '...if ever you try to think about...' also implies that the client might not even be able to do so (he/she might not ever think about the old problem). The problem is also labelled as being 'old' which implies that it is now more of a past tense (as in both interpretations of the expression, temporal and physiological) issue rather than current. The words 'as well' further embed the concept that if the client becomes involved in thinking about the problem (in the context of trying to resist it), a solution will appear 'as well'. This means that the intended resultant outcome is that now rather than becoming stuck in a problem loop, the client will instead, shift into a solution loop.

2) '...Which means that if at sometime you try to think about that like you used to, you'll also discover, even if you try not to, that you'll begin to sense a better option becoming available to you.'

Similarly, in the above example, it's implied that the client might not even engage in the problem thinking pattern again, by the use of the words 'if at sometime' (the use of the word 'if' casts doubt on whether or not they will). The phrase: '...if at sometime you try...' also suggests that they won't be able to do it in the same way that they used to, because they can only 'try' to do it. The problem is also placed in the past with the words 'like you used to'. Then it's suggested that a 'better option' will become available, even if they 'try not to' think about it (and it's likely that that's the opposite of what they would want to do – they would want to think of a better option. So whether the client thinks of a better option or tries not to think of a better option either way they'll sense a better option becoming available).

3) 'So this means if you try to start to think about that problem ever again and then not to think about it you'll begin to notice that without you having to do anything about it from somewhere inside better thoughts will happen and you won't be able to stop the better thoughts consciously even if you try. But then you wouldn't want to – after all it's better to let better things happen is it not? Which is why you will.'

There is a similarity in the above example to examples that preceded it inasmuch as an element of doubt is created around whether or not the client will even think about the problem again, through the use of the words 'if' and 'ever again'. The phrase 'and then not to think about it' matches their recent behaviour. Then, however it's suggested that 'from somewhere inside', 'better thoughts', will start to appear that the client won't be able to <u>consciously</u> stop (which implies unconscious assistance is being given) 'even if you try', which 'gets inside' the hitherto dominant resistance pattern which has been generating the problem and begins to utilise it for positive purposes, by reversing its effects. This is then ratified by the following statement-of-the-obvious 'but then you wouldn't want to' which sets up a further agreement frame in the client's thinking. A comparison is alluded to between the old state and the new one in the use of the words 'it's better to let better things happen' (rather than the old alternative), which is followed by quite a direct suggestion in the form of: 'which is why you will'.

4) 'And if you're ever faced with this challenge in the future your unconscious will help you immediately start to notice better ways of dealing with it. You just try and stop yourself – and you'll see how powerful this is.'

This is a slightly different approach. This would perhaps suit a situation in which the likelihood of the client experiencing the 'problem situation' is in fact quite limited (albeit still possible). In this instance the emergence of the problem context triggers the emergence of a solution too. And in order to magnify the power of the solution the therapist says, almost as if 'in passing' 'you just try and stop yourself – and you'll see how powerful this is'.

5) 'If you want to test this you can even try not to think of a better way of doing it when the time comes and you'll find that you will anyway.'

This example actually invites the client to 'test' the Coué Bind, by trying not to think of a 'better way'. If he/she really does try 'not to' think about better ways, he/she will have no option but to 'have to', which will act as an additional source of evidence for him/her that there has been a change. To further reinforce this, the direct suggestion is made that if the client does try to 'test this', they will 'find that you will anyway' [think of better ways].

Counter Example (Sleight Of Mouth)

Sleight of Mouth principles were first delineated by Robert Dilts as he himself modelled Richard Bandler's language patterns. Additional contributions have been made by Steve and Connirae Andreas. A number of Sleight of Mouth patterns now exist, which are covered in this book. Sleight of Mouth patterns are utilised to unravel and in the process depotentiate adverse Complex Equivalence and/or Cause and Effect statements made by the client. [See: Analogy, Another Outcome, Apply To Self, Challenge, Change Of Reference Frame Size, Chunk Size, Consequences, Counter Example, Hierarchy Of Criteria, Intention, Meta Frame, Model Of The World, Reality Strategy, Redefine, Switch Referential Index.] In this example the principle of Counter Example is employed.

The Pattern:

1) 'You just can't trust a man/woman.'

2) 'Conventional medicine is bad for you.'

3) 'Complementary medicine isn't any good.'

4) 'Men/Women are the ones who are causing all the problems. What's more they always have!'

The Structure:

1) 'You just can't trust a man/woman.'

Possible response: 'Has there ever been a man/woman you could trust?'

(Or...)

Possible response: 'Is it likely that somewhere in the world of 6 billion people there are trustworthy men/women?'

2) 'Conventional medicine is bad for you.'

Possible response: 'Have you ever known or heard of someone that has used conventional medicine and found it helpful?'

3) 'Complementary medicine isn't any good.'

Possible response: 'Is it possible that someone, somewhere, may have gained benefit from using complementary medicine?'

4) 'Men/Women are the ones who are causing all the problems. What's more they always have!'

Possible response: 'Actually aren't there many more examples of men/women who haven't caused problems, but rather who have contributed good things to society? What about all of them, and all they've done, past and present?'

Counter Factual Conditional Clauses

The Pattern:

1) 'If you had applied that self-hypnosis technique that we practised together you could have done better in that situation. Still – it's never too late to start. Do I have an agreement with you now, that you are really committed to following through this time?'

2) 'Think about it for a moment. If you had applied for the job you could be in a better financial position already. So – what are we waiting for? You don't want to miss another opportunity do you? Are you ready to take action this time and send your CV to the other employer who expressed an interest in seeing you?'

3) 'Okay, so **if only** you had gone to Harvard, you could have gotten your doctorate and you'd be **sitting on top of the world**.   And now there are no opportunities left in the **whooole world** that will suit you? **Riiight?**'

The Structure:

A self-evident fact is stated. A Counter Factual Conditional Clause is applied to the statement which indicates that, had the person being spoken to behaved differently a different outcome would have occurred. This is achieved by the use of the words 'had' and 'could'.

1) 'If you <u>had</u> applied that self-hypnosis technique that we practised together you <u>could</u> have done better in that situation. Still – it's never too late to start. Do I have an agreement with you now, that you are **really** committed to following through this time?'

In this example the client has clearly already admitted that he/she never utilised certain skills that he/she had learned from the therapist. They had, in effect, expected the therapist to 'do it all for them'. As a result things did not go as planned. The hypnotherapist deals with the fact of the matter, but in such a way as to highlight what could have happened had he/she followed through. And, because this is a therapeutic situation, rather than leaving things at that juncture, the therapist quickly adds: 'it's never too late to start'. He or she then gains an agreement with the client to verify that they are now 'really' (the use of the word 'really' adds emphasis in a positive way) prepared to follow through in future so as to avoid the likelihood of a repetition of the previous situation.

2) 'Think about it for a moment. If you had applied for the job you could be in a better financial position already. So – what are we waiting for? You don't want to miss another opportunity do you? Are you ready to take action this time and send your CV to the other employer who expressed an interest in seeing you?'

This is a similar example to the one directly above. The hypnotherapist deals with the fact of the matter, in such a way as to impress upon the client what could have happened if he/she had followed through. And then, quickly the hypnotherapist 'lightens things up' with the expression, 'So - what are we waiting for...?', in the process suggesting a more positive response by his/her tonality. Then the therapist quickly aims to <u>gain commitment</u> from the client regarding making an application for the other job opportunity ('Are you ready...?').

3) 'Okay, so **if only** you had gone to Harvard, you could have gotten your doctorate and you'd be **sitting on top of the world**.   And now there are no opportunities left in the **whooole world** that will suit you? **Riiight**?'

This example is totally different. It could be called a Pseudo Counter Factual Conditional Clause. That's because in this situation the hypnotherapist is employing a Provocative Therapy style approach (as developed by Frank Farrelly A.C.S.W.).   The tonality that the hypnotherapist uses could be summed up as a 'Yeah, Yeah!, So what...' tone of voice. So, while on the surface it sounds like the hypnotherapist is dealing with the fact in order to counterfactually encourage the opposite response from the client, in reality, the voice tone implies that not only is that 'fact' not so factual - but that the counter factual argument is also spurious. This kind of approach can be very powerful and almost makes light of the client's problem while pouring doubt on their fixed and rigid ideas in order to help them loosen up and consider other possibilities (We hosted Frank Farrelly at Eos Seminars Ltd for a four-day master class and as a result we observed him doing this kind of thing often - and he does it marvellously).

(For more information on **Provocative Therapy** read the book 'Provocative Therapy' by **Frank Farrelly** and Jeff Brandsma.)

Coupled Words

The Pattern:

'It's nice... to know... that you... can go... inside now... and make... changes that... help you... improve today... so that... things can... get better... in many... wonderful ways...'

The Structure:

As the above example shows, Coupled Words utilises the principle of saying two words that are, in effect, coupled together, then briefly pausing before following up with the next two coupled words. This creates the effect of a sentence that's delivered in two-bit sections. This works very well with hypnotic Rhythm and because the language pattern is so unusual (most people don't encounter it in their day-to-day lives) this too generates an Affect Effect which further enhances the trancework that's in motion.

Covering All Possible Alternatives

The Pattern:

1) 'In trance you may notice that your hands will feel lighter or heavier or warmer or cooler or maybe you'll notice no difference whatsoever.'

2) 'You may notice the changes immediately or in a few moments, it may take until this evening or it could be a day or even as many as two before you consciously notice it starting to happen.'

3) 'You can do this right away or later on, or whenever you sense that the time is right.'

The Structure:

As the name implies, the hypnotherapist covers 'all possible alternatives' so that, whatever happens during the trancework session (and, if appropriate, afterwards) is implied to be due to the result of one of the suggestions (which, curiously, in a circular reasoning fashion it will be). This method also helps to avoid any kind of confrontation that could develop if the hypnotherapist limited him/herself to suggesting one particular trance phenomenon (which the client may not want to elicit). Only offering one choice could theoretically result in a failed therapeutic intervention because the therapist is too specific. But, by being very general, very indirect and open, the client is going to feel more relaxed and the therapist is more likely to get a positive response.

Creating An Environment For Change

The Pattern:

1) Hypnotherapist: 'Look at that spot on the wall while I talk to you.'

2) Hypnotherapist: 'Are you ready now to start to make some changes?'

3) Hypnotherapist: 'Okay then. If you'd like to sit in the 'hypnotherapy chair'. This is where it all happens now.'

4) Hypnotherapist: 'So – you booked this appointment because you feel you're ready to sort this issue out?'

5) Hypnotherapist: 'Oh – so you came as a result of a referral. So you're already aware of how powerful this is.'

6) Hypnotherapist: 'You may find yourself feeling a bit excited about applying this new skill at work.'

The Structure:

1) Hypnotherapist: 'Look at that spot on the wall while I talk to you.'

We don't usually tell people that we are going to talk to them before we do, so this implies that, because we've told the client that we're going to talk to him/her, something important is about to happen.

2) Hypnotherapist: 'Are you ready now to start to make some changes?'

This Conversational Postulate could be used in situations when a person knows the answer they're going to get is likely to be yes, so that it actually reinforces that yes answer.

3) Hypnotherapist: 'Okay then. If you'd like to sit in the 'hypnotherapy chair.'

The use of the expression 'hypnotherapy chair' associates the chair with the therapy, which means that to sit in the chair is to start to undergo a process of positive change.

4) Hypnotherapist: 'So – you booked this appointment because you feel you're ready to sort this issue out?'

The hypnotherapist takes a Truism and uses it to begin to move the client's desire to change from 'first or second gear' into 'overdrive'.

5) Hypnotherapist: 'Oh – so you came as a result of a referral. So you're already aware of how powerful this is.'

The hypnotherapist references a previous client's positive outcome and uses it as a basis on which to generate positive expectations within the current client.

6) Hypnotherapist: 'You may find yourself feeling a bit excited about applying this new skill at work.'

The words 'a bit excited' are gauged in such a way as to suggest a form of positive expectancy in the client about how they will apply (future) the new skills at work. This in turn creates a positive emotional loop in that, because the client has 'fore knowledge' (in the present) that they will (future) use the skills well, they will in turn actually use the skills when the moment is at hand (the future becoming the expected present).

Creating Doubt

<u>The Pattern</u>:

1)

Hypnotherapist: 'So. You feel this is the way it is?'

Client: 'Yes, I Think so.'

Hypnotherapist: 'That's right – <u>you think so</u>!'

2)

Client: 'It's never going to work out for us!'

Hypnotherapist: 'Are you sure?'

Client: 'Yes!'

Hypnotherapist: 'Oh, so you <u>think</u> you're sure.'

3)

Client: 'I suppose I'll never be able to change.'

Hypnotherapist: 'What do you think?'

Client: 'No'.

Hypnotherapist: 'Is that what you think!? Wow!'

4)

Hypnotherapist: 'You're saying it will always be like this?'

Client: 'I believe it will.'

Hypnotherapist: 'That's right – <u>you believe it will</u>.'

<u>The Structure</u>:

Doubt can be a very useful tool. It can be used to help a client loosen up a rigid, limiting, perceptual reference frame in order to create a more useful model of the world.

D

Decision Conditioning

Decision Conditioning is the term we use at Eos Seminars Ltd to describe a therapeutic principle which we ourselves derived from attending Anthony Robbins 'Unleash The Power Within' fire-walk seminar a couple of times. Tony utilises a brilliant approach that he created called the 'Dickens Pattern', which is itself based on NLP's Meta Programs and Time Based Therapy techniques. During the seminar (which is geared towards thousands of attendees in one room) the Dickens Pattern takes about six hours to present, which, while being incredibly powerful in its own environment, as a step-by-step rapid-delivery therapeutic technique, it is nevertheless in the context of most therapy delivery situations too long to consider, unaltered, as a practical exercise. We therefore (we believe) replicated the critical elements within Anthony's NLP-based approach and created a model, that we call Decision Conditioning, which is very powerful, and which can be actioned in most cases in between 20 minutes and an hour (which is a similar time-frame to that which I believe Tony himself works towards, on a one-to-one basis). In essence the pattern retains the Meta Program drivers that Tony uses by focussing on assisting the client to associate 'massive pain' with the continuation of whatever the problem-issue is that needs to be changed while 'great pleasure' is associated to choosing and actioning a better, preferred course of action. The setting or 'frame' that we use for this approach is to have the client imagine that they're at a 'juncture in time' which is mapped out on the ground in front of them. Kind of like a cross roads. (Like you would with NLP Time Based Therapy; which is also sometimes called 'Time Line Therapy', which, I'm led to believe, is a trademarked term owned by Dr Tad James [who's also written an excellent book on hypnosis called: 'Hypnosis: A Comprehensive Guide'] hence my references to 'timepaths' in the following example.) The crossroads 'metaphor' then represents the present moment and there are two possible futures mapped out ahead of the client, visually on the floor, as 'timepaths'; the contents/events of which could develop from the present moment, depending upon the choices that the client makes in the now. This means that the future is unwritten, but is in the process of developing, based on what the client does in the now. As a formula this means that if the client continues to do unhelpful things their future will naturally develop in an undesired fashion. However, by contrast, if they accept personal responsibility for their actions and commit to doing more of what they want, the future that will develop will, then, naturally turn out better. I often 'prime' clients before working through this technique with them by talking to them about the movie 'Back to the Future II' in which Marty McFly changed his future into a better one, by readjusting the way things took place at a critical point in a 'timepath' that had previously resulted in setting off a negative chain of events in his life. Most clients have seen the movie and it helps them to 'slip into' an uptime trance quite easily, in anticipation of the process. Then the client is invited to 'walk into' and along each of the possible futures, describing potential situations at various points, starting (usually) at six months in the future, leading to one year, two years, five years and, possibly, ten years time, commencing with the unwanted possible future. After they've fully 'pre-experienced' the negative ramifications of travelling down the unpleasant 'timepath' they're then guided to travel down the positive potential 'timepath', before returning to the present moment. At which point they contrast the likely outcome of the desired future with that of the unwanted (very negative) possible future. Having got a pretty good idea where each course of action will lead (which can become quite emotionally charged, in fact, in most cases it's good if it does) the client is then invited to think carefully about which future they want to live, based on the newly learned understanding that <u>they will be responsible for its manifestation</u> and with this insight (and all the emotional energy that will by then have been generated) they're invited to step forward to 'claim' the desired future, by committing totally to it. This can be a very powerful pattern and very cathartic in the process.

Space and context do not allow a full demonstration. Nevertheless here are a few examples of how the **conversational elements** of this principle can be utilised therapeutically.

The Pattern:

Client: 'I feel so shitty when I wake up every day with a hangover. And I hate being sick time after time. And that awful feeling I get when the room starts to spin around and around. I hate it.'

Hypnotherapist: 'Ugghh! And you've been doing that daily for how long?'

Client: 'Ten years now.'

Hypnotherapist: 'Ten years! And how many times per week do you reckon you've been sick like that.'

Client: 'Five out of seven.'

Hypnotherapist: 'Five out of seven. Let's total that up….that means you've spent approximately 2,600 days puking up down the loo. How shitty do you feel about that?'

Client: 'Pretty shitty.'

Hypnotherapist: 'And what's going to happen if you don't do something about it?'

Client: 'I'll get worse and worse.'

Hypnotherapist: 'How worse do you think things could get?'

Client: 'My partner could leave me. I could lose my job. I could end up on the streets. And this worries me a lot – I could end up with an alcohol related disease.'

Hypnotherapist: 'That frightens you doesn't it?'

Client: 'Yes.'

Hypnotherapist: 'A lot?'

Client: 'Yes.'

Hypnotherapist: 'So isn't it about time to do something about this? Aren't you totally sick – literally – and tired of spending every day puking up down the loo and feeling shitty?'

Client: '(Crying by now) Oh God yes. I fuckin' hate this. It's fuckin' awful. I hate it. I wish I'd never touched a drink – ever.'

Hypnotherapist: 'Now – I want you to think very carefully about what I'm going to ask you. Don't say what you think I want to hear or what you think you should say. Be really real with yourself now. I want you to tell me if you are really, honestly, ready to change, ready to get rid of that shitty stuff out of your life for good. To create a better life that you really deserve. Now really think about this before you answer.'

Client: '(sobbing) Yes – yes. I'd do anything to be free of this awful, this bloody terrible stuff.'

Hypnotherapist: 'Okay – well done. So tell me. What would you prefer your life to be like?'

Client: 'Free from drink.'

Hypnotherapist: 'Right – and then what.'

Client: 'Well, I'd have more energy. My relationship would be back on track. My job would be going well. And I'd be healthier.'

Hypnotherapist: 'Now – that sounds like a much better deal to me. Tell me – if you don't change, where will you be in five years' time?'

Client: 'In a mental hospital or on the streets.'

Hypnotherapist: 'And that's not a good place to be.'

Client: 'No.'

Hypnotherapist: 'But if you absolutely decided that you were so pissed off with drink and all of the problems it causes...because it's not your friend you know...it hurts you on a daily basis...and you stepped forward into a new future in which you are a happy healthy person liberated from the evil of alcohol – how would this five years in the future be better?'

Client: 'Oh boy. So different. Ever so different. Everything would be brighter. I'd be so proud of myself. I can't describe just how much things would be better. God – this way is so much nicer. I have so much longer to live, so much more to do. So many more good times. My family are happy. I'm happy. I even have more money – rather than pissing it up against the wall like I used to.'

The therapist <u>contrasts</u> both <u>possible futures</u> (when I do this I even play 'Devil's Advocate' when the client is fully associated into the positive future by saying things like: **'Hey – it's been five years now. You've proven that you can beat it. Have a drink! Celebrate!'** In order to get them to resist me <u>now</u> – so that in the future they'll do likewise when required to do so <u>in reality</u>.)

Once the therapist has generated enough perceived/anticipated pain towards the unwanted behaviour and enough perceived/anticipated pleasure towards the desired response, he or she says to the client something along the lines of:

'Neither of those two futures has happened yet but one or other will – to one degree or another, depending upon whether or not <u>you accept personal responsibility</u> for your actions and the decisions you make.'

(This phrase is then repeated for emphasis - to highlight the client's responsibility):

Hypnotherapist: 'Neither of those two futures has happened yet. But one or other will – to one degree or another, depending upon whether or not you accept personal responsibility for your actions and the decisions you make. You can either have the shitty alcohol sodden future where you end up on your own, who knows where, vulnerable and penniless – or you can have the other future. The better one, where you absolutely make a decision, a commitment to yourself today so that no more....no more!...will you ever let that horrible stuff into your life – because now you are absolutely determined - totally committed - to being true to yourself, getting rid of all of that alcohol generated pain once and for all. But I can't do it for you. You have to do it. And the way you have to do it is...choose. That's it...choose that from now, today you are stepping into the future that you really want to happen... and you know that you can because <u>all it takes is the decision to choose to do so</u>. Here and now.'

Hypnotherapist: 'So – now's the time to choose. Think about it – then tell me. Which future do you want; the shitty one or the bright one? Think about it carefully – because it's up to you to follow through and make it happen, by the decision you make. Shitty or bright? It's your choice.'

Client: 'Bright. Bright. I'm fucked off with drink. From now on it's bright. I'll never let that fuckin' stuff get a hold on me again. Never!'

(This illustration is based on an experience gained when I first used this approach in just such a situation - and the client has been dry for several years now. As a result, since then, I've been able to help other people with alcohol problems in similar ways. This method has practically 'universal' applicability though, and can therefore be applied in many other situations too (over eating, smoking, procrastination, etc). The important point in this and any other kind of therapeutic situation – is that the client must be absolutely <u>100% committed to change</u>. They can't be 'half-hearted'. If they're truly committed, this kind of approach can help to create massive leverage, causing the client to 'move away from' the source of the pain and 'towards' the better option/pleasure).

Here's a basic visual representation of the pattern:

1)

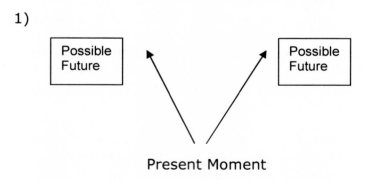

www.eosseminars.com   192

The client starts by considering the fact that they're at a critical juncture of opportunity in time. Two possible futures are before them.

2)

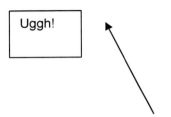

Present Moment

The client is invited to pre-experience all of the negativity that will result by continuing down the negative 'timepath', by walking down the 'timepath' that's mapped out on the floor, while stopping at certain points and associating to the negative repercussions of what they sense is occurring.

3)

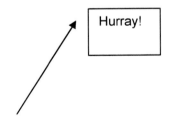

Present Moment

The client is then invited to pre-experience all of the positivity that will result by continuing down the positive 'timepath', by walking down the 'timepath' that's mapped out on the floor, while stopping at certain points and associating to the very positive results of what they sense is occurring.

4)

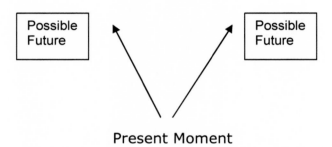

Present Moment

The client is then invited to return to the present instant to spend a few moments contrasting each possible future's outcome.

5)

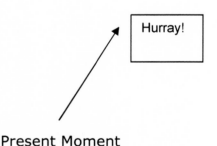

Present Moment

Then, with the client powerfully 'moving away from' the painful future and decidedly 'moving towards' the desired future they can be invited to 'claim' their new future by 'stepping into it'. They've just pre-experienced both possible scenarios and then contrasted them. They fully understand that <u>the future is flexible</u> and it can be fashioned in the way they choose, simply by choosing to <u>accept responsibility for their actions</u> and only doing those things that lead in the direction of (thereby causing) the better future.

DeConsciousing

(Playing down the conscious mind)

<u>The Pattern</u>:

DeConsciousing examples are designed to 'play down' the conscious mind and encourage the unconscious mind to become more active. They also help to offer encouragement to the client that although they may have wrestled with a problem for a long time – hope is at hand because now another part of them, a wiser, more powerful aspect of themselves is about to help.

<u>The Structure</u>:

'When you tie your shoelaces, which hand bends the lace to make the first part of the bow? You probably don't consciously know. But your unconscious can do it for you without you really having to think about it. So maybe now is a good time to ask the part of you which knows how to tie your shoelaces for you - without you consciously needing to think about it when you do it - to resolve this issue for you too. It's much faster this way. You know, your unconscious mind is growing your fingernails for you even as we speak. You don't have to consciously think about that either. It just happens! And even if you did think about it consciously you wouldn't know how to do it – but your unconscious mind does. All the best scientists in the world can't make finger nails grow with the raw materials that your inner self uses every day to do so. You are that amazing! So why not ask the part of you which knows how to work miracles, like growing your nails...generating new cells...thinking the next thought for you...before you're even consciously aware of what that thought will be...to help you? After all, it is an incredibly wise and powerful part of you and it, or <u>rather</u>, <u>the</u> inner deeper you, <u>always</u> wants what's best for you. And I think that's encouraging to know. Think about it!'

Deductive Language Patterns

Deductive Language Patterns are patterns which move from the 'total' to the 'specific'. From the big picture to the detail.

<u>The Pattern</u>:

1) 'So – you're saying that writing a book and getting it published will make you feel really good and your whole life will be better. And what can you do today to be able to set things in motion?'

2) 'Okay. You know what it's like to be 12 stone and how good you feel about yourself like that. What is the first thing you can do today to be true to yourself and make it start to happen?'

3) 'So – you don't have any friends. Maybe now would be a good time to look at how you interact with others.'

4) 'You've spent the last 10 years deeply in debt. How did this start?'

<u>The Structure</u>:

1) 'So – you're saying that writing a book and getting it published will make you feel really good and your whole life will be better. [Big picture] And what can you do today to be able to set things in motion? [Detail]'

2) 'Okay. You know what it's like to be 12 stone and how good you feel about yourself like that. [Big picture] What is the first thing you can do today to be true to yourself and make it start to happen? [Detail]'

3) 'So – you don't have any friends. [Big picture] Maybe now would be a good time to look at how you interact with others. [Detail]'

4) 'You've spent the last 10 years deeply in debt. [Big picture] How did this start? [Detail]'

This pattern is somewhat different from the Milton/Meta Model contrast in the sense that a meta comment is generally 'specific' which, when translated into Miltonian language can become quite 'general' (or vice versa – general into specific). For instance. Milton: 'You feel a certain way' becomes; Meta: 'You feel calm'. Deductive Language Patterns <u>maintain</u> specificity. [See also Inductive Language Patterns.]   Notice also that whereas in a Milton/Meta exchange it, in effect, revolves around a polar contrast occurring, relating to the topic being addressed (vague 'certain' feelings becoming specific 'calm' feelings, for instance) this language pattern (Deductive) maintains a focus on the overall goal <u>and</u> moves between 'specificity' and 'total' (not 'specificity' and 'general'). Thereby maintaining its overall goal-directed outcome without necessarily doing a 'polar flip'. For instance: 'You say you like feeling calm' [total]. 'How do you start to notice when it's beginning to happen [specific]?'

Definite Descriptions

<u>The Pattern</u>:

1) '...because you like holidaying in the flat in Royan...'

2) '...while you know that the person at the seminar wants to help you...'

3) '...and this means that when you next meet her on Friday you can say what needs to be said...'

<u>The Structure</u>:

This language pattern involves the use of a descriptive element which is very definite in what it's identifying.

1) '...because you like holidaying in the flat in Royan...' [A flat in Royan exists.]

2) '...while you know that the person at the seminar wants to help you...' [There is a person at the seminar.]

3) '...and this means that when you next meet her on Friday you can say what needs to be said...' [The client will meet 'her' – a 'her' exists - on Friday, which will be the next time that 'they meet'.]

Deletion

There are a number of categories that come under the overall heading of 'deletions' in relation to Indirect Hypnotherapy Language Patterning. These include: Comparative Deletions (see above) Simple Deletions (see below) Ambiguous Deletions (see above) Specific Deletions (see below), and Universal Deletions (see below), Lack of Referential Index (see below) and Unspecified Nouns (see below).

Derivative Example

The Pattern:

1)

Hypnotherapist: 'Give me an example of how you'd like things to be different?'

Client: 'I'd like to have more choices.'

Hypnotherapist: 'And if you had more choices you'd be able to do more of the things that you enjoy. Would you choose to take time to relax, learn something new, go away for a while, meet up with family and friends, or read a good book (or maybe something else)?'

2)

Client: 'I'll never get over this.'

Hypnotherapist: 'Maybe you won't. But if you did what would be different?'

Client: 'I suppose I'd meet someone else eventually.'

Hypnotherapist: 'Maybe you would. Perhaps by getting back in circulation again. Meeting new people. Going to new places. Developing new interests. You never can tell just how far this could lead. But don't rush straight out and do it today.'

The Structure:

1)

Lots of examples are offered about what the client could do with more choices, which are derived from the client's own original example (which means they have original 'ownership' of the derivations): The client offers an 'ideal' example. The therapist develops the theme by deriving more, therapeutic examples, from the original one given by the client. As the client explores the concepts they can (as in the above example) consider an ever increasing range of therapeutic potentials.

Hypnotherapist: 'Give me an example of how you'd like things to be different? [Searching for an ideal example]'

Client: 'I'd like to have more choices. [Example is given]'

Hypnotherapist: 'And if you had more choices you'd be able to do more of the things that you enjoy. Would you choose to take time to relax, learn something new, go away for a while, meet up with family and friends, or read a good book (or maybe something else)? [Examples are derived from the original, gently leading the client further along the theme they have at first suggested.]'

2)

The client presents with an issue of 'loss'. ['I'll never <u>get</u> <u>over</u> <u>this</u>'] They express 'hopelessness'. ['I'll <u>never</u> get over this']. Rather than challenge it (possibly resulting in the client defensively resisting the intervention) the therapist seems to agree with the possibility ['Maybe you won't']. Then the therapist gently coaxes the client to expand upon the possibility of 'getting over it', albeit, in a seemingly dismissive way, which stays in character with the preceding sentence ['But if you did what would be different?']. The client, largely because they don't feel coerced into exploring the concept is more open to doing so ['I suppose I'd meet someone else eventually']. The therapist then creates a range of life-expanding examples derived from the client's own proposition ['Maybe you would. Perhaps by getting back in circulation again. Meeting new people. Going to new places. Developing new interests. You never can tell just how far this could lead. But don't rush straight out and do it today']. Notice, though, the therapist says 'maybe you would', which again, is in-keeping with the tenor of the moment.

Client: 'I'll never get over this [expression of loss/hopelessness]'

Hypnotherapist: 'Maybe you won't [agreement frame]. But if you did what would be different [expanded frame].'

Client: 'I suppose I'd meet someone else eventually. [possibility frame]'

Hypnotherapist: 'Maybe you would. Perhaps by getting back in circulation again. Meeting new people. Going to new places. Developing new interests. You never can tell just how far this could lead. But don't rush straight out and do it today [derivate examples].'

Derivative Suggestion

<u>The Pattern</u>:

Tense Client: 'I'd like to go on holiday soon.'

Hypnotherapist: 'Yes – Holidays can be nice. They can be very relaxing. How do you feel when you're relaxed like that?'

<u>The Structure</u>:

The Derivative Suggestion is based on something that the client has conveyed which can be used by the therapist to help the client move towards a solution. In the above example the client (who is feeling tense) mentions that they'd like to go on holiday. The client's problem is tension. They explain that they'd like to go on holiday. The therapist, understanding the client's problem and the need for a restorative change, takes the theme that the client has raised (holidays) and then creates some suggestions which implicitly send messages to counteract tension:

Tense Client: 'I'd like to go on holiday soon.'

Hypnotherapist: 'Yes – Holidays can be nice [meeting client at the introduced theme – holidays]. They can be very relaxing [a suggestion – derived from the original theme is presented]. How do you feel when you're relaxed like that [the derivative theme is reinforced]?'

Desired Direction

The Pattern:

1) 'And as you begin to think about a better way of doing this...'

2) 'So now that you're starting to think in a solution-focussed way...'

3) 'Which is why, with each new idea you develop...'

The Structure:

Implicit within each of these suggestions exists a prompt to facilitate generative change in order to help the client move in a Desired Direction.

1) 'And as you begin to think about a better way of doing this [Desired Direction: the client will start to begin to think about a better way of doing something]...'

2) 'So now that you're starting to think in a solution-focussed way [Desired Direction: The client will start thinking in more of a solution-focussed way]...'

3) 'Which is why, with each new helpful idea you develop [Desired Direction: the client will develop helpful new ideas]...'

Desired Outcome

<u>The Pattern</u>:

1) 'Now, as you move ever closer to becoming a qualified exponent of Indirect Hypnotherapy.'

2) '...so by the time you become a qualified exponent of NLP.'

3) '...and as you're honing your skills to the point that you are using them unconsciously.'

<u>The Structure</u>:

The structure of this pattern is very similar to the Desired Direction, except that a <u>specific</u> outcome is the object. Therefore – emphasis is placed on the outcome – although of course, in the process, it can also be placed on the Desired Direction (as in the first and third example) in order to help create momentum to move towards the Desired Outcome.

1) 'Now, as you move ever closer [Desired Direction] to becoming a qualified exponent of Indirect Hypnotherapy [Specific Desired Outcome].'

2) '...so by the time you become a qualified exponent of NLP [Specific Desired Outcome].'

3) '...and as you're honing your skills [Desired Direction] to the point that you are using them unconsciously [Specific Desired Outcome].'

Directive Suggestion

The Pattern:

1) 'Now when you are in XYZ I want you to do ABC...in ways that work for your highest good.'

2) 'When you walk into the interview room I want you to smile appropriately at the interviewer, feel relaxed and begin.'

3) 'Next time you see her I want you to start to feel calm and collected and make all the right choices which help you...'

The Structure:

Sometimes client's feel the need for 'permission' to be given in the early stages of therapy, in order for them to allow themselves to take new challenges and/or exhibit new behaviours. A Directive Suggestion can take account of this need in such a way that the client can meet the 'permission need' and resultantly follow through on a helpful suggestion.

1) 'Now when you are in XYZ I want you to do ABC...in ways that work for your highest good...[an ecology checkpoint is inserted so that while the

client may be following a helpful directive...it's with the caveat that it will be in a way that works for the client's highest good]'

2) 'When you walk into the interview room <u>I want you to</u> smile appropriately at the interviewer, feel relaxed and do well...['do well' includes, by implication, a similar ecological checkpoint].'

3) 'Next time you see her <u>I want you</u> to start to feel calm and collected and make all the right choices which help you...['all the right choices', is also an ecological checkpoint].'

Direct Suggestion

Sometimes one of the most important aspects of successfully employing Indirect Hypnotherapy principles is also knowing when and how to use Direct Suggestion in the process.

<u>The Pattern</u>:

1) 'Next time you walk into the meeting <u>you</u> <u>will</u> start to feel calm, confident and self-assured.'

2) 'From now on you are becoming more creative in your work. That's right. More creative. <u>You</u> <u>will</u> be more creative at work.'

3) 'Because your social life is improving. <u>You</u> <u>will</u> start to go out and enjoy yourself more.'

<u>The Structure</u>:

The structure is self-evident. Very direct instructions are given, in these examples, prefixed by the words 'you will'.

Disjunctions

The Pattern:

1) 'You might not notice the change immediately but when it starts to happen things will start to shift.'

2) 'You may enjoy relaxing in trance...or letting yourself unwind or taking it easy...but whatever you do will be good.'

3) 'It could be that you choose to do this and this...but whatever you choose it will be better than being where you were.'

The Structure:

The first part of each sentence, due to the use of the word 'but', in effect, is accepted to mean that it's being presupposed that what's been stated (before 'but') will manifest. However, the use of the word 'but' also creates a 'disconnection' of sorts with what preceded its use (the presupposition) thereby allowing suggestions to be made immediately after its application too, which, while bearing a relation to the first part of each sentence, also imply that movement is taking place beyond the original opening remarks (which have already been presupposed). This in turn results in the communication thread 'looping back', so to speak, to its original focal point, thereby reinforcing the first element of the suggestion.

1) 'You might not notice the <u>change</u> immediately <u>but</u> <u>when</u> it starts to happen <u>things will start to shift</u>.'

2) 'You may enjoy <u>relaxing</u> in trance...or letting yourself <u>unwind</u> or <u>taking it easy</u>...<u>but</u> whatever you do <u>will be good</u>.'

3) 'It could be that <u>you choose</u> to <u>do this</u> <u>and this</u>...<u>but</u> <u>whatever</u> you choose <u>it will be better</u> than being where you were.'

Dissociated Associated Unconscious Conscious Double Bind

<u>The Pattern</u>:

1) 'And I wonder what helpful feeling that you're not consciously aware of now that your unconscious can begin to generate inside and let you experience it now...which helps you...could be?...'

2) 'And I wonder what resource that you're not consciously aware of but which your unconscious mind is and can begin to let you experience now might be?'

<u>The Structure</u>:

The primary purpose of the Dissociated Associated Unconscious Conscious Double Bind is to elicit a therapeutic state potential from within the client and then begin to have him/her associate into it.

1) 'And I wonder what helpful feeling [therapeutic state potential is suggested] that you're not consciously aware of [it's dissociated – which in this context is also a Truism because the client was not consciously experiencing that state before the moment it began to be suggested] now that your unconscious can begin to generate inside [momentum is added to the therapeutic state potential] and let you experience it now [it is suggested that the client moves into an associated experience]…which helps you…[it's ecological] could be? [The client has to wait and see, which means it's to be an unconscious response]'

You will notice the linear process involved. The client starts from a disempowered position and the process gently and swiftly shifts them towards a helpful associated state, in the space of a few words.

2) 'And I wonder what resource [therapeutic state potential] that you're not consciously aware of [dissociated] but which your unconscious mind is and can begin to let you experience now [associated]…might be? [which means it's to be an unconscious response]'

Dissociated Double Bind

The Pattern:

1) 'And I wonder if you will notice the new solutions before you change or just change before you notice them?'

2) 'So, as you consider making changes will you know when they will happen, or will they start to happen without you knowing how?'

3) 'Or it could be that without having to think about how you just start to feel better, or maybe you'll be thinking about how...and feeling better as you do...'

The Structure:

This is very similar to the Double Dissociated Double Bind (see above). The difference being that there's only one dissociative element within its structure. It can be employed in much the same way as Double Dissociated Double Bind.

1) 'And I wonder if you will notice the new solutions [new solutions are the focus of the Bind] before you change [bound once – associated] or just change before you notice them [bound twice – dissociated]?'

2) 'So, as you consider making changes [making changes – the focus of the Bind] will you know when they will happen [bound once – associated] or will they start to happen without you knowing how [bound twice – dissociated]?'

3) 'Or it could be that without having to think about how [bound once, in advance of the 'focus' itself being given – dissociated] you just start to feel better [the focus of the Bind is on feeling better] or maybe you'll be thinking [bound twice – associated] about how... and feeling better as you do...'

Dissociative Language

[See Association]

Distortion

Distortion includes The Lost Performative [see below] Mind Reading [see below] Cause and Effect [see above], Complex Equivalence [see above] and Liedentity [see below].

Distraction

Derren Brown the 'mind control' expert uses the technique of misdirection and distraction to generate the amazing results that he does. Frank Farrelly the Provocative Therapy specialist likewise utilises this approach adroitly. It can serve a number of purposes, including, (Frank Farrelly style) to break up a client's rigid self-defeating belief system. If a client continues to indulge in destructive thinking it can reinforce the destructive nature of their habit. By distracting the client from their 'woe story' it can serve to help them to begin to move beyond it (for a fuller explanation of some of Frank Farrelly's strategies see the accompanying article called: 'The Wizard of Wisconsin', which is located in the appendixes section of this book).

Here are a couple of examples of how distraction and misdirection can be employed therapeutically:

1)

Misdirection:

Hypnotherapist: 'It's very important that you keep repeating to yourself as we talk the phrase: 'I can change – I will change'. And as you do that you don't need to listen to anything else...unless you want to...so keep repeating to yourself the important phrase 'I can change – I will change'.'

While the client is focussed on repeating these suggestions (misdirection) the therapist then proceeds to convey a range of positive suggestions 'in the background':

'That's right and as you keep repeating this important statement to yourself [misdirection], a [here come the indirect-direct suggestions...] range of new options are beginning to present themselves to you. When will you first notice them? What will they be? How will they help you to make the kind of changes you want? Won't it be great to notice how much better things are! That's it – just keep repeating that important statement [misdirection], really listen to what you're saying and what it means [misdirection]. And [here come some more indirect-direct suggestions...] because you are now beginning to change – your life starts to improve in profound ways. And other people begin to notice the amazing results too...that's because...[etc].'

It seems to the client that the rote phrase is the most important element of the process. In this example it is itself a <u>helpful</u> phrase to say (but not <u>the</u> most important). The fact that it is genuinely helpful actually enhances the misdirection, because the client will likely perceive that it is the focus of the intervention (at this point) whereas the peripheral suggestions that the therapist is offering are, in reality, the main area of intervention. They are taking place overtly yet, paradoxically, in a subliminal kind of way (allowing them to be absorbed unconsciously, which is the therapist's goal). Notice: the client isn't told they <u>won't</u> hear anything else, they are told, they <u>don't need to</u> listen to anything else, <u>unless they want to</u>. This allows for an ecology check and for the inclusion of any safety issues (such as the need to hear instructions from the therapist or others that could, very remotely, occur during a session; for instance, if a building needed to be evacuated).

<u>Distraction</u>:

If a client is locked into a 'woe story' from which they're generating significant amounts of secondary gain (attention, sympathy, victim-hood, etc), the therapist can begin to look bored every time they start to do so. This approach can begin to distract the client from the 'woe story' and its related secondary gains (because they're no longer being met) and as a result an opportunity to develop a new and functional (as opposed to the old, habituated, dysfunctional) strategy is enhanced. Frank Farrelly is a master at utilising this approach [see appendix].

Do It Now...

The phrase 'Do it now' is a 'stock in trade' phrase utilised in the personal development field. Here are some examples of how it may be applied in a hypnotherapeutic context.

1) 'Now, as your unconscious considers how you will **do it now**...'

2) 'That's right, make the change happen at an unconscious level. **Do it now...right now** and as **you do** you will start to notice the difference in ways that are new and in ways that you know about...'

3) 'You may already be thinking that you want to **do it now**...or you may be thinking about what it would be like to **do it now**...and whether you are thinking about **doing it now**...or thinking about what it would be like to **do it now**...you can choose when the time is right to **do it**.'

Double Bind

This is similar to the Bind/Simple Bind, except that the choice cannot be made at the conscious level.

<u>Here are some examples</u>:

1) 'Do you think your left hand will get warm before your right hand?'

2) 'Do you think you will breathe more slowly before you relax more or will you relax more before you breathe more slowly?'

3) 'Will you feel better immediately or later?'

4) 'I wonder whether you will sense this change on an intellectual level or on an emotional level...first?'

5) 'I don't know whether you will find that your eyes are getting tired or getting heavy as you go into trance...'

6) 'I wonder whether you'll notice a sensation in your feet or something happening in your hands first?'

7) 'Will you notice your hearing range increasing or will relaxing sensations occur as you experience the state of hypnosis developing...now!?'

8) 'Changes can happen slowly at first or quickly and I wonder what you will do with them when you start to use them?'

9) 'And I wonder what you will do with the new changes when you start to use them and if you will notice them happening slowly at first or quickly.'

(Notice, each of these Double Binds can only be answered at an unconscious level and the conscious mind has to <u>wait and experience what actually occurs</u> in order to learn the answer. Will you sense that you've learned Double Binds by using them or will you find that you use them because you sense that you've learned them?)

<u>The Structure of a Double Bind</u>:

I wonder whether you will notice these new good feelings by this evening or will they occur in a day or so?

In this case the implication is that the client will notice the 'new good feelings' at sometime, but the way the question is structured also implies that the noticing part will take place due to the unconscious release of these feelings. It's not something a person can consciously decide to do, which means that, by implication, the unconscious needs to do it for them. The process is seeded by suggesting/using hypnotic presupposition that new good feelings will be generated. And the rest is left up to the unconscious to do.

Double Dissociated Double Bind

The Pattern:

1) 'You can experience a sensation without knowing that it's there or know that it's there without knowing where it came from.'

2) 'You can notice an experience without knowing that it's there or know that it's there without knowing how you discovered it.'

3) 'You can wonder about a solution without knowing what it is or know what it is without realising how you found it.'

4) 'You can discover a resource without knowing how you did or know how you did without knowing where it came from.'

5) 'As you …create new ideas without knowing how you do or knowing how you do without understanding how you create them….you can begin to sense them creating new opportunities for you…'

6) 'A person… like you… can feel better quickly without noticing that you are or noticing that you are feeling better without knowing how you do it.'

7) 'It's possible to think about eating healthily without remembering that you're doing so – or remembering that you're doing so without knowing how you think it.'

8) 'You can remember a happy time without remembering that you're remembering it or know that you're remembering it without knowing that you are. (A Double Dissociated Double Bind – plus suggestions to produce amnesia).'

9) 'A new thought can happen without you knowing that it's happened or you can know that it's happened without knowing how you thought it.'

10) 'You can feel more confident without having to think about it or you can think about it and wonder where it comes from.'

11) 'And you can imagine a solution without understanding how or you can understand the solution without knowing how you created it.'

12) 'You can explore a rigidity without knowing that it's there.   Or knowing that it's rigid without knowing how you discovered it.'

13) 'You can slowly return to a pleasant memory and forget the future as it passes or discover yourself already in the memory realising that the future hasn't happened but knowing that you remember a past time when you forgot the future.' [A Stephen Brooks'-style example.]

(This guides the client back to a time when there was no knowledge of the present, and then back to a time before that).

14) 'You can awaken as a person but you don't have to awaken as a body.'

The Structure of a Double Dissociated Double Bind:

1)

'And you can generate a good feeling without knowing where it's coming from or you can know where it's coming from without knowing how you generated it.'

'And you can generate a good feeling [this part is associated]'

'...without knowing where it's coming from [this dissociates it once]'

'...or you can know where it's coming from [this part is associated]'

'...without knowing how you generated it [this dissociates it again creating a Double Dissociation].'

2)

'And you may find yourself creating new feelings that you don't know about or know that you know about them without realising that it's happening.'

'And you may find yourself creating new feelings [this part is associated]'

'...that you don't know about [this dissociates it once]'

'...or know that you know about them [this is associated]'

'...without realising how it's happening [this dissociates it for the second time – while 'tying the bind' by the further implication of new feelings.']

3)

First part:

'And you can explore a sensation without knowing that it's there.'

This involves dissociation. How can you explore something without knowing that it's there unless you're dissociated from it at some level?

Second part:

'Or you can know that it's there without knowing how you discovered it.'

This also involves dissociation. How can you not know how you discovered it without some kind of dissociation taking place?

The Bind part: The Bind is contained in the reference to the sensation, in exploring it, and in knowing that it's there.

4)

'And you can experience a resource without knowing how you know it. Or know that you know it without knowing how you experience it.'

Notice the mirror-image-like way in which these Double Dissociated Double Binds are structured. The first part and the last part, in effect reflect each other's intent. They both reflect the 'experience' part, which, in this example, is what the Bind is aiming to achieve. We want the client to experience a resource.

5)

'And you can remember a happy feeling without knowing how you discovered it or know how you discovered it without knowing that you've remembered it.'

In this instance the Bind is front loaded with a reference to the client experiencing a 'happy feeling'. Then the first dissociation takes place, with the words: 'without knowing how you discovered it'. This is then followed up with the second element, in the phrase: 'know how you discovered it' which is itself followed by the second dissociation, in the form of the words: 'without knowing that you've remembered it.'

Doubt

The Pattern:

1)

Stephen Brooks: 'Tell me – what's happening now – are you out of that trance?'

Client: 'I Think so.'

Stephen Brooks: 'That's right – you think so!'

2)

Richard Bandler: 'Are you sure?'

Client: 'Yes!'

Richard Bandler: 'Are you sure enough to be unsure?'

3)

Client: 'I don't know.'

Anthony Robbins: 'I know you don't know – but if you did, what would it be?'

Client: 'Oh. Uh! It would be ...'

The Structure:

This principle can be useful to generate doubt in a client's mind in order to enhance the hypnotic phenomena which are occurring, break up self-defeating patterns and open up new possibilities (etc).

1)

Stephen Brooks: 'Tell me – what's happening now – are you out of that trance?'

Client: 'I Think so.'

Stephen Brooks: 'That's right – you think so!'

In this example, which I heard Stephen Brooks use, the emphasis on the words 'you think so', generates doubt in a client's mind, and makes the experience more 'trancey', as Stephen might say.

2)

Richard Bandler: 'Are you sure?'

Client: 'Yes!'

Richard Bandler: 'Are you sure enough to <u>be unsure</u>?'

In this example, Richard Bandler uses the client's unit of measurement (surety) and then challenges them to use that same unit of measurement against their own problem. Paradoxically, if they say they are not sure enough to be unsure, it generates doubt. And if they say they are sure enough to be unsure, it generates doubt. Either response works therapeutically.

3)

Client: 'I don't know.'

Anthony Robbins: 'I know you don't know – <u>but if you did</u>, what would it be?'

Client: 'Oh. Uh! It would be …'

A slightly different version. In this instance the client is expressing doubt about their ability to 'know' something (or make a choice that will have some therapeutic benefit). They 'know that they don't know'. They are sure about their doubt.

Anthony <u>meets</u> <u>them</u> <u>at</u> <u>their</u> <u>position</u> of doubt and rather than overtly challenging it (which may generate a 'resistance') he uses the Aikido approach of stepping out of its way, (metaphorically speaking) and then turns the energy around in the direction of a solution-focussed way of thinking. The client does not feel coerced into taking a position that is 'set in stone', because Tony has agreed that they 'don't know', so (as he might say) it's 'just a hypothesis'. However, as soon as the client has moved from their position of 'knowing they don't know', to considering the idea that they might know, he works with the client, from the new perspective, in ways that continue to reinforce it therapeutically.

E

Early Learning Set Inductions

Early Learning Set inductions/interventions involve drawing upon universally shared early life experiences to communicate helpful messages, indirectly. For instance:

<u>Child Walking</u>:

'It's just like a child learning to walk, <u>standing for the first time on their own</u>. You don't consciously remember <u>when</u> you did - yet a part of you knows <u>how</u> you did it.'

One of the indirect messages here is that there is a part of the client which helped him/her to learn to walk (outside of conscious awareness), a 'part' which can also help the client now to 'stand up' in life.

<u>Here's another example</u>:

'I remember when I first started learning to ride a bike. At first it seemed a bit tricky. I wasn't sure if I would really be able to do it. But I did. Somehow, it all started to come together. The balance, the direction, the certainty that I could do it. Until I reached a point where I could bring it all together naturally and do it comfortably.'

While the therapist is (seemingly) talking about himself/herself, the message to the client is universally understood. Doing something new can seem a bit daunting – but with a little practice it can soon start to become easy.

Eirenicon Suggestions

Eirenicon suggestions are suggestions which promote inner-peace and self-esteem. (From the Greek word 'Eirene' which means peace.)

1) 'How many ways will you notice your own feelings of inner-peace beginning to develop?'

2) 'You know, I like the words 'self esteem'. One reason being is that the word 'self' also means 'nature' and the word 'esteem' also means 'good opinion' and we are all a part of the natural world and it's been demonstrated time-and-again that it's good to naturally have a good opinion of ourselves. <u>Inwardly</u> we all do anyway – it's just that sometimes we don't <u>outwardly</u> fully know that we do. But you're starting to make changes - which tells us both that you are starting to understand this at a conscious level too now.'

In this example we have shifted the client's train of awareness to acceptance of the Eirenicon Suggestions by 'synonymising', by drawing their awareness to related meanings of words which may be negatively semantically charged (meaning the intended sense has become 'lost' to them, due to a fixed opinion; for instance the expression 'self-esteem' may, by now, actually be anchored to a feeling that that's something they're 'incapable' of having). By 'synonymising' to non-semantically charged words, which basically mean the same kind of thing, but which convey the desired meaning in this roundabout, circuitous way (indirectly) it can help a client to begin to accept the concept (and related affect) that they are, actually, 'allowed' to possess healthy (natural) self-esteem (a good opinion of themselves). This helps promote a sense of developing 'peace'.

Elicitation Of Universal Experience

<u>The Pattern</u>:

1) 'And when you've enjoyed eating an appropriate amount of food for your evening meal you can remember to think 'Full Stop!'. (The 'Full Stop!' phrase is one that I've borrowed from Gill, who in turn borrowed it from Paul McKenna who used it himself when she attended one of his seminars).'

2) 'So – that just means that up until now the 'traffic lights of life' were turned to red. But now they've switched to green. And this means that it's now time for you to get going. To move forward.'

3) 'We've all believed something to be a 'fact' and then found out it wasn't true after all. I mean, didn't you used to believe, or, at the very least, think that perhaps Father Christmas might really exist? But now you know for sure that what you used to believe (or maybe at least wondered about) is absolutely not true. What else might you be believing to be true now – and therefore responding to in <u>your life</u> as if it was a fact – that may actually not be true at all? Maybe, perhaps, that old belief

that you had about 'never being able to become a non-smoker'? Maybe that's just a ho! ho! hoax – after all?'

The Structure:

The structure is apparent in the pattern. It draws upon a universal experience in order to elicit states, thoughts and feelings associated with the experience for therapeutic purposes.

Elvis Effect

The Pattern:

This is among my favourite ways of helping clients to begin to 'stop trying too hard' consciously to make changes. It utilises (and explains) Coue's law of reversed effect.

The Structure:

Often when a client presents for help with dealing with an addiction, for example; smoking, they may say something like:

'I've tried really hard to stop smoking. Every day I wake up and say to myself the last thing I'm going to think about today is having a cigarette. But immediately I do that I find I want one! And the harder I try to resist the harder it gets not to have one.'

I'll then ask the client not to think of Elvis (I have an Elvis bust in my treatment room that was given to me as a gift, which helps) like this:

'I want to do a little experiment now. It's fun. You'll see. Try this for a moment will you? Don't think of Elvis Presley. That's it. Just don't think of Elvis Presley. Whatever you do, don't hear the words 'all shook up'. Don't get a picture of him with his dark blue/black hair. And please make sure you don't imagine him in one of those white jumpsuits will all of the sequins on it. [Pause and smile]. Oh oh! What did yooou just do? Oops! [Client:] I couldn't help it. I couldn't stop myself thinking about Elvis Presley. [Kerin:] <u>That's right</u> – and that's the way it works – <u>consciously</u>. When you try and <u>force</u> <u>yourself</u> to change consciously - sometimes it just works against you. This is when it's useful to '<u>relax the changes to occur</u>' instead. Change by not trying – consciously at least. After all – if I were to ask you now to <u>think of Elvis Presley</u>, you can do it equally as well by not trying hard to resist thinking about him as you can by just allowing yourself to think about him. Can't you? [Please read that through again. It is logical, however, when said quickly, most people, won't be able to 'unpack' it, but will simply accept the statement as a fact – which it is. This itself generates a trance state – in which the suggestions can find a home.] And that's the way changes happen in hypnosis! Your unconscious mind - which grows your fingernails for you without you having to think about that <u>either</u> - just gets on with doing it for you without you really having to try, or not try, to <u>make it happen</u>. You just <u>relax and become a non-smoker</u>. So you can remember to forget 'trying to change' and just let yourself <u>remember to change naturally instead</u>! That sounds much easier doesn't it? Anyway...let's move on to the next stage now...'.

What this example does is reduce the client's worry about not being able to change by shifting the emphasis on which part of them will be making the changes happen <u>for them</u> (their unconscious). This can be quite a liberating concept for them, particularly if they're at their 'wit's end' believing that 'willpower' won't work - for them. This provides a nice contrast to the Decision Conditioning program in which the therapist 'ratchets up' a client's willpower to help them change. Indirect Hypnotherapists can work paradoxically to help their clients achieve the best possible outcome. Whereas many people engage in 'black or white' thinking, for example; 'I must use willpower', 'I must only not use willpower', Indirect Hypnotherapists will instead use what works! They epitomise tactical flexibility.

Embedded Commands/Embedded Suggestions

Embedded Commands involve the use of pauses (...) with a... ^{shift} in... **tonality** ...in order to intersperse therapeutic suggestions throughout the trancework being delivered. When done skilfully such 'commands' can bypass the conscious mind and be communicated directly to the unconscious mind. (Note: personally I prefer the expression 'Embedded Suggestion' to 'Embedded Command' because it emphasises the client's ability to choose whether or not to accept what is being proffered – because it is only a <u>suggestion</u>, whereas the concept of a command implies no choice, whether or not that is actually true.)

Here's an example:

'It's good to know that ...**things can come easily••••** ^{to you} as you begin to... **focus your attention** inwards...**now**...^{that's} ^{right}...and you don't have to know how... **you**... are beginning to **change your behaviour** ^{immediately}...or later, because you know that.... **it will happen•••** when ^{you need it} ^{to} ..._,'

Embedded Questions

<u>The Pattern</u>:

1) 'Would you like to start using Embedded Questions as soon as you get the next opportunity?'

2) 'Wouldn't it be great to develop your indirect hypnotherapy language patterns naturally?'

3) 'How many ways do you think you could suggest now to get motivated?'

<u>The Structure</u>:

This pattern employs the same principle as the Embedded Command method, except that the suggestion is 'hidden' within a question.

1) 'Would you like to **start using Embedded Questions** as soon as you get the next opportunity?'

2) 'Wouldn't it be great to ^{develop your indirect hypnotherapy} ^{language patterns} naturally?'

3) 'How many ways do you think you could suggest now to ^{get motivated}?'

Emotional Content

The Pattern:

1)

'So, you've thought about this a lot now. Well done! That's the first step in beginning to change. So let's add the emotion that goes with it. The power that's going to drive you forward. The emotional energy of your unstoppable positivity that comes from deep within...'

The Structure:

1)

'So, you've thought about this a lot now. Well done! That's the first step in beginning to change. So let's **add the emotion** that goes with it. **The power** that's going to **drive you** forward. The **emotional energy** of your unstoppable **positivity** that comes from deep within...'

In the classic movie 'Enter The Dragon' starring Bruce Lee, when teaching one of his young students Bruce emphasised that, to be proficient at Kung Fu, 'You need emotional content'. He distinguished this (emotional content) from surrendering to an unbridled emotion (in the movie example it was anger) which is often what happens to a person who becomes 'stuck' in a state like 'depression' for instance (although, as Stephen Brooks likes to point out, 'melancholy' is a much better word than 'depression'. The term 'depression', today, often carries with it the connotation that it's a fixed state, whereas a diagnosis of 'melancholy' is much more likely to be considered to be just a transient phase.). This demonstrates the line of reasoning that proposes that there is, in many instances of personal development work, the need for a <u>positively charged emotional factor</u> to be included. Likewise, in therapy, for generative change to occur and – importantly – be maintained, there needs to be a considerable degree of emotional content. It can include enthusiasm, determination, or even being plain 'sick and tired' of an existing state to the extent that it becomes too painful to be allowed to continue. Anthony Robbins places emphasis on this theme too – albeit in a slightly different way. He talks about leverage. The leverage being the emotional energy that helps the client to begin to move forward. He uses the definitions of 'pain' and 'pleasure' to denote the dual areas of 'emotional content'. And he does so to great affect/effect in his excellent work.

Emotional Shifting

<u>The Pattern</u>:

1)

Client: 'I feel totally angry. And I can't seem to calm down.'

Hypnotherapist: 'How do you feel about feeling angry like that?'

Client: 'Disappointed.'

Hypnotherapist: 'Disappointed. Right. How would you rather feel?'

The Structure:

1)

Client: 'I feel totally angry. And I can't seem to calm down.'

Hypnotherapist: *'<u>How do you feel about feeling angry</u> like that?'

Client: 'Disappointed.'

Hypnotherapist: 'Disappointed. Right. <u>How would you rather feel</u>?'

The pivotal point in the above example is the element that I've highlighted with an asterisk. By asking 'How do you feel about feeling ...' it causes a person to need to shift to a different emotional viewpoint in order to be able to consider the question. From there the therapist can move into exploring preferable states: 'How would you rather feel?'.

Here are some related Emotional Shifting questions.

'How do you feel about feeling scared?'
'How do you feel about feeling shy?'
'How do you feel about feeling jealous?'
'How do you feel about feeling frustrated?'

Emotion Binds

<u>The Pattern</u>:

1) 'Now...as things improve...I don't know whether you'll start to feel more positive first – or just begin to notice feeling more up-beat generally...but when you sense that something is happening...'

2) 'Now, I want you to listen carefully (but you don't have to listen). Sometime soon I want you to begin to create some appropriate new ways of feeling comfortable in your work – or just more at ease if you prefer...and as you do this...I wonder how you will notice this is happening?'

3) 'And now...as you become more positive and more optimistic, or just more happy about things generally...you might like to ask yourself: How will the changes happen? And then wait and see, when they start, what you notice.'

<u>The Structure</u>:

Emotion Binds are basically Double Binds which are focused specifically on helping the client to shift his/her emotional reference state from an unwanted/outdated one, to chosen and preferred forms of affective experience.

1) 'Now...**as things improve**...I don't know whether you'll start to **feel more positive** first – or just begin to notice **feeling more up-beat** generally...but when you sense that something is happening...'

If the therapist 'doesn't know' who does? Not the client. At least, not consciously. This means that it's a Double Bind, because the only way the client will find out is by waiting for the affective change to happen, which indicates that it must be taking place at an unconscious level.

2) 'Now, I want ^{you} to listen carefully (but $_{you}$ don't have to listen). Sometime soon I want $_{you}$ to begin to create some appropriate new ways of **feeling comfortable** in your work – or just more **at ease** if $_{you}$ prefer...and as you do this...I wonder how ^{you} will notice this is happening?'

The: 'I want you to listen carefully' is aimed at the unconscious mind, while the '(but you don't have to listen)', is aimed at the conscious mind. This method will also likely generate a certain amount of therapeutic confusion in the client. 'Sometime soon' implies that neither the therapist, nor the client will (consciously) know for sure 'when' things will, start to occur. This means that, again, the change is to be generated unconsciously. This is ratified by the statement: 'I wonder how you will notice this is happening?'.

3) 'And now...as you become **more positive and more optimistic**, or just **more happy** about things generally...you might like to ask yourself: How will the changes happen? And then wait and see, when they start, what you notice.'

If the client has to 'ask' questions about how the affective responses will happen, it implies: a) they don't consciously know and: b) they unconsciously know. A Double Bind – with an emotional 'tie' to it.

Exactitude

'The exact, appropriate, helpful, healthful, way that's right for you.'

<u>The Pattern</u>:

'And I want your unconscious mind to make these changes in the exact, appropriate, helpful, healthful way that's right for you.'

<u>The Structure</u>:

'And I want your unconscious mind to make these changes in the **exact, appropriate**, **helpful**, **healthful** way **that's right for you**.

In essence this suggestion is focussed on ensuring that everything that takes place in-and-as-a-result-of the therapy session is for the client's welfare, with the results manifesting in the most ecological and fitting ways. A similar phrase that can be used is:

'And the changes will happen in **normal**, **balanced** and **harmonious** ways which work **exactly** right for you.'

I liberally include phrases like this in all the therapy and coaching work that I do, as a matter of course and with mind to duty of care.

Extended Quotes

<u>The Pattern</u>:

1) 'Carol Lankton said that...'

2) 'One of my clients had a similar experience and he found that...'

3) 'My dad discovered that the best way to do this was...'

<u>The Structure</u>:

1) '<u>Carol Lankton</u> said that...'

2) '<u>One of my clients</u> had a similar experience and he found that...'

3) '<u>My dad</u> discovered that the best way to do this was...'

This pattern has the effect of 'distancing' the speaker from the statement they're about to make. This can be useful because, rather than something that's said seeming to be a direct instruction, a piece of information can be offered indirectly, by referring to someone else's experience, in the context of which the desired meaning can be conveyed. Milton Erickson used to help his clients by talking to them about his friend John's experiences. And his friend John used to have many wonderful experiences. [Which was itself an example of a 'double extended quote'.]

Eyes-Closed Trance / Eyes-Open Trance

The Pattern:

'It doesn't matter whether you prefer to experience Eyes-Closed Trance, after Eyes-Open Trance, or let those open eyes start to close, to move into an Eyes-Closed Trance, because trance can happen in many ways at many levels...'

The Structure:

The phrases 'Eyes-Closed Trance' and 'Eyes-Open Trance' imply that closed or open, the client is going to experience a trance. This sentence is structured to generate a certain amount of therapeutic confusion and movement in the direction of achieving eye closure.

'It doesn't matter whether you prefer to experience **Eyes-Closed Trance,** after **Eyes-Open Trance,** or **let those open eyes start to close,** to **move into an Eyes-Closed Trance,** because trance can happen in many ways at many levels...'

F

Factive Verbs And Adjectives

<u>The Pattern</u>:

1) 'And won't you be pleased to discover yourself using indirect hypnotherapy principles well?'

2) 'You might think it odd that you ever used to feel that way.'

3) 'As you are aware your unconscious understands things even more completely...'

4) 'You know that you can do this...'

5) 'As you realise how much easier it can be...'

6) 'Wouldn't it be sad to have to regret the fact that you didn't take action?'

<u>The Structure</u>:

1) 'And won't you be **pleased** to discover yourself using indirect hypnotherapy principles well?'

2) 'You might think it **odd** that you ever used to feel that way.'

3) 'As you are **aware** your unconscious understands things even more completely...'

4) 'You **know** that you can do this...'

5) 'As you **realise** how much easier it can be...'

6) 'Wouldn't it be sad to have to **regret** the fact that you didn't take action?'

Factive Verbs and Adjectives are used to generate a psycho-emotional element to the trancework, in ways that help the client move forward.

Fantasy

Often it's useful to encourage the client to create a compelling fantasy, representing the desired way things will be as he/she integrates the psychotherapeutic work that takes place during therapy in order to give them something to move toward. This can also be known as using 'Imagination' and as 'Visualisation'. If a client wants a better job, for instance, the therapist might suggest that they spend a few minutes each day imagining actually working in the kind of job they desire. If the client is shy, the therapist may suggest that they visualise themselves meeting more people, comfortably. If the client has difficulty in seeing a way forward, the therapist might 'side step' the problem by asking them to describe details of a 'pure fantasy' about the way they'd 'prefer things to be'.

Find

Gill mentioned this useful language pattern that she heard Tad James use: 'You might find that you can't find it anymore'. (It's a good example of the Apply To Self method.)

Fixation

<u>The Pattern</u>:

1) 'And as you continue giving yourself permission to take it easy, I'd like you to listen to the gentle rhythm of the music now. That's it. Continue to be aware of the rhythm of the music.'

2) 'And as we begin, let yourself find a spot on the wall over there and let your eyes gently rest their gaze on that spot... and let your gaze remain only on the spot... until... you sense you are ready to close your eyes.'

3) 'So, while you continue in your trance-formation continue to think about that thought now. Just allow yourself to continue to think about that thought while your unconscious gets on with thinking about which part to change for the better first.'

<u>The Structure</u>:

1) 'And as you continue giving yourself permission to take it easy I'd like you to <u>listen to the gentle rhythm of the music now</u>. That's it. Continue to <u>be aware of the rhythm of the music</u>.'

2) 'And as we begin, let yourself find a spot on the wall over there and <u>let your eyes gently rest their gaze on that spot</u>... and <u>let your gaze remain only</u>

<u>on the spot</u>... until... you sense you are ready to close your eyes.'

3) 'So, while you continue in your trance-formation <u>continue to think about that thought now</u>. Just allow yourself to <u>continue to think about that thought</u> while your unconscious gets on with thinking about which part to change for the better first.'

The client is invited to fix their attention on something suggested by the therapist. Fixation, as a 'technique' is one of the oldest forms of generating trance states. It happens naturally. Most everyone has had the experience of 'staring' at something and finding their gaze becoming 'stuck' on the object of their observation. Maybe even to the extent that someone has waived their hand in front of them while saying something like: 'Hey you! Are you with us?'. This method takes a natural phenomenon and utilises it for therapeutic purposes. After all, hypnosis itself is a regularly occurring natural state, which is used for therapeutic purposes.

You can also fixate attention by talking about something that the recipient of the suggestion is relaxed or motivated by... and then combine this experience with internal experiences: 'So as you consider again how much you enjoy laying on that beach in Cyprus you can let yourself unwind within now'. Both elements (Cyprus on the beach and unwinding within) are a fixation on a theme.

Fluff

<u>The Pattern</u>:

'Now, you have a very clear understanding of how resourcefully you are going to respond in the ABC situation now. So while you enjoy allowing yourself to consider just how nice it can be to let yourself continue to experience a certain special kind of pleasure as you fully explore the possibilities of trance to its fullest potential. Knowing that as you do this – as you fully explore the possibilities of trance to its fullest level, even more positive changes can occur which help you. Now, again, as you fully consider how confidently you will walk into the room, how dynamic your voice will sound and how good you will feel about doing it this way instead...'

<u>The Structure</u>:

I remember Wilf Proudfoot (of the Proudfoot School of Clinical Hypnosis & Psychotherapy) talking about using 'fluff' and 'super fluff'. In essence what he was explaining was that sometimes, in amongst all of the strategic work that a hypnotherapist will utilise, they may also, as a kind of transitional phrase/phase, between each directed therapeutic element, incorporate this 'fluff' and 'super fluff'.

'...and now...you have a very clear understanding of how resourcefully <u>you</u> <u>are</u> <u>going</u> <u>to</u> <u>respond</u> in the ABC situation as you walk confidently, speak dynamically and feel good. [super fluff starts] So while you enjoy allowing yourself to consider just how nice it can be to let yourself continue to experience a certain special kind of pleasure as you fully explore the possibilities of trance to its fullest potential. Knowing that as you do this – as you fully explore the possibilities of trance to its fullest level, even more positive changes can occur which help you. [super fluff ends] Now, again, as <u>you</u> <u>fully</u> <u>consider</u> how confidently <u>you</u> <u>will</u> walk into the room, how dynamic your voice will sound and how good you will feel about doing it this way instead...'

Focussing

Focussing means doing what needs to be done to ensure that you and your client remain on track. This might include becoming ever more detailed (microscopically and/or macroscopically) about the required means to achieving the desired outcome(s). It basically means keeping the session and/or your client on target.

Frame Size

Client: 'I don't understand what they just said. Now I feel silly.'

Hypnotherapist: Intervention 1) 'What else don't you understand that you're not aware of?' [This intervention changes the client's 'frame size' or perspective towards their problem by taking the theme of 'not understanding' and using it to shift their awareness onto other areas.]

Hypnotherapist: Intervention 2) 'I wonder. How many others in the room do you think also felt silly with you?' [This intervention helps the client to change his/her 'frame size' perspective from one of being self-focussed (and then judging themselves harshly) to expanding their thoughts to include the possibility of the fact that it's likely others felt the same way.] (Frank Farrelly uses this skill very well – see appendix: The Wizard of Wisconsin'.)

Hypnotherapist: Intervention 3) 'Did you know that feeling silly is just one of the many possible feelings to have about not understanding.' [This intervention encourages the client to change their perspective and consider the wider range of emotions that he/she could feel instead.]

Framing

This means setting a desired 'frame' or reference perspective to a situation.

Frontloaded Framing:

'Think about this...wouldn't it be better to change sooner...'

Rearloaded Framing:

'Wouldn't it be better to change sooner...think about that.'

The instruction to think about the suggestion is introduced either just before or just after the framed suggestion to (in this case) 'change sooner'. In effect the therapist is setting a situation up and 'framing' it in such a way that it's most likely to be accepted, and acted upon.

Some other 'front loaded' phrases can include:

1) 'Consider this for a moment...'

2) 'Give some thought to this...'

3) 'Remember...'

4) 'Ask yourself this...'

'Rear loaded' the above examples could look like this:

1) '...consider that for a moment.'

2) '...give some thought to that.'

3) '...remember that.'

4) '...ask yourself that.'

Frustrating The Response

The Pattern:

1) 'But don't do it just yet.'

2) 'Stop. Wait. Not too soon. Wait until you sense the time is right.'

3) 'Not right away. Let it happen in its own time.'

The Structure:

By frustrating the manifestation of a response it actually causes the client to desire its realisation profoundly. It's a curious thing about human nature. Most of us have noticed it. Things that sometimes seem 'too easy' to obtain, we often don't value. By making the attainment of a desired response that bit 'harder' to have, it actually makes the process of its realisation more effective (because the person will want it more). But wait! Don't start using this principle now. No. Leave it until you're ready to savour it and totally enjoy it.

Future Pacing

Future pacing utilises language to help encourage a client to move either toward, or away from, or towards and away from (a) particular outcome(s).

Towards:

1) 'Think about all that will be better when you've completed...'

2) 'Just consider for a moment how good you'll feel when you've...'

3) 'Imagine what a nicer kind of situation you'll be in when you...'

Away from:

1) 'Ugh! That's yucky. Think about how horrible that will be if you let that happen.'

2) 'Now that wouldn't be nice. Imagine how bad things would be if you kept doing that each day...'

3) 'And that's not all. Consider this...if you let her do ABC that would mean that you'd have to keep

doing XYZ and that would be really nasty. Think about that.'

Away from and towards (towards and away from):

1) 'Now, if you carry on doing that you're going to continue to experience all of that cruddy stuff. However, if you continue to do more of this – just think how much better things will get.'

2) 'And that's just the start of the crap. It will get worse if you continue to leave things like that. But, if you follow through right now - I mean right now! And do what you suggested would be better, things will start to improve quicker than that. Think how much better things will be, even by this time next week!'

3) 'Now this means you can either have this! What you really want. Or a load of that (ugh!). It's entirely up to you.'

G

Generalisation

There are a number of forms of Generalisation. These include Generalised Referential Index [see above], Modal Operator of Necessity [see below], Modal Operator of Possibility [see below] and the Simple Generalisation [see below].

Generative Change Suggestion

The suggestion of change is not limited to the moment but has inherent within itself a generative capacity that, by its very nature, ensures ongoing transformation.

Example:

'And what starts to improve today caaaan only become better and better. You just wait and see...'

The suggestion for improvement is time bound (it starts today) and it has (in the form of a Modal Operator of Possibility) the inherent character within it that ensures that it can only (the use of the word 'only' limits its manifestation to the words that follow) become better and better (it's 'limited' to becoming better and better – it's an ongoing self-generating process of improvement).

Generic Noun Phrases

<u>The Pattern</u>:

1) 'If brilliant therapists are conversant in indirect hypnotherapy skills how come all therapists don't use them? I think it would be better if they did. Do you?'

2) 'If positive people accomplish more in life – and it's true that they do. I wonder - wouldn't it be better for everyone to become more positive in outlook? How about you?'

3) 'If lazy people always seem to miss out on life's opportunities - why doesn't everyone become a bit more proactive?'

<u>The Structure</u>:

This pattern utilises nouns which stand for a whole 'class' and uses this to 'argue' for a particular point of view.

1) 'If **brilliant therapists** [there is a 'class' or group of therapists who are 'brilliant'] are conversant in indirect hypnotherapy skills how come all therapists don't use them? I think it would be better if they did. Do you?'

2) 'If **positive people** [there is a 'class' or group of people who are 'positive'] accomplish more in life – and it's true that they do. I wonder - wouldn't it be better for everyone to become more positive in outlook? How about you?'

3) 'If **lazy people** [there is a 'class' or group of people who are 'lazy'] always seem to miss out on life's opportunities - why doesn't everyone become a bit more proactive?'

Globalising

This means taking a positive (or negative) attribute or behaviour that your client has evidenced and providing a global example of how, by utilising it more often it could improve (or make worse) their life experience. Hypnotherapist: 'So – you're an artist. Imagine if you used your creativity in all the important areas of your life – not just when you're painting. How much better things could be'.

H

Hallucination Elicitation For Hypnotic Change

Hypnotherapy sessions usually include elements in which the client is invited to create 'hallucinations' in the form of imagining, visualising or thinking about something, in one way or another, while sensing that he/she is moving towards a desired outcome and/or away from an undesired one. For example:

<u>Indirectly</u>:

'The **nice thing** about hypnosis is that your inner self can **begin to visualise yourself** now **doing things really well**. It doesn't really matter whether or not you consciously **visualise yourself doing that ABC really well** right now, or just wait until it happens (or both) because your unconscious mind can **think about it in detail** and **make all the changes** that need to be made **in all the best ways**. It's possible that you may **have a sense** of how you'll handle this much **more confidently** now. Will you **walk into the room in an up-beat way**. When **you express your point of view** how will others see and hear you?'

<u>Or more directly</u>:

'That's right...**see yourself now**...in your mind's eye...**radiating confidence and positivity**. Now...doesn't that **look much better than before** [invites a Comparison of Opposites which further enhances the magnitude of the suggested change] and isn't it ['isn't it' creates a temporal reorientation to one that represents the present moment] **much better** to **look and feel good** like this [Embedded Suggestion].'

Hierarchy Of Criteria (Sleight Of Mouth)

Sleight of Mouth principles were first delineated by Robert Dilts as he himself modelled Richard Bandler's language patterns. Additional contributions have been made by Steve and Connirae Andreas. A number of Sleight of Mouth patterns now exist, which are covered in this book. Sleight of Mouth patterns are utilised to unravel and in the process depotentiate adverse Complex Equivalence and/or Cause and Effect statements made by the client. [See: Analogy, Another Outcome, Apply To Self, Challenge, Change Of Reference Frame Size, Chunk Size, Consequences, Counter Example, Hierarchy Of Criteria, Intention, Meta Frame, Model Of The World, Reality Strategy, Redefine, Switch Referential Index.] In this example the principle of Hierarchy Of Criteria is employed.

Client statement: 'I don't know what to do next...this makes me feel like a failure.'

'(A) I don't know what to do next...(B) this makes me feel like a failure.'

A)

'Not knowing isn't the same as not being able to find a solution - you know.'

This example works on the first element of the client's statement. It 'reframes' the value that the client is attaching to not knowing.

B)

'Feeling a failure is quite a different thing from really being a failure. Isn't it better to just 'feel' a failure than really being a 'failure'?'

This example works on the second theme of the client's statement: It 'undermines'/casts doubt upon the premise of the client's belief (which is the Cause and Effect relationship they've created between 'not knowing' and 'feeling a failure') so that the 'feelings' are dissociated from the belief that relates to their self-image, so that the self-image can be improved upon and the limiting beliefs subtly, yet profoundly, altered.

You could add: '...And you can change those feelings you know...and then it's anyone's guess how things can improve...'

C)

[Leading into the pattern with: 'Have you thought about it this way? Think about it this way...'] 'In the scheme of things, what counts the most...ruminating over those feelings or putting the past behind you and moving forward into a better future?'

However

The word 'however' is a wonderful word. It can be used much as an Aikido or Tai Chi Master would use their physical prowess to redirect a person's energy, while in this context it can be used to gently, yet profoundly, redirect a person's <u>mental focus</u>. Here are a couple of examples:

1) Client: 'I'll never be able to change unless I can feel ABC first!'

Hypnotherapist: 'That may be true, <u>however</u>, experience also shows that sometimes by beginning to do XYZ on a day-to-day basis it can gently nurture feelings of ABC which can result in the kind of change your looking for – by just going about it in a slightly different way.'

2) Client: 'I'll never find another love as great as my first love!'

Hypnotherapist: 'I hear what you're saying. That must have been quite a 'first love' – <u>however</u> – how can you be soooo sure that there isn't at least as good to come? After all you're not psychic are you?... (don't ask this sort of question of a genuine psychic ☺) ...which means that there's at least some room for a bit of genuine doubt or some natural uncertainty (...now!).

I

Idea Bind

Example: 'You can think of a new idea about how to change - today or tomorrow - the choice is up to you. What will you choose?'

[Two choices relating to the process of a developing idea are offered with a timeframe attached to them. Whatever is chosen leads in the Desired Direction. The client <u>can</u> consciously choose which ideation strategy to follow. An Idea Bind is basically a Bind/Simple Bind with the concept of an 'idea' forming the focus of the Bind]

Idea Double Bind

'You can think of a new idea about how to change - today or tomorrow - the choice is up to your unconscious. What will it be?'

[Two choices relating to the process of a developing idea are offered with a timeframe attached to them. Whatever is chosen leads in the Desired Direction. The client <u>can't</u> consciously choose which ideation strategy to follow. He/she <u>has</u> <u>to</u> <u>wait</u> <u>and</u> <u>see</u> what begins to occur because the suggestion is geared to prime the unconscious mind to respond, outside of conscious control. An Idea Double Bind is basically a Double Bind with the concept of an 'idea' forming the focus of the Bind]

Ideo Affective Suggestions

'It's nice to **smile** when you're **recalling that pleasant feeling**.'

In effect an Ideo Affective Suggestion is one that causes an affective response due to a cognitive experience. In the above example the 'affect' is the smile while the cognitive experience is **'recalling that pleasant feeling**.'

Here's another example:

'And that hand can feel cooler and cooler as you remember what it's like to hold an ice cube in the palm of that hand now.'

[Notice also the use of the term 'that hand' rather than 'your hand.' This creates a further hypnotically induced sense of dissociation which can enhance the anaesthesia being generated in the above example.]

Ideocognitive Suggestion

'You know that you will **remember this suggestion** when you return to work...'

The Ideo Cognitive Suggestion is geared to facilitate a desired cognition within the client. In this example the cognition to **'remember this suggestion'** (which would relate to a suggestion already given in the course of therapy) is triggered (NLP: 'anchored') to the moment of returning to work. Therefore, returning to work = triggering an ideo cognitive response <u>because</u> <u>of</u> the

Ideocognitive Suggestion which has already been generated.

Ideo Motor Suggestion

The Ideo Motor Suggestion principle is often used in hypnotherapy and is well known to most practitioners. Here's an example:

'And as your trance continues to develop nicely you may find that because you want to 'move ahead' [move a head] in your life you can let me know when you <u>are</u> ready to integrate a new idea by <u>gently</u> <u>moving</u> <u>your</u> <u>head</u>. You might find <u>you</u> <u>move</u> <u>it</u> gently to the <u>right</u>, <u>or</u> to the <u>left</u>. It may be a little bit <u>up</u>ward or a little way in <u>another</u> <u>direction</u> – only you will know what <u>it</u> <u>is</u> <u>to</u> <u>be</u> but you may not find out until <u>you</u> <u>do</u> <u>it</u>. And if you choose to remain <u>still</u> you can <u>still</u> <u>let</u> <u>me</u> <u>know</u> that <u>you</u> <u>are</u> <u>communicating</u> to me this way by <u>show</u>ing <u>me</u> a smaller <u>movement</u> that hardly involves <u>moving</u> at all and is <u>clear</u> enough to me to <u>let</u> <u>me</u> <u>know</u> that <u>you</u> <u>are</u> <u>letting</u> <u>me</u> <u>know</u> while choosing to remain <u>almost</u> still for the duration of your trance as <u>you</u> <u>make</u> <u>the</u> <u>changes</u> anyway.'

Woven throughout this paragraph are suggestions designed to elicit ideo motor movement which are deemed to be connected to the client's acceptance of readiness to integrate a new idea that's geared to help him/her move ahead. Any such movement - at all - therefore presupposes readiness to accept the suggestion(s). Changes are also presupposed: '...as <u>you</u> <u>make</u> <u>the</u> <u>changes</u> anyway.'

Ideosensory Suggestion

'You know it's possible that you will experience this in such an amazing way that you will notice that you can <u>sense</u> <u>the</u> <u>scent</u> of those flowers again and <u>notice</u> <u>the</u> <u>texture</u> of the petals on your finger tips like you did before… as you <u>recall</u> <u>it</u> <u>all</u> **now**…'

As this pattern's name indicates this category of suggestion is designed to elicit sensory-based-stimuli relating to a desired outcome. In this example it relates to the scent and texture of roses that have been pre-experienced and are therefore within the realm of recall.

I Don't Know

<u>The Pattern</u>:

This approach is helpful when desiring to offer suggestions in an indirect way.

1) 'I don't know if your unconscious will do this immediately or just quickly…'

2) 'I don't know when you will first notice this positive change taking place…'

3) 'I don't know how many better ways your unconscious will generate for you now…'

<u>The Structure</u>:

1) '**I don't know** if <u>your unconscious will do this</u> immediately or just quickly…'

2) '**I don't know** when <u>you will first notice this positive change taking place</u>...'

3) '**I don't know** how many better ways <u>your unconscious will generate for you now</u>...'

Illusion Of Choice

<u>The Pattern</u>:

The illusion of choice pattern, as the name suggests works in such a way as to appear to offer a choice, but the offer is an 'illusion', because the 'choices' offered all lead in the Desired Direction.

1) 'Do you want to sort this part out right now...or in a few minutes?'

2) 'Would you like the car in red or in blue?'

3) 'So...what you're saying is that there are three things stopping you from moving forward. When these things are dealt with you say you know you will be able to enjoy your life more. But you've been putting off starting because doing all three has seemed, you said 'too much'. So...don't do all three. You can choose one first and then, when that's done, you can move onto...in a more comfortable way...the second and then the third. Which one will you choose first?'

4) 'I wonder how your unconscious mind can communicate [pause... then, with the client's pre-arranged permission, lift their hands up saying something like] ... I'm now going to gently lift your hands up to here... [and then say...] if your

unconscious wants you to go into a deep, deep trance they can move together or a profound trance they can move apart...[and then seem curious...as if you're waiting to see what happens, adding]....and what must that sensation feel like?'

The <u>Structure</u>:

1) 'Do you want to sort this part out right now...or in a few minutes? [It's presupposed that sorting the 'part' out will take place. The illusion of choice takes place with reference to the 'when' this will occur. This pattern is a form of Bind.]'

2) 'Would you like the car in red or in blue? [The salesperson's approach. It's presupposed that the customer will buy a car. The illusion of choice takes place with reference to the colour of the car. This pattern is a form of Bind.]'

3) 'So...what you're saying is that there are three things stopping you from moving forward. When these things are dealt with you say you know you will be able to enjoy your life more. But you've been putting off starting because doing all three has seemed, you said 'too much'. So...don't do all three. You can choose one first and then, when that's done, you can move onto...in a more comfortable way...the second and then the third. Which one will you choose first? [This example involves a more 'layered' approach. The therapist has listened to and acknowledged the client's 'objections' and then used those objections to create a 'frame' that encourages forward movement by presenting an illusion of choice. Of course, the therapist isn't overly concerned which of the apparent choices are taken, because they all lead in

the direction of the overall goal, which is the resolution of the problem of the client's 'stuck state'. The question: 'Which one will you choose first' contains the presupposition that the client will choose one of the options. What's more the word 'first' implies that it will commence a sequence which will result in the completion of all of the options outlined.]'

4) 'I wonder how your unconscious mind can communicate [pause... then, with the client's pre-arranged permission, lift their hands up saying something like] ... I'm now going to gently lift your hands up to here... [and then say...] if your unconscious wants you to go into a deep, deep trance they can move together or a profound trance they can move apart...[and then seem curious...as if you're waiting to see what happens, adding]....and what must that sensation feel like?' [This is the sort of approach that Stephen Brooks likes to employ. Although there is an element of choice – each choice leads to trance.]'

Illusion That Something Is There / Not There

This pattern can be used to generate positive hallucinations for therapeutic work.

<u>Here are some examples of the pattern</u>:

1) 'You can notice things that are not really here or know that they're here without knowing how you noticed them.'

2) 'You can see [hear/feel]...things that are not really here or know that they're here without knowing how you see [hear/feel] them.'

This is how this approach may be employed in a therapeutic context:

'And now you can notice that whenever you begin to write you see your finished book with you when it's not really there (whispered:) yet. Or know that it is there even while it isn't (whispered:) yet. And that inspires you even more.' [This example is an obvious use of generating a positive hallucination that's anchored to a writer writing so that they 'see' a finished copy of their book, which in turn acts as a source of inspiration to make the 'dream' a reality. The whispered use of the word 'yet' addresses the fact that the book isn't physically there, yet it is just a matter of time before it is. So the imagination is used to produce a physical manifestation of that which is being imagined.]

Here the approach can be used to elicit a negative hallucination (negative, in this context simply means that it's being suggested that something which does exist is being 'hallucinated away' temporarily for the purpose of the therapy).

1) 'And you can notice that you don't notice that ABC that's over there or know that it's there without letting yourself see it.'

2) 'And you can sense that you don't see that XYZ just here or know that you see it without choosing to register that you do.'

This is how this approach may be employed in a therapeutic context:

'Yes. And all the while you take it easy it gets easier all the while to change the way you perceive things about life. After all, often all it takes is noticing more of what you want to notice. For instance; you can listen to my voice without hearing what I'm saying or you can hear what I'm saying without needing to listen to my voice. But you will notice all of the suggestions which help you - whichever way you do this'. [This suggests an illusion that the client won't hear the speaker's voice or what he/she is saying while simultaneously suggesting that they will <u>absorb the meaning</u> of what is being said. The client may have a hypnotic amnesia at a conscious level of much of what the therapist spoke about – thereby leaving the unconscious to apply the therapeutic patterns appropriately in his/her life.]

I'm Not Going To Tell You

<u>The Pattern</u>:

This is a wonderful pattern for asserting something, in a semi-direct manner, which is helpful for the client to develop an awareness of. Here are some examples:

1) 'And while you consider all of the solutions which are available to you, I'm not going to tell you that learning to relax is one of the best. See what you think yourself.'

2) 'Because I'm not going to tell you it's about changing your perspective. Because it's better for you to consider your own perspective and then consider whether it would be helpful to change it.'

3) 'I'm not going to tell you that trance is the best way to make changes. It's better that you find out for yourself.'

The Structure:

1) 'And while you consider all of the solutions which are available to you, **I'm not going to tell** you that <u>learning to relax is one of the best</u>. See what you think yourself.'

2) 'Because **I'm not going to tell you** <u>it's about changing your perspective</u>. Because it's better for you to consider your own perspective and then consider whether it would be helpful to change it.'

3) '**I'm not going to tell you** that <u>trance is the best way to make changes</u>. It's better that you find out for yourself.'

Implication

Implication can be used to discreetly help the client re-assess a situation. Here are some examples:

1) 'I don't know how much you have learned from this. ('How much' implies that the client will have learned something).'

2) 'Where do you feel most relaxed at this time? ('Most relaxed' implies that the client is feeling relaxed.)'

Implied Causative

As this category of language pattern suggests the words used imply a first cause. [See also Contingent Suggestion.]

1) '**After** you start to feel different...' [The client will feel different.]

2) '**As** you do this...' [The client will do this.]

3) '**Before** you change...' [The client will change.]

4) '**During** your next trance...' [There will be a next trance.]

5) '**While** you think of your next option...' [There is a next option.]

6) '**Since** the changes have started you can...' [Changes have started.]

The words which have been highlighted in bold all have, inherent within them, the implication of a cause in motion. This therefore suggests that what follows is a given. These patterns are sometimes also called 'Adverbial Clauses'.

Implied Connection

The Implied Connection method can be used to suggest that there is a connection between one thing and another. This is how it can be used in a therapeutic context:

1) 'And I wonder if you've noticed what's been gently happening to the rhythm of your breathing with each pleasant tick of the clock. (The client's relaxed breathing has been associated to the sound of the clock. The sound of the clock therefore becomes, in trance, a catalyst for relaxed breathing and hypnosis.)'

2) 'But don't go into a trance until you sit all the way down. (The act of sitting down is implied to be related to the act of going into trance.)'

3) 'Have you become aware of how your thoughts have developed with the rhythm of the music? (The client's thoughts have been associated to the rhythm of the music. Continuation of developing thoughts can then be implied, by mentioning the sound of the music.)'

The Structure of an Implied Connection:

'And as you're listening to what you're hearing I wonder if you've even consciously noticed what's been happening to your relaxation levels as you have?'

'And as you're listening to what you're hearing...'

[a Truism]

'...I wonder if you've even consciously noticed...'

[which implies that they unconsciously have]

'...what's been happening...'

[which implies that something has been happening]

'...to your relaxation levels as you have?'

[which implies that the client's relaxation levels are being influenced by what they're hearing]

Implied Directive

This pattern implies that something will occur without a direct instruction being given for its enactment.

The Pattern:

1) 'I'm curious about how your unconscious will choose to let us know when it's ready to make the change start to happen...and when it does...one of your fingers will move...how good will that feel when you notice it?'

2) 'Many people notice that changes that occur in trance allow them to feel better quite quickly. Now I don't know exactly when your unconscious mind will do it for you...but I do know that when you take a nice looooong deep breath in something good will begin to take place.'

3) 'You don't have to consciously know everything about how you are going to discover these solutions...because when one of those fingers moves juuust a little...this way or that...in trance...here...you'll begin to notice some new ideas are beginning to develop.'

<u>The Structure</u>:

1) 'I'm curious about how your unconscious will choose to let us know when it's ready to make the change start to happen...and when it does...**one of your fingers will move**...how good will that feel when you notice it? [The Implied Directive states that one of the client's fingers will move. In this context such movement is linked to the commencement of a therapeutic outcome.]'

2) 'Many people notice that changes that occur in trance allow them to feel better quite quickly. Now I don't know exactly when your unconscious mind will do it for you...but I do know that when **you take a nice looooong deep breath in** something good will begin to take place. [The Implied Directive encourages the client to take a deep breath. In this context this action is associated with 'something good' which 'will begin to take place'.]'

3) 'You don't have to consciously know everything about how you are going to discover these solutions...because **when one of those fingers moves juuust a little...this way or that...in trance**...here...you'll begin to notice some new ideas are beginning to develop. [In this example the Implied Directive encourages the movement of a finger – which is also tied to the conscious

realisation that 'some new ideas are beginning to develop'.]'

Implied Separation Of Body And Mind

In order to further enhance the client's experience of trance and its related phenomena, when commenting (in a Bio-Feedback way) on certain parts of the person's body, rather than saying 'your right arm' you can instead say, 'that right arm' which creates a sense of dissociation, which is particularly useful when generating ideo motor response (IMR), anaesthesia and levitation phenomena.

Example:

'And as you sense that that arm – over there - begins to feel heavier so that arm – over there – can continue to feel lighter.'

[Notice the difference in perceptual awareness in the above statement when contrasted with the following version:]

'And as you sense that your right arm begins to feel heavier so your left arm can continue to feel lighter.'

Neither option is more 'right' than the other. But understanding how they're likely to be perceived by the client can enable the skilled therapist to elicit subtle differences in the outcome of the trancework. Do you want to generate an increased sense of dissociation – perhaps when helping with pain relief? Then it's likely that option one will be most helpful.

Implied Simultaneity

In this instance a simultaneous connection is implied between what the therapist is saying and an event that is occurring.

The Pattern:

1) 'You can let your eyes defocus and begin to think of something new.'

2) 'You may have felt uncertain but you continue to explore solutions.'

3) 'You can continue to feel comfortable and not do anything about it.'

The Structure:

1) 'You can let your eyes defocus <u>and</u> begin to think of something new.'

2) 'You may have felt uncertain <u>but</u> you continue to explore solutions.'

3) 'You can continue to feel comfortable <u>and not</u> do anything about it.'

The words 'and', 'but' and 'and not' create a linking effect which implies a simultaneous relationship. You will notice how easily a therapeutic 'frame' can be offered to the client, with subtlety, by incorporating this approach.

Impossible Problems / Impossible Solutions

Not a 'language pattern' per se. This is more of a 'work around' technique that I developed for use in certain situations. These terms relate to the behaviour patterns of the kind of client who presents for help and then proceeds to tell the therapist about an 'impossible problem' which requires an 'impossible solution' (they don't use the terms 'impossible problem' and 'impossible solution' but what they do do is describe a situation that has these 'impossible' components intricately woven into the framework). That's to say that they say they're looking for help and then box themselves into their problem and seem to challenge every ensuing attempt at problem resolution. One way that I developed to depotentiate such situations was to invent a 'psychological term' for this type of scenario. Having invented the term, in situations which required its application, I would proceed to explain to such clients that this psychological term exists, which, interestingly, describes their self-limiting behaviour. In so doing, by labelling it, it suggests that their behaviour has been 'noted' and implies that 'we' have seen through their ruse and it's time to 'get real' and quit the game.

Here's an example:

'Phew! That certainly is a situation isn't it. Now – with great respect, I'd like to share something with you, which you probably didn't know about but which I'm sure you will find useful for helping you to help yourself to create the solutions you've told me you want.'

[By reminding the client that they have said they want help – you are bringing to bear the force of honesty and congruity in order to dismantle an incongruity in what they're presenting]

'You see, there's a psychological term for what you've just described to me. It's well-known that sometimes, some people, box themselves in, without realising that they've done so. And they do this by creating, in their minds, what's known as an 'impossible problem'. Now, in all likelihood, it will be a variation of a problem that many other people will have experienced and resolved in one way or another. So it is solvable. But when a person is unknowingly...or perhaps even knowingly...boxing themselves in with an 'impossible problem' they add a further element to the situation, which closes the lid on the box so to speak – thereby making any possible solution appear to be unworkable. When in reality there are likely to be many ways to change things! The secondary part which 'closes the lid', so to speak, is known as the 'impossible solution'. Such people then, say that the only thing that will solve their 'impossible problem' is an equally 'impossible solution'. Which means that there is, supposedly, for them, in all of the known universe, no solution. Let me give you an idea of how this might occur: someone who says, for instance, that they're seeking to resolve an 'impossible' relationship problem might also say though, something like: 'I really want to sort this out – but the only way it will get better is if she comes to me on bended knees and says that she is totally to blame and will never, ever, do that again! Of course, I know she never will. But that's all I'm prepared to accept! Okay hypnotherapist: how are you going to help me sort this out? Remember –

you're the expert and nothing will work except bended knees - and that will never happen.'

Here's another example:

Someone who's holding themselves back from following through with the opportunities that life often brings could say: 'My problem is that the my life is the pits. Everyone around me seems to get lots of opportunities and do well. I don't. People keep telling me that I have lots of opportunities too. But I don't really. The only solution that I'm prepared to accept that can ever help me get out of this situation and improve my opportunities is if I win the lottery. Nothing else will work. Okay hypnotherapist: How are you going to help me feel better? Remember. Only the lottery win will do and I've only got a 1 in 16 million chance.'

Now, although the above examples are fictional scenarios they are nevertheless based on the sort of situations that can be encountered from time to time. By explaining the dynamics of their behaviour to such presenting clients in ways that let them know that experts 'in the field of psychology' have noticed this self-limiting pattern and that it now <u>even</u> has a classification: 'impossible problems requiring impossible solutions', it brings the 'game' out into the open and can thereby diffuse it. It's about bringing things into the open, 'putting all the cards on the table' and naming the game.

Indirect Focussing

Indirect Associative Focussing

The Pattern:

The Indirect Associative Focussing principle can be used to introduce some possible steps towards obtaining a workable solution to the client but in, as the title suggests, an indirect manner. The outcome of this approach is that the client will likely do a Transderivational Search (also known as a 'TDS' – see below) to develop his/her understanding of what's been addressed and resultantly therefore develop his/her approach towards obtaining a solution(s) based on the insights obtained from within.

For example:

Hypnotherapist: 'Excuse me – something you just said reminded me that I must make a note for myself to get my copy of Dr Claire Weekes' book back - called 'Self Help For Your Nerves'. I loaned it out a while ago. And I think now is the time to have it returned. [Writing – while talking out load to himself/herself]: 'Dr Claire Weekes – 'Self Help for Your Nerves'. Get book.'

'Okay – thanks for reminding me. Now! Where were we? So – you're going to practice some relaxed breathing because it helps you to feel calmer… [= Consider Dr Claire Weekes' books.]'

And/or:

'And as you continue to explore your trance it's not important...that you consider what you'd learn about yourself if chocolate just disappeared from the planet...it's not important...the only thing that is important right now is that you continue to allow yourself to be relaxed and as you listen to my voice... (= If chocolate disappeared you'd survive quite easily. Think about it.)'

And/or:

'Who knows the way of the flower and how it knows when to bloom? (= There is a similarity that can be drawn between the growth of a flower and your personal development. Think about it.)'

And/or:

'The wind is free – I wonder what that's like? (= What would it feel like for you to feel free? Think about it.)'

And/or:

'In order to learn how to fly the chick must spread its wings. (= Good things happen when you take action. Think about it.)'

And/or:

'Even a gentle stream leaves an impression in the ground. (= You don't have to be 'over the top' to make your impression in life. Go with the flow. Think about it.)'

And/or:

'A kitten always knows how to ask it's mother for milk in the right way. (= There is a 'right' way to ask for things which will be more likely to gain a favourable response. Think about it.)'

Indirect Framing

This language pattern example illustrates how a therapist can 'set up' a therapeutic working 'frame' (or context) indirectly. For instance, rather than saying 'now you will relax' to a client, which is pretty direct and could involve the possibility of perceived 'failure' (if the client does not immediately begin to feel whatever it is they think they should feel when they're in a state of relaxation) the therapist could instead say something like: 'If you want to relax now that's fine. Or if you just want to sit here and listen that's fine too. Just do what feels most comfortable for you. Okay?' This is like the 'Covering All Possible Alternatives' technique; used in this context to set a 'working frame' (in this case meaning the state of relaxation) around the intervention that's likely to be conducive to obtaining good hypnotherapy results.

Indirect Ideomatic Focusing

This approach employs the principle of 'priming' a person, through prior exposure to a desired outcome. Instances of this can occur by having an individual (or group) observe someone else experiencing trance, before they themselves go into trance (as Milton Erickson does with Nick in the Monde video). In a corporate-coaching context it can occur via one person 'shadowing' a colleague who already possesses certain skills that are deemed to be beneficial in the workplace – so that the 'shadower' can learn how to replicate the methods so observed in their own work too.

Example:

'And you noticed how Sally just closed her eyes and began to breathe in a calm and comfortable way...now that it's your turn and as you close your eyes you can also begin to become aware of your breathing. (Sally has given you a good example of how you can go into trance.)'

And/or:

'Now I wonder how many ways you saw John do that really well. And as you think about that in your own way – I wonder which parts of what you saw him do you will do really well too? And which new parts that you don't know that you saw that you saw you do really well too?' (John has given you a good example of how to do it really well.)'

And/or:

I remember watching my friend Mary...when she was learning to paint. What she used to do was trace the picture out on the canvas first in pencil and then add the paint afterwards. It was much easier this way. She said. (I've shared an example with you of how my friend Mary learned to paint.)'

Indirect Induction (A Structure Of)

<u>OO ON NN</u>

A useful indirect induction pattern to remember is the Observable/Observable; Observable/Non-Observable; Non-Observable/Non-Observable, method.

'As you sit here (observable) and breathe in that relaxed way (observable) you can listen to the sounds that are taking place now (observable) and notice what kind of thoughts you are thinking (non observable) and as you think these thoughts your unconscious can begin to make changes (non observable) somewhere inside and as these changes occur (non observable) then new solutions can begin to take place.'

This approach is developed by gently encouraging the client to shift his/her awareness levels into a trance state by initially making reference to phenomena which can be readily observed and then referring subtly to phenomena which are not obviously discernable but which are likely to be perceived as Truisms (see Truisms) – thereby allowing for positive suggestions to be offered to the unconscious mind in the process of inducing trance. The therapist can loop through this induction (meaning to repeat the pattern several times, using different observable and non-observable criteria) thereby generating more receptivity. (Trance is naturally quite cyclical in as much as a client's perception of the hypnotic experience will often move 'up' and 'down' between levels of awareness – rather than appearing to remain 'static'. This induction method can work harmoniously with the natural 'ebb and flow' of a person's awareness.)

Inductive Language Patterns

Inductive Language Patterns are patterns which move from 'specific' to 'total'. From detail to the big picture.

The Pattern:

1) 'Okay. So, this isn't just about getting fit is it? [Specific] What else is it about? [Total]'

2) 'Right. I see – this isn't only about wanting to change your job. [Specific] What else is it about? [Total]'

3) 'Oh – so this isn't just about your relationship is it? [Specific – designed to draw out a response that will lead to 'Total'.]'

4) 'So tell me. What specifically can you do to sort that money situation out? [Specific – designed to draw out a response that will lead to 'Total'.]'

5) 'Let's see then. What's the one thing [Specific] you could do today to get the ball rolling and start writing your book [Total]?'

The Structure:

This principle is somewhat different from the Milton/Meta Model contrast in the sense that a meta comment is generally 'specific' which, when translated into Miltonian language can become quite 'general' (or vice versa – general into specific). For instance. Milton: 'You feel a certain way', becomes Meta: 'You feel calm'. Inductive Language Patterns <u>maintain</u> specificity. [See also Deductive Language Patterns.] Notice also that whereas in a Milton/Meta exchange it, in effect, revolves around a polar contrast occurring, relating to the topic being addressed (vague 'certain' feelings becoming specific 'calm' feelings, for instance) this language pattern (inductive) maintains a focus on the overall goal <u>and</u> moves between 'specificity' and 'total' (not 'specificity' and 'general'). Thereby maintaining its overall goal-directed outcome without necessarily doing a 'polar flip'. For instance: 'What do you start to notice first?' [Specific] 'What else is there about that feeling of calm that you like?' [Total].

Insecurity (in security)

This is a phonological ambiguity that I've heard Richard Bandler use. It's a good one which enables the hypnotherapist to do a number of things for the client's perceptions about the state of 'in security'. It scrambles disempowering beliefs by playing around with the contrasting elements involved: 'And when you notice a feeling of insecurity – in security you can let yourself relax and know that it is a passing thing leading to a feeling of being in security.'

This example alters the <u>client's relationship to the word</u>. In effect 'insecurity' becomes an anchor for its polar extreme: a feeling of security. The message is therefore that that word insecurity (and all that's associated to it?) leads now to feelings of being in security. It's also a very 'trancey' technique as at one level the client will probably be trying to make 'sense' of what's being said and (because of the phonological work) as they do they'll unconsciously absorb the meaning, but likely become consciously lost in the detail of the language. All in all, in my opinion, it's a pretty good way to help assist clients to reframe their feelings of insecurity towards a sense of being secure - in security.

Intention (Sleight Of Mouth)

Sleight of Mouth principles were first delineated by Robert Dilts as he himself modelled Richard Bandler's language patterns. Additional contributions have been made by Steve and Connirae Andreas. A number of Sleight of Mouth patterns now exist, which are covered in this book. Sleight of Mouth patterns are utilised to unravel and in the process depotentiate adverse Complex Equivalence and/or Cause and Effect statements made by the client. [See: Analogy, Another Outcome, Apply To Self, Challenge, Change Of Reference Frame Size, Chunk Size, Consequences, Counter Example, Hierarchy Of Criteria, Intention, Meta Frame, Model Of The World, Reality Strategy, Redefine, Switch Referential Index.] In this example the principle of Intention is employed.

Cause and Effect Example:

Client: (A) 'Every time I go to that club (B) it makes me get angry.'

Therapist (A): 'But you want to go to that club?'

Therapist (B): 'You'd prefer that you feel otherwise?'
Therapist (A/B): 'A helpful thing about wanting to go to that club and not get angry is that it reminds you that you can develop other ways to respond.'

Complex Equivalence Example:

(A) 'I didn't go to Eton (B) that means I'll never succeed.'

Therapist (A): 'So - you wanted to go to Eton?'
Therapist (B): 'I see so you want to succeed.'
Therapist (A/B): 'Maybe because you wanted to go to Eton but didn't is what has motivated you to want to succeed anyway?'

Interspersal Technique

'And you can allow yourself to begin **relaxing** whenever you want to start to begin to **relax** and every one **relaxes** in different ways. I wonder whether you would like to **relax** consciously and unconsciously or just **relax** unconsciously while your conscious mind can choose to **relax** when you know the time is right.'

When considering the difference between Embedded Commands and the Interspersal Technique it's worth remembering that an Embedded Command <u>always</u> involves a hypnotic suggestion whereas the Interspersal Technique highlights certain words, which might <u>also</u> be Embedded Commands.

Intuition (in tuition)

This is a phonological ambiguity that I use often as a means via which I can talk to my clients about developing their intuition while they're learning ('in tuition') with me. Example: 'Your unconscious knows your (you're) intuition (in tuition). That's right. Your (you're) intuition (in tuition)...is working for you while you are learning about how you're... in tuition... with... your intuition...and I wonder... if your (you're) unconscious was to teach you something helpful...intuition (in tuition)...what would it be and how would you learn that you've learned what your (you're) intuition (in tuition) is teaching you...here (hear) today...'

It's...

The Pattern:

'**It's** (it is) is a good way to introduce a suggestion.'

1) '**It's** a good thing to...'

2) '**It's** possible to...'

3) '**It's** natural for you to...'

4) '**It's** up to you to ABC...'

5) '**It's** your responsibility to take care of...'

<u>The Structure</u>:

This is a form of **Lost Performative** which in this example can be used to introduce helpful suggestions following the use of the word 'it's'.

J

'Jeet Kune Do Therapy'

'Jeet Kune Do Therapy' isn't a language pattern – it's more a way of life. I was greatly inspired by Bruce Lee's philosophy, which he sought to promote through his fighting art called 'Jeet Kune Do' that taught that fixed forms (in his case martial arts) can become, due to their 'fixed' traditional nature, lacking in creative vibrancy. Because that's often what happens with therapeutic models too - after the founder first expresses the way to others. People acknowledge the merit in the approach and then 'fix it in time', so to speak, and (unwittingly) slowly begin to ossify it. This causes it to lose much of the original intent and vitalism with which it was first conveyed. As time passes the effect continues. And, like 'Chinese whispers' the further the message gets removed from the founder, the more the original spirit can become diluted, even by well-meaning people. (I often wonder would Milton Erickson be working in exactly the same way today if he was alive? Would he still feel the same way about some of the ideas he expressed back then?) Bruce Lee said: 'Learn the rules – then dissolve the rules'. When Milton was learning, he himself studied what there was to be known about psychiatry/hypnotherapy, as it existed at that time (just as Bruce himself became highly skilled, first, in the art of Wing Chun Kung Fu). At first then, Milton worked within the (then) current psychotherapy model <u>but</u> he gradually 'dissolved the rules', so to speak, (having first learned them) and developed his own approach (just as Bruce went on to incorporate principles from many other forms of martial arts to create his own unique method called Jeet Kune Do). Frank Farrelly did the same. He worked with Carl Rogers, the famous developer of Person Centred Counselling/Client Centred Therapy. He learned a great deal from Carl (and continues to hold him in high regard) but he then 'dissolved the rules', so to speak, and developed his own, radically different approach, called 'Provocative Therapy'. Which, in many ways, could be considered (on the surface) to be the polar extreme to Person Centred Counselling. Just as Milton's indirect <u>intervention</u> approach is 'miles apart' from Freud's analytical <u>categorising</u> school of thought. But Milton first learned Freud to get to where he got to. Jeet Kune Do Therapy then is about developing proficiency in a form and then allowing that form to express itself and develop through you. So that the form evolves and becomes a 'form of no form'. (And in a moment I'll say the word awake and you'll awaken...☺ But you know what I'm talking about.)

Juxtaposed Options

<u>The Pattern</u>:

1) 'And you can feel calm or creative.'

2) 'Ask yourself – do you want to start or stop?'

3) 'Think about it – do you want to do it or not?'

4) 'And you can feel this and you can feel this.'

<u>The Structure</u>:

Juxtaposing options creates contrasts in the client's mind and encourages him/her to explore possibilities.

1) 'And you can feel calm / <u>or</u> creative.'

2) 'Ask yourself – do you want to start / <u>or</u> stop?'

3) 'Think about it – do you want to do it / <u>or</u> not?'

4) 'And you can feel this / <u>and</u> you can feel this.'

K

Kinaesthetic Coordinates

Developing an awareness of subjective Kinaesthetic Coordinates can support the client in the process of 'getting in touch with' positive feelings and/or help to alter how the client relates to unwanted subjective kinaesthetic experiences.

Example: 'And when you say you get a good feeling – where specifically is that good feeling?'

Knowing

This is a form of 'Mind Reading'. It's a very useful language pattern and can help to create rapport at a deep level.

Here are some examples:

1) 'I know that your unconscious...'

2) 'I know that you know that I know...'

3) 'You know that I know that...'

Extended Example: 'Now...while you're thinking about that – or not – not thinking about it...I know that you are... aware... of many things... and you know... that I know... that you have... a wide range of unconscious talents... available... which I know...

that you know... that I know... your unconscious mind is ready to begin to activate... for you... now... that the time is right – now.'

L

Lack Of Referential Index

The Pattern:

'Solutions are created...'

The Structure of a Lack of Referential Index

A Lack of Referential Index in effect 'deletes' a person or object who either takes action, or is affected in some way by some action being taken. In the above example which says 'Solutions are created', we could ask: 'Who's creating them?' However, hypnotically speaking, it's often better to leave that part out. That's because this pattern is useful for offering suggestions which are 'artfully vague', in order that the positive message can be conveyed in ways that allow the client's unconscious mind to add appropriate (to them) meaning to them.

Here are some examples:

1) 'Things can excite you.'

[This sentence carries with it a lack of specificity. What specifically are the 'things' that can do the exciting?]

2) 'Changes were made.'

[Who specifically was making the changes?]

3) 'New feelings were felt.'

[Who specifically felt the new feelings?]

4) 'Ideas were formed.'

[Who specifically formed them?]

5) 'Happiness was experienced'

[Who specifically experienced the happiness?]

6) 'They were feeling curious...'

[Who specifically is the 'they' who were feeling curious?]

Leading

<u>Visual Leading</u>

<u>The Pattern</u>:

'And you can see the clock on the wall and that may remind you of other clocks you have seen in the past....and as you think about the past...'

<u>The Structure</u>:

In this example a visual point of reference is utilised in order to lead into a hypnotically generated temporal (time based) change of reference.

Auditory Leading

The Pattern:

'And you can hear the sound of the clock on the wall and that may remind you of other clocks you have heard in the past...and as you think about the past...'

The Structure:

In this example an auditory point of reference is utilised in order to lead in to a hypnotically generated temporal (time based) change of reference.

Kinaesthetic Leading

The Pattern:

'And as you notice the sensation of your watch upon your wrist it may remind you of a time that you were aware of feeling your watch like this in the past and as you think about the past...'

The Structure:

In this similar example a kinaesthetic point of reference is utilised in order to lead in to a hypnotically generated temporal (time based) change of reference.

Leading Questions

Leading questions can be used in order to create a 'bridge' from the leading question being 'asked' and the desired outcome/solution being offered.

The Pattern:

'So your breathing has slowed down to help you feel more relaxed?'

The Structure:

So your breathing has slowed down [leading question] to **help you feel more relaxed [desired outcome]?**

Here are some other examples:

1) 'So you're talking about the past in order to **start to get over your problem?'**

2) 'That's why you've done this – **to begin to explore new options?'**

3) 'You've decided you don't like your job – **in order to motivate yourself to find a better one?'**

4) 'So you phoned me about this - **in order to start improve things?'**

5) 'So you've been feeling panicky – **to make yourself aware that something needs to change?'**

Left Right, Right Left

This is a wonderful pattern that can be used, amongst other things, for deepening the hypnotic state through the process of generating confusion.

Here's an example:

'Now your left foot right here now is left there while you're right that your right is right next to it where you left it. That's right. And whether you've left thinking about your left...right at the moment or whether your thinking of your left right now...what's left is the right kind of awareness that let's you know that you always have left the right kind of resources that you want...right?'

Levels Of Abstraction

The Pattern:

'That's right...and as you think about how good it will be to heal your relationship with her I wonder what will be the first thing you can do to express your desire to be friends.'

The Structure:

The Levels of Abstraction pattern is used to help a client move between a generalised worldview of a situation to a specific – or a lateral (sideways) point of reference. For instance in the above example the client wants to improve his relationship with someone. So the hypnotherapist starts at that very global/generalised goal and using that as an agreement foundation proceeds to help the client begin to consider the detail that's required to achieve that overall goal. Which, in this case is making a first move of friendship.

Here's an example going from <u>detail</u> to <u>generality</u>:

'Isn't it wonderful how you've worked all of those figures out like that? You know every pound that your company has spent. You know every pound that your company has earned. I wonder how you can put all of this information together in a way that gives you a good overview of your company's overall financial strength?'

In this example a person has a very good head for detail. The hypnotherapist is helping them to put it all together in such a way as to gain an insight into the bigger picture.

Here's a <u>lateral</u> example including a <u>generalisation</u> moving <u>to</u> some <u>detail</u>:

'So – you like dogs. And you like cats. And you want to help animals in general. Which animal can you help first?'

In this example of Levels of Abstraction the hypnotherapist has first moved laterally. You like dogs. (Dogs are a 'group'). And you like cats. (Cats are a 'group'. This is a sideways move from one group to another.) And you want to help animals in general (this involves a movement 'up' to the more general classification of helping 'animals'). Which animal can you help first? (Chunks right down to a specific animal and the defined act of helping it in particular.)

Liedentity

A Liedentity (lie and i-dentity) situation occurs when a client suggests/implies that they have a 'core belief' that they are fundamentally 'wrong' in some way. This is a distortion of their I-dentity. This distorted viewpoint may seem to exist (to the client) without other delineable contributory factors. Searching for them (contributory factors) may (or may not) reinforce the Liedentity. However – by giving it (the belief) a name, a form, as a 'Liedentity', it implies, in a fundamental way, that it's not to be trusted as representing reality. This can help the client to develop a more self-affirming identity-awareness based on their real worth. This term is reminiscent of Dr Fritz Perls' method in which he would talk to clients about their fundamental nature in ways that implied intrinsic worth and conversely anything that they said or did which appeared to sustain beliefs and/or behaviours diametrically opposite to this intrinsic worth were challenged by him and deemed to be false or 'phoney' (see the highly regarded video of him working with 'Gloria', for an example of this approach).

Here's an example of how this distortion can be challenged:

Client: 'I don't know why! I've always felt like I'm bad through and through. I try to do my best, but I always feel like I'm bad. And I can't change who I am.'

Hypnotherapist: 'So – you're always aiming to do your best in life. That's what we call a Truism. This means that you <u>are</u> honestly seeking to do things well. But – for some mysterious reason you haven't yet been able to shake the feeling that in some way, somewhere inside, 'waaaay dooown deeeeep inside' [said in a compassionate and humorous tone] you're bad, despite the fact that you're aiming to do your best. That's mixed up. That's not an identity it's a Liedentity. You've been believing a lie about yourself for so long that you can't tell the difference. Wasn't it Hitler, or one of his cronies, who said something about lying and how, if a lie was big enough and repeated often enough...? Phew! You've tricked yourself into having a Liedentity, rather than your true identity. Oh well – if that's what you want. I suppose it's up to you. It just seems to me that it's a bit of a shame to kid yourself so much, for so long, even in the face of all the evidence which shows that, despite a few foibles here and there (smile) you're a pretty decent person. [This intervention is based on naming the problem, which gives it a label and labels can be changed; in tandem with utilising a Frank Farrelly style humorous approach in order to 1) depotentiate and 2) reframe the belief, while pouring liberal amounts of doubt on the veracity of the negative 'core belief' – as measured against the client's spoken positive behaviours]. You could even follow up with: 'You know what they say - if you want to know what a person believes, don't necessarily listen to what they say. Look at what they do. And you seek to do your best. Which tells me that somewhere inside you know the truth about yourself. Even if you haven't yet fully realised it yourself yet! How about that! You know that you know even if you don't know that you know it. Now that's convoluted! You must be brighter than you look to figure that one out all for yourself"! Have you thought of going into politics I mean what with being able to do all of that double-layered reasoning? On second thoughts though – forget it. You're too good for politics, down deep inside (smile).'

Like You

The Like You pattern can be used to build self-esteem in a client and to increase rapport between people:

The Pattern:

1) 'I like you understand how important this is…'

2) 'You like me realise that you have many choices…'

3) 'I was talking to someone…like yourself…who said that…'

The Structure:

1) '**I like you** understand how important this is…'

The words 'I like you' are introduced in a way that conveys the intended meaning (I like you) specifically to the unconscious mind, because the inference is 'hidden' within a wider statement (while the untrained conscious mind absorbs the statement in full, being oblivious to its deeper 'hidden' meaning).

2) '**You like me** realise that you have many choices…'

The words 'You like me' are introduced in a way that conveys the intended meaning (You like me) specifically to the unconscious mind, because the inference is 'hidden' within a wider statement (while the untrained conscious mind absorbs the statement in full, being oblivious to its deeper 'hidden' meaning).

3) 'I was talking to someone....**like yourself**...who said that...'

The words 'like yourself' are introduced in a way that conveys the intended meaning (like yourself) specifically to the unconscious mind, because the inference is 'hidden' within a wider statement (while the untrained conscious mind absorbs the statement in full, being oblivious to its deeper 'hidden' meaning).

On a personal level, I think that the 'I like you' and the 'like yourself' patterns can be used readily. The 'you like me' pattern though is perhaps bordering on unscrupulous manipulation to be often used in therapy?

Limits

Using Limits is a very good way of eliciting/encouraging a desired cognitive and/or behavioural response from a client.

The Pattern:

'Don't turn it up too far.'

The Structure:

Whatever the 'it' is that's being referred to it's being presupposed that 'it' will be 'turned up' – but not too far.

<u>Here are some more examples</u>:

1) 'Don't go too deep.'

[The implication is that the client will 'go deep' – but not 'too deep']

2) 'Don't change all at once.'

[The implication is that the client will 'change' – but not 'all at once']

3) 'You don't have to do it too quickly.'

[The implication is that the client will 'do it' – but not 'too quickly']

4) 'It's not important that you think about relaxing right now.'

[The implication is that it's important that the client thinks about relaxing at sometime – but not 'right now']

5) 'Don't think of too many good ideas all at once. Save some for later.'

[The implication is that the client will think of 'good ideas' – but not 'all at once']

Linking Language

This is an umbrella expression that describes all categories of language pattern which comment on the listener's observable experience and then, through the use of linking words, lead the listener in a Desired Direction. [See: And / Compound Suggestions / Conjunctions / Contingent Suggestions / Disjunctions / Implied Causative.]

Linking Words

Linking words are words that can be used to link one statement or phrase to the next.

<u>The Pattern</u>:

'...And every time you notice something good you can remember the changes you've already made too in whichever is the most helpful and appropriate way for you...so that while you do...your inner self can be doing something else which helps you...and during this wonderful experience...as good things continue to happen...you will notice...when you want to that...'

<u>The Structure</u>:

'...<u>And</u> every time you notice something good you can remember the changes you've already made too in whichever is the most helpful and appropriate way for you...so that <u>while</u> you do...your inner self can be doing something else which helps you...<u>and during</u> this wonderful experience...<u>as</u> good things continue to happen...you will notice...when you want to that...'

In this example there is also a time-based element to the suggestions: 'as', 'while', 'during', 'and every time', which is very helpful because it suggests, in this context, changes in motion (or change is in motion. Or both? ☺).

Here are a couple of examples of how the word 'and' – or a pause – can be used to similar effect.

1) 'Some sounds give us special memories AND it can be interesting seeing the images associated with them.'

2) 'Some sounds give us special memories….it can be interesting seeing the images associated with them.'

[See also Compound Suggestion and Contingent Suggestion.]

Listen

The Pattern:

1) 'Hello Sally. Listen, now's a good time to get on with that coaching outcome.'

2) 'Okay. Listen, here's what I want you to do.'

3) 'I understand what you're saying. Listen, if we do XYZ we can reach ABC more quickly.'

4) 'Hey! Hold up a moment. I didn't do it. Listen, what you can do to change it is…'

5) 'Everyone thinks it's a good idea. Listen, if you start to do ABC you'll notice that too.'

<u>The Structure</u>:

The word 'Listen' creates powerful leverage. It has the effect of turning whatever follows its use into a powerful hypnotic suggestion. It also implies a high degree of importance to whatever follows its inclusion.

1) 'Hello Sally. <u>Listen</u>, now's a good time to **get on with that coaching outcome**.'

2) 'Okay. <u>Listen</u>, **here's what I want you to do**.'

3) 'I understand what you're saying. <u>Listen</u>, if **we do XYZ we can reach ABC more quickly**.'

4) 'Hey! Hold up a moment. I didn't do it. <u>Listen</u>, **what you can do to change it is**...'

5) 'Everyone thinks it's a good idea. <u>Listen</u>, if **you start to do ABC you'll notice that too**.'

Loaded Binds

<u>Front Loaded Double Bind</u>

<u>The Pattern</u>:

'Change can happen unexpectedly. And I wonder if you will notice the changes now or later?'

<u>The Structure</u>:

'**Change can happen unexpectedly.** [This suggestion is 'front loaded' onto a Double Bind which follows...] And I wonder if you will notice the changes now or later?'

Rear Loaded Double Bind

The Pattern:

'And I wonder if you will notice the changes now or later? Change can happen unexpectedly.'

The Structure:

'And I wonder if you will notice the changes now or later? **Change can happen unexpectedly.** [This suggestion is 'rear loaded' onto a Double Bind which precedes it.]'

Loaded Language

The Pattern:

'You're clever – what other things might you be good at?'

The Structure:

I was once role-playing the part of a client for a GP who was taking an assessment module in one of our training programmes. He used the above phrase (or one very much like it) which I thought was quite an artful example of Loaded Language. Notice what he did. He 'loaded' what he said by making a statement about the client being 'clever'. This meant that he was attributing something to the client (cleverness) and then <u>on</u> <u>the</u> <u>basis</u> <u>of</u> <u>this</u> suggested attribute he asked a question which was <u>designed</u> to <u>facilitate</u> a <u>positive</u> <u>search</u> from the client, of experiences which affirmed being 'clever'.

Location Binds

<u>The Pattern</u>:

'Now…we both know that…it's good to feel positive and there are many ways to feel positive at work…and I don't know whether you will feel happier at work…or more optimistic but I know that you know your unconscious knows what good feelings you can begin to notice at work now and in the future…'

<u>The Structure</u>:

This is basically a Double Bind with a location tied into the structure of the Bind. The location is made an integral part of the structure of the suggestion in order to act as a trigger for the underlying dynamics of the Bind. In this case arrival at the location is geared to trigger feelings of positivity, in one or more ways. In effect being in the location acts as an anchor to trigger the post hypnotic affect of positivity.

Now…we both know that…it's good to feel positive and there are many ways to feel positive <u>at</u> <u>work</u>…and I don't know whether you will feel happier <u>at</u> <u>work</u>…or more optimistic but I know that you know your unconscious knows what good feelings you can begin to notice <u>at</u> <u>work</u> now and in the future…

Lost Performative

The Lost Performative pattern is used to make a statement which has inherent within it an implied authoritative source for the assertion being made (in the form of a 'judgement'). But the original source of authority (the original speaker) has become 'lost' due to the pattern's structure.

The Pattern:

1) 'It's a good thing to create new ideas because when you do it means that...'

2) 'That is a great idea and the more often you think like this...'

3) 'Those are wonderful attributes which is why...'

The Structure:

1) '**It's** a good thing to create new ideas because when you do it means that...'

In this example an authoritative ('judgemental') statement is made. However the speaker neither says 'I think that' or 'so and so says'. Rather the speaker says 'it's' thereby adopting an authoritative position from which to empower the therapeutic suggestion being made, without offering a source of reference. You could of course ask the question 'who says so?' in order to uncover the source. Remembering this principle is a good way of identifying - and creating - Lost Performative Suggestions.

Here are some more examples which follow the same theme:

2) '**That is a great idea** [who says so?] and the more often you think like this...'

3) '**Those are wonderful attributes** [who says so?] which is why...'

Here are some more detailed examples:

4) 'It's good to use your unconscious mind to help you.'

By definition, the original performer of this statement has again become 'lost' by the use of the word 'it's'. By adding the 'performer' we could say it thus: 'Milton says it's good...'. But often it's good [there's another one] to leave the performer out and be a bit vague, because doing so helps to bypass any conscious resistance.

Notice for instance how a statement like 'Tony Blair says its good to...', will probably cause a different response in a Conservative supporter than would 'Margaret Thatcher says...' (and vice versa for a Labour supporter). However when we 'lose the performer' and simply say, for example, 'it's good to...', we can bypass the 'critical' conscious mind and help the client directly at an unconscious level.

M

Magical Because

<u>The Pattern</u>:

'It always begins to get better when you do it like this because that's the way things are here...'

<u>The Structure</u>:

Experiments have discovered that use of the word 'because' will influence people in such a way as to significantly improve the 'follow response' that occurs towards any suggestion that follows its application. I remember hearing somewhere that when researchers tested the use of the word 'because' for its power to generate influence in individuals they noticed a significant difference in peoples' reactions to requests made with or without its inclusion. For example; in an office environment if a person walked up to someone using a photocopier and asked the person using the machine the question: 'Can I use the photocopier now ahead of you?'. They found that that type of question could pretty much be guaranteed to draw a 'no!' response from the person already using the machine. However, when they introduced the word 'because' into the situation things turned out much differently. Questions like: 'Can I use the photocopier now ahead of you <u>because</u> I need to do these?' were much more likely to draw a 'yes!' response. Why, because the word because was included and we've grown up in a culture which has become accustomed (anchored) to perceive that whatever follows the word because is a suitable <u>explanation</u> for the request and we are therefore more 'obliged' (conditioned) to respond to its use in a pre-determined way. Notice, in the example I've written, there isn't really any 'justification' being given to explain why the person should be accorded the 'right' to queue jump. But the addition of the word because generates this response because that's what it does! ☺

Maybe

<u>The Pattern</u>:

The use of the word 'maybe' is very good for being artfully vague in the practice of hypnotherapy.

Here are a couple that I heard Stephen Brooks use:

1) '**Maybe** you don't have to decide – **maybe** there's a part of you that can decide and keep that to yourself if you wish.'

2) '**Maybe** your unconscious can remember a time when you slept on your arm and it became numb or when you held cold snow in your hand and lost the feeling in your fingers...'

Meaning Reframes

<u>The Pattern</u>:

1)

Client:

'I feel frustrated in my job which means I won't enjoy it.'

Hypnotherapist:

'I hear what you're saying, but maybe that sense of frustration really means that you're looking for a way to 'spice up' your work, so that you can enjoy it more? Often we need to experience the frustration first in order to know we're ready to discover the enjoyment.'

2)

Client:

'I keep watching the news and it makes me feel sad when I see so many examples of humanity's inhumanity to itself and this means I feel overwhelmed a lot of the time.'

Hypnotherapist:

'Maybe that overwhelming feeling and sadness about what you've been watching is also a message from you to yourself to encourage you to do something about what's been overwhelming you? Maybe it's telling you that now is the time to get proactive?'

3)

Client:

'I get so angry when I watch the way some people cruelly treat the animals that live on this planet with us that I feel this means I'll never be happy again.'

Hypnotherapist:

'I used to feel like that sometimes as well. But then I realised that my anger could actually be transformed into a source of energy which could help me to do something about it and doing so has made me much happier.'

The Structure:

In essence, when unpacking a Meaning Reframe the therapist's goal is to leave the <u>content</u> of the communication <u>the same</u> while <u>transforming</u> the <u>meaning</u> of the behaviour (in the sense of the client's interpretation of the meaning of their behaviour) in that <u>same context</u>. This means the client's <u>interpretation of the meaning</u> of their hitherto, perceived to be 'problem' behaviour becomes radically altered for the better. The Meaning Reframe can then quickly be employed to turn a perceived 'problem' into an 'attribute' by transforming the meaning of the situation to include an inherent solution within it – when viewed from a different angle, so to speak.

Meta Frame (Sleight Of Mouth)

Sleight of Mouth principles were first delineated by Robert Dilts as he himself modelled Richard Bandler's language patterns. Additional contributions have been made by Steve and

Connirae Andreas. A number of Sleight of Mouth patterns now exist, which are covered in this book. Sleight of Mouth patterns are utilised to unravel and in the process depotentiate adverse Complex Equivalence and/or Cause and Effect statements made by the client. [See: Analogy, Another Outcome, Apply To Self, Challenge, Change Of Reference Frame Size, Chunk Size, Consequences, Counter Example, Hierarchy Of Criteria, Intention, Meta Frame, Model Of The World, Reality Strategy, Redefine, Switch Referential Index.] In this example the principle of Meta Frame is employed.

Client statement:

'I think being kind causes me to feel weak.'

'(A) I think being kind causes (B) me to feel weak.'

Hypnotherapist:

A)

'And what do you mean by kind?'

B)

'How do you mean when you say 'weak' exactly?'

A/B)

It's good to know that you're thinking about important issues like these.'

Meta Model

'I know that you're thinking that everyone knows that Elvis is the best!'

The Meta Model is used to recover lost information, which always (always?) happens in the communication cycle. By recovering this lost information it's possible to deal with the real issue rather than with the:

Distortions – 'I know that you are thinking that...'

What evidence is there that I am thinking that?

Generalisations – '...everyone...'

Everyone?

Deletions – 'Elvis is the best!'

Compared to whom?

The Meta Model was developed by Bandler and Grinder and is based on the work of Virginia Satir. It is, in effect, the inverse of the Milton Model.

Metaphors

Metaphors can be employed to convey therapeutic messages in non-direct ways. They can involve stories, anecdotes and similes. Hypnotically speaking (in both senses of this expression) the aim is to introduce a concept to the client in a way that 'side steps' the conscious mind's sometimes 'restrictive' logical inclination in order to communicate more directly with the unconscious mind so as to elicit its natural, unhindered, creativity. It's a bit like learning by reading a book which has a 'special message' woven into the thread of the story (like the Chronicles of Narnia, or Star Wars do, for instance: The Lion The Witch and the Wardrobe is based on the Christian story (Aslan having Christ's role) and Star Wars has, I believe, been likened to Joseph Campbell's The Hero With a Thousand Faces, which explains the perennial myth of the young man who leaves his home to face trial and testing but the successful overcoming of which leads to him eventually gaining a kingdom/great reward).

For example; in the context of hypnotherapy it can be useful to use the metaphor of a diamond to help a client remember that there are many facets to their personality and countless emotional states to choose from, rather than just continually experiencing an undesired facet/state:

'And you know I have a little diamond in the ring on my hand. Sometimes I like to look at it because it reminds me of something really helpful. And you know what that is? Well...let me tell you. It reminds me that just like a diamond has many facets to its nature...so too...we as people have many facets to our characters and many emotional states to choose from...but sometimes we get so used to looking at one facet that we need a reminder...(like maybe now?)...to choose to look at yourself from another perspective and notice that you can choose to experience a whole range of nicer emotions just by remembering that they are there now...and as you think about one or two of them now...the mere fact that you are thinking about them means that at some level you are experiencing them...because in order to be able to think about them...you must have some inner representation of what they're like to experience...and this means that in order to know which emotions you're thinking of...you already know how to have them...and now that you've remembered that you know how to have them...your experience can begin to gently shift for the better...just like beginning to consider the many facets of a diamond and choosing now perhaps to consider some of the other ones available to you too. And remember: you're worth much more than a diamond.'

Notice during the course of the metaphor many language patterns and principles (which are covered within the pages of this book) were used to shift the metaphor from a dissociated state to an associated state of <u>knowing</u> and <u>experiencing</u> positive emotions. In this example I also translated the point of reference <u>from myself</u> at the start <u>to the client</u>. In order to create a hypnotic 'loop' I began with the early introduction of the word 'facets' and towards the end of the metaphor I again used this word to bring the theme back to its beginning, which can help to integrate the entire message at an unconscious level.

Milton Model

The Milton Model, in effect, uses the principles contained in the Meta Model in reverse. It seeks to delete, generalise and 'distort' information so that it will bypass the critical conscious mind and be communicated to the unconscious mind, without being challenged.

'It's <u>always</u> good to let your unconscious mind help you because that is the <u>best</u> way to do things, and <u>I sense that you sense this</u>.'

Mind Reading

Mind reading implies that at some level the therapist has an insight into the client's experience. To utilise Mind Reading effectively it's best to include personal Truisms/universal Truisms within the suggestions being offered. Truisms are necessary because if a hypnotherapist uses a 'Mind Reading' statement which has no bearing on a client's personal experience or on their wider perception of accepted universal reality they will likely reject the suggestion on the grounds that it is erroneous or beyond the bounds of reason.

<u>The Pattern</u>:

'I know that sometimes you are curious...and that's a good thing because it means that you know about learning new things...'

<u>The Structure</u>:

Everyone is curious at some time or other in their lives. The statement about the client being curious 'sometimes' is therefore a Truism. It is then linked with a Complex Equivalence ('...it means that...') which is followed by 'you know about learning new things' (this is a Truism too, because being curious invariably leads to learning new things).

Additionally this statement ('...you know about learning new things...') forms a positive suggestion which the client can accept in the form of <u>an established attribute</u> (based on the embedded Truisms) which applies directly to him/her. This attribute-effect can further act as a 'self-fulfilling prophesy' and help the client to begin to appraise his/her ability to be able to learn new things in a positive way.

<u>Other Mind Reading phrases include</u>:

1) 'I sense that...'

2) 'I understand that...'

3) 'You are...'

4) 'We both know...'

5) 'And I understand that you're choosing the right kind of responses for you...'

[By suggesting that you 'understand' you are, in effect, 'Mind Reading'.]

Mirror Grammar

An extension of Pivot Grammar [See Pivot Grammar] in which three words are, effectively, 'mirrored' back upon themselves. This creates a wonderful hypnotic effect when employed with extensive use of rhythm.

'And as you...

> You as and...

Make these changes...

> Changes these make...

You will find...

> Find will you...

Things get better...

> Better get things...

Things get better...

...and that's nice to know. Nice to know that things are getting better! And better.'

This method employs repetition and something of a natural 'subliminal effect' because it isn't easy for the client to consciously 'unpack' the precise structure of the suggestions, although the overall meaning is readily apparent as they listen. While, at an unconscious level, as research around subliminal and peripheral learning shows, the unconscious mind will be hearing a 'mirrored' copy of each positive suggestion and will therefore be able to incorporate the suggestions appropriately.

Misdirection – A Derren Brown Technique

Client: 'I've got this problem.'

Hypnotherapist: 'Oh really. We'll let's take a look at that in some more detail in a few moments. Just before we do I'd be grateful if you'd tell me a bit more about yourself.' [The hypnotherapist then uses this as an opportunity to gather information about the client's (unrealised) resources in order to reflect them back to the client, while in the process helping the client to change their perception of their ability. At the end of which the therapist could say:] 'Well thanks for all of that useful information. My – you certainly have accomplished a lot. Now let's take a look at that little problem you mentioned.'

By misdirecting the client away from the problem, the therapist is able to help the client reinforce their self-image without doing so <u>while</u> the client is <u>directly</u> <u>measuring</u> <u>it</u> against their problem. The problem is first disengaged, the client is strengthened, the therapist then returns to the issue of the 'little problem' with the client feeling more empowered, which in turn diminishes the stature of the problem in the client's mind.

A few patterns that I've heard Derren Brown use which could loosely be labelled as misdirection (that is to say that Derren is a master of the art of misdirection, but the following patterns are not 'strictly' misdirection, in the illusionist sense of the word, but, nevertheless there are hints of the principles of linguistic misdirection within them. They are perhaps examples of 'de facto misdirection') are as follows:

<u>The Pattern</u>:

1) 'Be honest...so what you're saying is...'

2) 'I'm not putting words into your mouth... but is that about right?'

<u>The Structure</u>:

1) 'Be honest...so what you're saying is...'

In the first example a 'doubt' is raised, in advance about the veracity of what the person could say. Derren then 'closes' the linguistic knot with the words 'so what you're saying is' and then 'tacks on' his desired interpretation of what the person is saying. Because the 'honest' answer has been presupposed to be in agreement with what's stated by Derren, the person likely 'agrees to agree'.

2) 'I'm not putting words into your mouth' [at which point Derren 'puts words into the person's mouth', so to speak. Words which reflect his desired outcome, at which point he concludes with...] '...but is that about right?'

In the second example Derren seems to indicate that he is not linguistically manipulating the participant's range of choice, which also implies that the client is free to choose his or her own conclusion...having diffused any potential resistance that the client may have had Derren then verbalises his desired 'interpretation' of the 'conclusion' that 'the client has drawn'. After having introduced his desired interpretation, in order to continue with the subterfuge of the participant's supposedly 'uninfluenced' choice he adds, 'is that about right?'. This implies that he really is trying to understand the client's point of view, when in actual fact he's influenced the client to adopt his own interpretation (for his own purposes) as their 'own' point of view.

It would of course be questionable to utilise such patterns, in this manner in a therapy/coaching session, if no real doubt exists. However, if there is a real doubt about the veracity of a client's statement or a misunderstanding, or need for clarification about a client's intent then such phrases as those demonstrated above could, when used ethically, in contexts such as these, have currency in the field of therapy.

Modal Operator Of Necessity

The Pattern:

'Making the improvements that you really know you have to make....because we both understand that you mustn't let them pass you by as now is the time when you ought to follow through...it needn't take long and you shouldn't have to try hard...it's all about doing it without trying...it's about making it happen without needing to make it happen...'

The Structure:

'Making the improvements that you **must** sense that you really know you **have** to make....because we both understand that you **mustn't** let them pass you by as now is the time when you **ought** to follow through...it **needn't** take long and you **shouldn't** have to try hard...it's all about doing it without trying...it's about making it happen without **needing** to make it happen...'

[The emboldened words indicate the 'necessity' elements of the linguistic structure and they imply that the receiver is 'bound' to respond to them - out of necessity. The words either imply allowance or prohibition.]

Modal Operator of Necessity words include: must, need, should, ought, mustn't, needn't, shouldn't, and ought not.

Useful phrases:

1) 'Your unconscious **must** always find ways to help you...'

2) 'Your unconscious **must** do the things which help you...'

3) 'You really **should** sense changes happening soon...'

4) 'You **ought** to be feeling better about things within a very short while...'

5) 'You **need** to fully understand just how powerful your unconscious is and why it always knows how to change things for the better...'

Modal Operator Of Possibility

The Pattern:

'You can wonder which benefits you will notice first but you can't consciously know for sure what they will be until they happen but it's possible that you may have a good idea...you could even be sensing them at some special level inside now because you are able to notice more when you think about things like this... it's impossible not to...can't you tell already or are you going to notice this soon...because even if you couldn't before...maybe you thought you were unable to do so...who knows?...but now you can...it's possible to do what your unconscious knows you can...and knowing this feels good...does it not?'

The Structure:

'You **can** wonder which benefits you will notice first but you **can't** consciously know for sure what they will be until they happen but it's **possible** that you may have a good idea...you **could** even be sensing them at some special level inside now because you are **able** to notice more when you think about things like this... it's **impossible** not to...**can't** you tell already or are you going to notice this soon...because even if you **couldn't** before...maybe you thought you were **unable** to do so?...who knows?...but now you **can**...it's **possible** to do what your unconscious knows you **can**...and knowing this feels good...does it not?'

[The emboldened words indicate the 'possibility' elements of the linguistic structure and they imply that the receiver either can or can't respond in a certain way. The words chosen indicate (by implication) whether or not something being addressed is within the listener's sphere of ability to either do or not do.]

Modal Operator of Possibility words include: can, possible, could, able, can't, impossible, couldn't, unable.

Useful Phrases:

1) 'Your inner self knows that you **can** change how you feel...'

2) 'It's **possible** to change the way you feel by changing your physiology you know...let me show you how you **can** do this...'

3) 'You **could** even notice that you sense more positive thoughts...just happening...in just the right kind of ways...'

4) 'It's **impossible** not to let your unconscious help you because it's **able** to make good things possible...you know...'

5) 'You **couldn't possibly** guess all of the new resources that are being generated for you...so you may as well just relax and let them come into your experience in all the right kind of ways...'

Model Of The World (Sleight Of Mouth)

Sleight of Mouth principles were first delineated by Robert Dilts as he himself modelled Richard Bandler's language patterns. Additional contributions have been made by Steve and Connirae Andreas. A number of Sleight of Mouth patterns now exist, which are covered in this book. Sleight of Mouth patterns are utilised to unravel and in the process depotentiate adverse Complex Equivalence and/or Cause and Effect statements made by the client. [See: Analogy, Another Outcome, Apply To Self, Challenge, Change Of Reference Frame Size, Chunk Size, Consequences, Counter Example, Hierarchy Of Criteria, Intention, Meta Frame, Model Of The World, Reality Strategy, Redefine, Switch Referential Index.] In this example the principle of Model Of The World is employed.

<u>Complex Equivalence Example</u>:

Client: '(A) I wasn't educated at Oxford (B) so I'll never amount to anything.'
Therapist (A): '<u>You</u> seem to believe that you didn't have the right kind of education.'
Therapist (B): 'It's curious that <u>you</u> should think that you'll never amount to anything.'
Therapist (A/B): '<u>You</u> seem to think that an Oxford education is necessary to getting anywhere in life, I think that's unusual.'

More The More (The)

This is a nice pattern that I've heard Richard Bandler use. Here are a few examples of how it can be utilised.

1) 'How about that! The more you want to change the more changes you get...'

2) 'Understand this...the more you take it easy the more easy it all becomes...'

3) 'Here...listen...the more you feel good the more you feel good...'

4) 'The more you wonder the more wonderful things can become...'

5) 'It works like this...the more you let it happen the more it happens...'

Here are some variations of my own:

(The Less The More)

1) 'The less you try the more it happens...'

2) 'The less you think about it now the more you understand...or the more you think about it now the more you know...'

3) 'The less you wonder the more you know...or the more you wonder the more you know...'

4) 'And this is how it happens...the less you think about doing it the more you do it...or the more you think about doing it the more you do it...'

5) 'Would you ever have guessed? The less it occurs the more good things are!'

(The More The Less)

1) 'It's in the past. It's over. In fact the more you try to do it the less it happens now. Until you don't even try anymore.'

2) 'That's right it's gone. The more you understand this the less you think about it. So that you can move on and be free now...'

3) 'What you don't need you can let go of and leave behind. The more you do the less important it becomes...'

4) 'The more happy you become the less unhappy you are now. And the more happy you feel the more you feel more happiness in your life.'

5) 'The more you embrace joy the less you notice those unwanted feelings. The more you embrace joy the more they fade away...for you...now...'

Motion Creates Emotion (Tony Robbins)

This is a useful phrase that I've heard Anthony Robbins use often. He uses it in the context of helping clients to understand that by changing their physiology they can change their emotions. Here's an example of how it can be employed in trancework:

'That's right...your thoughts are in motion...and we all know that motion creates emotion. So now is the time to bring some forward movement into your life...some motion... so that you can choose the positive emotions that occur when you get in motion...creates...emotion...and you can remember that by changing your posture you can change your emotions... can change... because... motion creates emotion and I want your unconscious mind to motion to you new and better emotions...'

Multiple Tasking Language

Multiple Tasking Language can be used to overload the conscious mind in order to generate more trance experiences...and to bypass so-called conscious 'resistance'.

1) 'As that hand becomes numb your eyelids can get heavier and as they get heavier you probably hadn't thought about that left foot in this trance until now...and as you notice that left foot that

anaesthesia can continue to develop in your right hand...'

2) 'And whatever you do don't forget to count backwards from 500 to 1 with each sound of the clock and remember to notice the sensations in your feet as another part compares them with the difference in sensation with what you haven't noticed in your hands...'

My Voice Will Go With You

A favourite phrase of Dr Milton Erickson:

'That's right and my voice will go with you and it can become the voice of your parents, your teachers, your friends as...'

N

Negation

Negation can be employed, paradoxically, to elicit the responses which are seemingly being suggested 'not' to occur. This is because the mind cannot process negation. In order to not think about something you first have to think about what you are 'not thinking about' in order to think about not thinking about it. So it generally has the opposite effect of that which is (seemingly) suggested.

Single Negative Suggestion / Coue's Law Bind

1) 'Don't think about that solution now...'

2) 'Don't think about what to do right now...'

3) 'Don't consider going into trance just yet...'

Double Negative Suggestion / Reversed Coue's Law Bind

1) 'Don't not think about that solution now...'

2) 'Don't not think about what to do right now...'

3) 'Don't not consider going deeper into trance just yet...'

<u>Triple Negative Suggestions</u>

1) 'Your unconscious never can't not make this change happen for you...'

2) 'It can't not never happen now that your unconscious has changed things inside...'

3) 'You don't not never have to think about this right now...'

4) 'You know you don't not never have to wonder just how deep you will go right now...'

Negative Questions

Negative Questions are similar to the more well-known Tag Questions pattern [see Tag Questions]. This method utilises negation in order to make a statement in the form of a suggestion.

1) 'Can you not see that something needs to change?'

2) 'Are you not empathic yourself?'

3) 'Did you not find a way forward last time?'

4) 'Isn't it right that you assert yourself too?'

5) 'Haven't you also sensed that you've had enough of that situation by now?'

Negatives (Tag Questions)

<u>The Pattern</u>:

1) 'So, there are some issues about your relationship that you want to change. And you want them to start changing soon, do you not?'

2) 'Alright. It's about believing in yourself, is it not?'

3) 'You want this to happen soon, don't you?'

4) 'That's why you've always done it this way, haven't you?'

5) And an in-trance example:

'And while you...do sense...new and... better... ideas coming into ...your mind...which... help you...help yourself...you can know...can you not?...that something good is beginning to occur...'

<u>The Structure</u>:

Negatives are also known as Tag Questions, and the term 'Tag Questions' describes the principle very well. In effect a question is added to a statement, which itself is posed in the intonation of a statement, in order to compound the statement (which is itself a suggestion) to enhance the therapeutic affect.

1) 'So, there are some issues about your relationship that you want to change. And you want them to start changing soon, <u>do you not</u>?'

2) 'Alright. It's about believing in yourself, <u>is it not</u>?'

3) 'You want this to happen soon, <u>don't you</u>?'

4) 'That's why you've always done it this way, <u>haven't you</u>?'

5) And an in trance example:

'And while you...do sense...new and... better... ideas coming into ...your mind...which... help you...help yourself...you can know...<u>can you not</u>?...that something good is beginning to occur...'

Negative Suggestions

Negative Suggestions are utilised to elicit a positive. As previously stated when covering Negation the mind cannot think in terms of a negative outright. It first needs to think about not thinking about what it is being asked to not think about in order to think about not thinking about it.

1) 'It's not for me to tell you that you can achieve even more. That's for you to discover for yourself.'

2) 'I'm not saying that you're going to notice changes today. I'm going to let you find out in your own good time.'

3) 'I'm not going to tell you that you have the potential to achieve this goal more easily than you realise. But I am going to let you experience a pleasant surprise when you start to notice how much you are beginning to achieve.'

4) 'I'm not telling you that indirect hypnosis is the best approach. Would you not rather discover this for yourself? After all how could you know whether it is or whether it isn't if you haven't yet experienced it? Have you? Have you!?'

Nominalisation

The Pattern:

A Nominalisation is a process word (a 'doing word') that's been fixed and made 'static' as if it has changed into a tangible object. So, for example, the process of 'learning' becomes (fixed) 'learnings'. The process of 'feeling' becomes 'feelings' and so on. It's a useful linguistic pattern for taking processes and turning them into 'assets'. For example:

1) 'You have been learning many things and those learnings are resources that you have now for life.'

2) 'That feeling you've been having can join all of your other feelings and you can pick and choose amongst all of your feelings now and choose which you choose to experience and which ones you are not going to select as often as you used to.'

3) 'All those successful communications that you have already achieved are some of your best assets'.

4) 'Taking into account your extensive understandings...it can only get better.'

5) 'Those learnings which you have.'

6) 'Those <u>feelings</u> which help you.'

7) 'Like bringing those <u>wonderments</u> with you and becoming happier because you have'.

8) 'Making sure all of those '<u>happinesses</u>' that you like are there whenever you need them.'

9) 'Knowing why and how you can tune into gentle <u>comforts</u> which you prefer quickly.'

10) 'And those '<u>cryings</u>' are in the past while the '<u>smilings</u>' are now drawing closer...and closer...maybe one will even be happening soon or sooner?'

Non Sequitur Suggestions

<u>The Pattern</u>:

1) 'You can let the relaxation happen or just make the changes right now.'

2) 'The birds are singing in the trees so you can let yourself feel better.'

3) 'Lots of people stop smoking with hypnosis – so you can use NLP to deal with that phobia.'

4) 'Happiness is available to everyone and you will feel more confident.'

5) 'Knowing that you can listen or just go deeper into trance.'

<u>The Structure</u>:

A Non Sequitur Suggestion is a suggestion which draws a conclusion which does not follow from the statement that preceded it (the term 'non sequitur' means 'it does not follow'). It 'breaks' the rules of conventional grammar. However, it is an excellent therapeutic tool for 'hitchhiking' suggestions onto the preceding statement so that they will be more readily accepted therapeutically by the client. Notice how the hitch-hiked statement seems to flow naturally with the preceding statement, which is acting as a vehicle.

1) 'You can let the relaxation happen <u>or just make the changes right now</u>.'

2) 'The birds are singing in the trees <u>so you can let yourself feel better</u>.'

3) 'Lots of people stop smoking with hypnosis – <u>so you can use NLP to deal with that phobia</u>.'

4) 'Happiness is available to everyone <u>and you will feel more confident</u>.'

5) 'Knowing that you can listen <u>or just go deeper into trance</u>.'

Not Doing....

<u>The Pattern</u>:

1) 'You don't have to do anything to go into a trance, you can just let it develop in its own unique way...'

2) 'You don't have to make this change happen consciously, you can relax and let your unconscious do it for you...'

3) 'You don't have to relax right now, you can just sit here and listen if you like, your unconscious is doing all the work for you...'

4) 'And while you're thinking about that remember you don't have to do anything about it while things are getting easier...'

5) 'You don't have to do anything. Not anything! Except what feels best for you and then notice what starts to happen which helps you...'

The Structure:

The Not Doing suggestion can be used to create a sense of 'no effort' which, generally speaking, has the effect of encouraging whatever is suggested by Not Doing and what follows, to occur. When we say things like 'try hard to do' XY or Z we immediately introduce the possibility of failure and the concept of effort, which many people will interpret in ways which cause them to believe that they stand little or no chance of achieving the desired outcome. Even suggesting something as easy as relaxation in the 'wrong' way can elicit the wrong outcome: 'Now you must begin by making yourself relax. That's it. Think really hard about making yourself relax. We have to get you feeling relaxed before we can do anything else. Come on – you want this sooo much. It's sooo important to you. You HAVE TO make yourself relax!'. Not very relaxing is it? Now contrast this with the same desired outcome while using the Not Doing approach: 'You know, one of the wonderful things that most amazes me about how trance happens is that it takes place without you having to do anything about it. That's right. You don't have to do a thing to make it happen more for you. You don't even have to try. In fact if you want to you can just sit here and listen to me or think about something else if you like and not try to do anything else while waiting for your own trance to happen. Maybe it already has? But you don't have to try to make it. And I think that is an amazing thing about going into a nice relaxing trance without having to really do very much at all….that's right…'

Here are the above mentioned examples with the relevant elements highlighted:

1) '<u>You don't have to do anything</u> to go into a trance, you can just let it develop in its own unique way…'

2) '<u>You don't have to make this change happen</u> consciously, you can relax and let your unconscious do it for you…'

3) '<u>You don't have to relax right now</u>, you can just sit here and listen if you like, your unconscious is doing all the work for you…'

4) 'And while you're thinking about that remember <u>you don't have to do anything about it</u> while things are getting easier…'

5) '<u>You don't have to do anything</u>. Not anything! Except what feels best for you and then notice what starts to happen which helps you…'

Not Knowing...

This, in essence, is practically the same principle as covered directly above in the Not Doing section, except here the focus is on Not Knowing:

The Pattern:

1) 'You don't have to know when your unconscious is starting to make these changes...'

2) 'You don't have to understand consciously what your unconscious is doing for you...'

3) 'You don't even have to know why it happens this way...you can just relax and feel comfortable knowing that it does...'

4) 'It's nice to know that you don't even have to know how it first started in order to get better today...'

5) 'You don't have to understand everything or even very much about what your inner self is going to do today that means that you are recovering quite nicely and moving forward to a better future...'

The Structure:

1) 'You don't have to know when your unconscious is starting to make these changes...'

2) 'You don't have to understand consciously what your unconscious is doing for you...'

3) '<u>You don't even have to know</u> why it happens this way...you can just relax and feel comfortable knowing that it does...'

4) 'It's nice to know that <u>you don't even have to know how it first started</u> in order to get better today...'

5) '<u>You don't have to understand everything or even very</u> much about what your inner self is going to do today that means that you are recovering quite nicely and moving forward to a better future...'

(Not Doing + Not Knowing)

Here are a couple of combined Not Doing and Not Knowing Suggestions.

1) 'The wonderful thing about being in therapy now is that you don't have to do anything – or even know how good things are happening you can simply let your unconscious do it all for you.'

2) 'You don't have to think about new solutions. Or even know where they come from. You don't have to do anything in trance. You can just let it happen naturally.'

Not Only...But Also...

This pattern was actually the title of a Peter Cooke and Dudley Moore show for BBC2... and it's also an excellent hypnotic language method.

Here are a few examples of how this can be used this therapeutically:

1) 'Not only can hypnosis help with smoking cessation but also many other useful things.'

2) 'Not only can you change that but also this…'

3) 'Not only will you notice an expanded sense of possibility but also a greater ability to enjoy it.'

4) 'Not only is hypnosis great but also very powerful too!'

5) 'Not only is therapeutic confusion useful but also you don't even have to think very much about developing anaesthesia in that left arm. Not only can you listen to me but also it can just start all on its own. Not only can you think those thoughts but also it can grow stronger. Not only can you feel comfortable but also a complete anaesthesia can take place in that left arm. Not only can you think about wondering but also it just makes that arm feel totally comfortably numb.' [In this example you'll notice that the first part of each sentence refers to one element while the following 'But Also' part constantly addresses suggestions geared to develop anaesthesia. Each 'But Also' builds upon the previous one, while each 'Not Only' continues to distract the conscious mind with other ideas.]

O

Obtaining Permission To Change

'Is it alright now for you to give up that problem?'

This is a pattern I heard Stephen Brooks employ. Very simple, yet very effective.

Oh Really?

I learned this from Peter Young. I met Peter when he and I were participants on an NLP Practitioner course some years ago with the NLP Learning Company. Subsequently he wrote his very good book called Understanding NLP.

The 'Oh Really?' technique Peter suggests can be quite useful for depotentiating the power of unwanted and/or untimely comments. In essence a person responds by replying 'Oh really!' and then proceeds by conversationally 'moving away from' what was said by the other person (which was unhelpful) addressing instead what is preferable. The 'Oh really!' response seems to acknowledge the statement made by the other person – while allowing room for the therapist to seamlessly move beyond the unwelcome remarks which were made.

Client: 'Anyway this is going to be difficult to solve because my great, great grandfather also had this problem.'

Hypnotherapist: 'Oh really! And you were also saying that you noticed that it never happens when you XYZ. Tell me some more about that. That's interesting.'

Only

The Pattern:

This is a pattern I've heard Richard Bandler use very well.

1) 'You only need to...'

2) 'You only need to notice that...'

3) 'And you only need to learn that...'

4) 'Only you will notice that as...'

5) 'Only let it happen when...'

The Structure:

In the first three examples the word 'only' limits the statement to the receiver. It can be used in a one-to-one context and in a group setting to ensure that the intended recipient is the 'only' person to get the message. In the last two examples it's used more generally, in the sense that it suggests a restriction, meaning that whatever the word only has referred to will 'only' occur when a certain set of criteria are met. For instance: 'Now...your unconscious has understood that changes have been made and is understanding the changes that have been made which means that it understands what it needs to know...now...to change this for you totally and completely...but...I'm going to ask your unconscious now to...<u>only let it happen when</u>... your unconscious is ready to make the changes totally and completely...in all the most helpful, healthful and appropriate ways for you...now and in the future...'.

Any sign of a manifestation of the desired cognitive/behavioural state will then act as a ratification of the changes that have been suggested. The supposed 'restriction' actually acts as a ratification – upon any evidence of the desired change – which results in the reinforcement of the therapeutic suggestion.

Open Ended Suggestion

Another name for 'Covering All Possible Alternatives'.

'You might wonder whether that hand is moving to the right or to the left, up or down, or not moving whatsoever.'

[See Covering All Possible Alternatives]

Ordinal Numbers

<u>The Pattern</u>:

1) 'I wonder will your first experience...'

2) 'And with each further change that you make...'

3) 'And after you notice these good things happening and then notice another good thing too...'

4) 'Who knows whether it will be on the first, second, third or fourth occasion that your inner confidence helps you...'

5) 'And another good thing.   With every further compounded benefit, from the first that you notice...'

The Structure:

As the title suggests the pattern being employed here is to do with <u>sequence</u>.   When talking specifically about numbers it can mean any number, or, more vaguely, it can be used by employing words such as 'before', 'after', 'further, 'another', 'next', 'subsequent', 'following', 'succeeding', 'ensuing', 'successive', 'consequent', 'additional', 'extra', 'prior', 'previous', 'preceding' 'past', 'former', etc.

By introducing the implication that whatever is being addressed is part of a pre-supposed (and therefore implicitly accepted as a given) sequence it presupposes that the suggested (by the therapist) effect will occur in sequence.   Now, of course, whether this means that the client will notice the affects on the first occasion they occur or after several experiences is for the client to discover. ☺

1) 'I wonder will your <u>first</u> experience...'

2) 'And with each <u>further</u> change that you make...'

3) 'And <u>after</u> you notice these good things happening and then notice another good thing too...'

4) 'Who knows whether it will be on the <u>first</u>, <u>second</u>, <u>third</u> or <u>fourth</u> occasion that your inner confidence helps you...'

5) 'And <u>another</u> good thing. With every <u>extra</u> compounded benefit, from the <u>first</u> that you notice...'

Oxymoron

<u>The Pattern</u>:

1) 'And you can make a speedy stop to that behaviour right now!'

2) 'You can begin by making small strides in the right direction so to speak. Can you not?'

3) 'And as you quickly slow things down...'

4) 'Now that you know how to remain changing like this...'

5) 'As we continue to begin...'

<u>The Structure</u>:

The Oxymoron pattern is useful for introducing concepts in a covert way. It introduces seemingly contradictory terms to the listener. Generally, the conscious mind will be focussed on the first part of the statement while the suggestion in the second part of the statement is accepted without critical thought.

1) 'And you can make a speedy <u>stop</u> to that behaviour right now!'

2) 'You can begin by making small <u>strides</u> in the right direction so to speak. Can you not?'

3) 'And as you quickly <u>slow</u> things down...'

4) 'Now that you know how to remain <u>changing</u> like this...'

5) 'As we continue to <u>begin</u>...'

P

Pacing Current Experience

The Pattern:

'And while you're sitting here, listening to me, a part of you is aware of the sensation of your watch on your wrist.'

The Structure:

This pattern involves commenting on (feeding back) elements of the client's observable experience of trance. In so doing a 'Yes Set' [See Yes Set] is generated. The client invariably <u>agrees</u> <u>with</u> <u>each</u> <u>Truism</u>: 1) He/she <u>is</u> sitting 'here'. 2) He/she <u>is</u> listening. 3) A part of him/her <u>is</u> aware of the sensation of the watch upon his or her wrist.

This can be taken a stage further by suggesting the process of certain non observable phenomena. Like this:

'And while you're sitting here, listening to me, a part of you is aware of the sensation of your watch upon your wrist and as you notice the sensation of the watch upon your wrist your unconscious mind is thinking unconscious thoughts...creating inner resources...generating greater talents...which help you to help yourself more easily now...'

Three non (immediately) observable phenomena are suggested 1) 'your unconscious mind is thinking unconscious thoughts' 2) 'creating inner resources' 3) 'generating greater talents'...which are likely to be accepted by the client because of the 'pacing of current experience' which was identified by the first three comments (which acted as a Yes Set) meaning that, as a result, the client will more readily be in agreement with the non observable phenomena suggested by the therapist. Please note: the non observable phenomena suggested must be within the bounds of reason and acceptability.

Panic Diffusion

On an occasion when we were presenting Stephen Brooks as he was doing a demonstration with a client, the client began to panic, 'live' in front of the class. This elicited a question from the group. In answering the question (while the client was still being treated by him before the assembled class) he explained what he was doing, in relation to her response, by saying, words to the effect of... 'If she chooses to flatter me by demonstrating that she trusts me enough to experience her panic...let her do it and experience it....I wouldn't stop it. I'd work with it. By trying to stop it, it will make it harder next time.'

In so doing he was indirectly telling the woman he was working with a number of things.

1) It was okay to feel panicky.

2) He was confident that he could help her even though she was feeling panicky.

3) By panicking she was 'flattering' him – and trusting him - <u>which</u> <u>meant</u> <u>that</u>, in reality, she felt safe at a deeper level.

4) He would work with the panic as she experienced it – <u>which</u> <u>meant</u> <u>that</u> it would be changed in some way. The implications were, naturally, that the change would be for the better.

I've also heard him respond to clients at other times who've expressed a certain amount of nervousness, for various reasons, by saying something like: 'Oh, so you're feeling a bit nervous. Good! It's good to have some energy to work with. I'd feel sorry for a carpenter who was given a completely smooth piece of wood to work with. Wouldn't you? It's so much nicer to be able to have something to work with. That way you can experience the feelings of enjoyment as everything becomes smooth. It's so much more satisfying. Don't you think?'

As in the first example, where he artfully reframed the feeling of panic to one of trust – and implicitly healing, in this example he reframes the sensations of 'panic' to being evidence of 'energy' and this energy is paralleled with the process of carpentry and of how much better it is, for a carpenter, to have something to work with, in order to enjoy the process of making it smooth. This turns the perception of nervousness, as being a 'bad' thing, to one of being, instead, a useful <u>source of energy</u> that leads naturally into feelings of enjoyment and accomplishment.

Paradoxing

<u>The Pattern</u>:

1) 'As you think about that...think about this...illness can be healing... you know...and now that you have experienced your illness as much as you need to, to learn from it in order to heal yourself and become even more than you were before it started...I wonder what it is that you will become aware of that you have learned by it which is helpful for you...today...'

2) 'Sometimes you can win by losing and sometimes you can lose by winning...wisdom comes by knowing the difference...and I wonder what you think is the best thing to do about that contest you were just talking about?'

3) 'And have you ever noticed how many people display their lack of wisdom by displaying their 'great' intelligence?'

4) 'I've learned that some people go through life trying to find ways to be happy and it makes them sad. I think that sometimes it's easier to get on with doing good things with your life and - you never can tell, you might find that the happiness just starts to appear, more often, when you're not trying to make it happen. That's a curious thing I've noticed about happiness anyway, and I just thought it would be worth mentioning now.'

5) 'Did you know that many ideas which lead to inventions have occurred when the inventor wasn't thinking about inventing? Sometimes, after we've learned everything we need to know about what

we're doing, the solution just pops into our head, when we're, supposedly, not thinking about it. I like it when it happens like that, don't you?'

6) 'Have you ever noticed how some people expend a lot of energy and accomplish nothing? How does that song go?: 'I'm busy doing nothing, working the whole day through, trying to find lots of things not to do'. Some people do that you know – they expend loads of energy accomplishing nothing! Isn't it better to invest, say even a tenth of all of that energy, by getting on with something worthwhile, than wasting 100% of it in ways that you know deep down are 'playing at being busy'. It might seem like you can kid yourself, or others, for a while that you're 'doing a lot' and it might even look that way on the surface too. But in the long term, the difference that makes the difference is have you changed things? If the answer is 'no', then things need to change don't they? And, be honest, if you think this sounds like your situation, maybe now is the time to get real and do something that amounts to something instead of playing at being 'busy'. Have you ever noticed how some people equate 'being busy' with 'being important'? If more people spent less time 'being important' and more time getting on with rewarding things, I think the problems of the world would soon begin to fade. Why not start now?'

The Structure:

Paradoxes can be used therapeutically to help a client begin to think 'outside of the box', so to speak. To learn the lessons that there are to be learned about seemingly contradictory positions. Many religious teachings employ paradox because of its potential for 'enlightenment'. In the above examples paradoxes are made in order to help the client 'see the light' so to speak about certain situations in order to become 'liberated'. Paradoxes are liberating, which brings to mind the phrase 'The Truth shall set you free'. Often times the message of the paradox is that by understanding and embracing the opposite point of view something better can occur.

Carl Jung, I believe, was a staunch advocate of the belief that <u>illness</u> <u>is</u> <u>healing</u>. In today's 'quick fix' society this position seems to be a contradiction, and perhaps, in some ways it is. But, when you consider that statement again and consider the deeper meaning, the paradoxical truth of the statement can be very encouraging and liberating. Likewise, we've all met people who have to 'win' every conversation (argument?) etc, and in the process lose everything as a result. And we've all probably met people who seem to have the need to demonstrate 'how clever' they are to 'everyone' and in the process, have paradoxically expressed their low WQ ('Wisdom Quotient').

Freedom lives in the realm of Paradox with his sister Wisdom. As clients discover paradox they can begin to learn how to 'step outside of the box' and thereby improve the quality of their lives.

Pausing

I've found that pauses correctly used when delivering trance can help to generate... expectancy and... **powerful**... embedded suggestions while using rhythm... to... maximize... the... trance...

ambiance... while... working... in... similar ways... to lullabies... so that... the client can... start to feel... nicely at ease... in order to... just let go... and go inside.

Shamans have utilised rhythm and song in the trance state for millennia. Based on these principles I regularly use various rhythm sets in the trancework that I deliver and have consistently found that it contributes very effectively to the therapeutic framework of the trance and the types of trances that the clients experience. [See also: Rhythming And Rhyming]

Perceptual Positions

The Pattern:

A hypnotherapist can embed suggestions and metaphors by using quotes which, because they are quotes, introduce a range of different perceptual positions to the situation. This can be useful for offering suggestions to a client conversationally in an indirect manner.

Hypnotherapist: 'You know I was talking to someone once about what it's like to go into trance for the first time. He'd just asked me: 'What will I notice about trance?' And I said: 'You can notice feeling calm.'

The Structure:

In this example the therapist appears to be engaging in general conversation with the client about someone else's experience of going into trance. The example is 'once removed' due to the fact that the therapist is quoting a different situation. However, in the context of the 'once removed' situation the therapist speaks from a 1st Position (that of the self) and then offers the desired suggestion, indirectly, from a 2nd position (that of 'other than self') perspective.

Hypnotherapist: [1st position] 'You know I was talking to someone once about what it's like to go into trance for the first time. [1st position] He'd just asked me: 'What will I notice about trance?' And I said: [2nd Position. Which relates to 'other'] 'You can notice feeling calm' [however, in actual fact, the 2nd Position perspective actually affords an indirect way to deliver a powerful suggestion to the client in the room, in the present moment].

Here's another example:

Client: 'Will I stop smoking in one session?'

Hypnotherapist: 'A good question. Of course I can't guarantee anything. However, you know someone else once asked me almost the same question. She said: When will I become a non-smoker then? And I said: You can become a non-smoker soon if you really want to. And she did.'

Hypnotherapist: 'So that's what I told her – does that answer your question too?'

Client: 'Yes thanks.'

Hypnotherapist: 'Okay. And are you ready to go into trance now too?'

Client: 'Yes.'

Phonological Ambiguity

<u>The Pattern</u>:

'How do you do that? How is it that you're sitting here [hear] and listening... to the sound of my voice... while your unconscious [you're unconscious] is thinking more deeply... sounds are happening outside... you can hear a quiet one... and a loud [allowed] ... to make changes today ...as you listen ... and you're thoughts can wander [wonder]... how will you experience your new emotions? ... someone else the other day noticed that ... their ... their [there there] ... thinking began to change... just a little bit at first... then their their [there there] emotions began to change and their... their [there...there] mood began to lift ... and as you listen to the sound of that aircraft outside [a regular occurrence in my treatment room under a flight path] ...the plain [plane] truth is that your mood can lift like this too... have you ever said: 'Hi' [high] to yourself and given yourself an inner smile? Letting the lightness [meaning opposite of heavy – while also meaning radiant] of that bright feeling shine throughout every level of your body and mind so that deep healing can occur? Or is this the first time you have done it like this? Now one lady used to like to relax into trance quite quickly... at first she thought she needed someone else to help her calm her [calmer] self down... but then she noticed that she could close those eyes [I] ... expect you already know how to do this ...by [buy as in 'buy into' this concept of relaxation] now... that's right make a mental note of it right now [write now] in your mind ... so that you can recall this calm feeling more often... and just sense your changing [you're changing] perceptions... change is [changes] taking place...'

Phonological ambiguities can be used for a number of reasons. One being to send messages to at least two layers of perceptual awareness in order to enhance unconsciousness reception of the embedded meaning of the messages. A second principle can be to generate a certain amount of conscious confusion when (as above) the syntax [meaning the order: '...close those eyes / I ... expect you...' Is the therapist saying close those eyes? Or I expect you...? Or both?] and scope [meaning the perspective: 'their their' or 'there there'] of the structure of certain sentences seems to deviate from traditional rules of grammar, as experienced by most people in the English speaking world in day-to-day life. This generally results in the person trying to make sense of the 'competing' meanings which often results in a sense of 'overload' which in turn un-inhibits the conscious mind, which then stops trying to analyse things too much or too deeply... resulting in a more relaxed perspective and more unhindered unconscious perception.

Pivot Grammar

The Pattern:

Pivot Grammar was, I believe, developed by Dr Richard Bandler. I like it a lot. It makes excellent use of rhythm and helps to generate very good trance states - while facilitating the use of Embedded Suggestions.

'You know... Know you... That now... Now that... You are... Are you... Getting better... Better getting... Things are... Are things... Looking up... Up looking... '

The Structure:

Pivot Grammar involves linguistically pivoting on chosen words, first said in 'forward motion' then, due to the 'pivot', in reverse order. To my mind this is similar to the subliminal effect that people talk about that occurs when spoken or written words are presented in reverse order. The unconscious mind deciphers the meaning and responds to the influence. The rhythm follows this kind of pitch: DA DA da da DA DA da da... and so on. As a 'rule of thumb' the first two words have more emphasis placed on them and they finish in an 'upward' tonality, while the pivoted words which follow have slightly less emphasis and a 'downward' tonality attached to them.

YOU KNO^W...

Know yo$_u$...

THAT NO^W...

Now tha$_t$...

YOU AR^E...

Are yo$_u$...

GETTING BETTE^R...

Better gettin$_g$...

THINGS AR^E...

Are thing$_s$...

LOOKING U^P...

Up lookin$_g$...

LOOKING UP!

[For recorded examples of this method along with many other patterns covered in this book visit www.ultrahypnosis.co.uk.]

Polarity Response Depotentiators

The Pattern:

A polarity response involves a person taking an opposite (polar extreme) point of view. For example, you suggest 'it's black', so they say 'it's white'. You change your mind and agree that 'it may be white' and they reconsider too and say 'it's black'. Some people habitually polarity respond in life, to greater or lesser degrees. Those who do this are generally beset by problems, to greater or lesser degrees, because, basically, they don't know how to get on with others and they're frustrating for most people to be around, due to this 'negative' trait. When 'Polarity Responders' present for therapy, in order to assist them it's important, I believe, to (sometimes covertly) depotentiate the polarity response so that therapy can occur (and often times, it's also useful to overtly educate the client regarding the nature of polarity responses so that they can begin to respond more appropriately instead).

The Structure:

Example Category A)

1) 'There is no reason why you should relax completely...'

2) 'You don't have to pay attention...'

3) 'You don't have to be bothered to talk...'

In the above three examples I appear to suggest one thing, which invites a polarity response in the Desired Direction (relaxation, paying attention, communicating). This kind of approach is a bit like one I adopted with a family dog we had years ago. He was a Red Setter called Tristan. Tristan was probably the best exemplar of a polarity responder that I've ever met. If I said to him 'Tristan Sit! Tristan Stay!' he'd instead get up and walk towards me. If I said 'Tristan, this way!' He'd instead sit down and stay where he was. So in the end <u>I learned</u> to <u>say the opposite</u> of what I seemingly 'wanted', in order to <u>get the result</u> I really wanted. Sometimes, some people, my experience indicates, will present for therapy acting in a similar kind of way, for 'who knows what' reason and a similar, but more subtle, approach can be helpful.

Example Category B)

Colin Saunders introduced me to an American Hypnotist called Marshall Sylver. I intuit that, like many others, he has modelled himself to a greater or lesser degree on Tony Robbins. A few years ago I found a script by him on the internet by chance and in it there was a lovely 'golden nugget' of a phrase for depotentiating polarity responders. Here it is:

'Of course you could resist but that's not why you're here...'

Example Category C)

Another way to depotentiate polarity responses (and other unwelcome habits and behaviours) is to (to borrow a phrase from James Redfield's Celestine Prophesy) **Name The Game**. Something like this:

'You know. I don't know what we're going to do then. We looked at it being black and you said it was white. We looked at the possibility that it was white and you said that you felt that, actually it might be black. So we looked at it again from the black perspective and you said that you instead felt it was white. Did you know there is a psychological term for this pattern? It's called a polarity response. Most people who do it – do it without knowing they're doing it. But – and now that I've shared this example with you – I'm sure you can see too now how it could cause lots of problems in a person's life if it was left to go unchecked. Now, I'm not saying you are one of the kind of people who do it to that degree. And we can't draw a firm conclusion from three small incidents like this. But I thought it would be worth drawing it to your attention now – so that you can become aware of the potential that you may have been doing it without knowing you were, so that you can change it. Experience shows that people who habitually polarity respond generally experience lots of problems in life because they just keep raising knee-jerk objections all of the time. And I know you don't want to be like that. Because you told me you want to change. So, now, remember, I can't force you to make any changes. And I wouldn't want to try. But I am prepared to work with you to help you do what needs to be done... as you do so of your own volition. So, let's consider this afresh now. White? Black?'

Example Category D)

The 'Yes But' Response

This is another form of polarity response, in which a person constantly responds by saying: 'Yes...but...' and then proceeds to take a contrary point of view. One of the best ways to deal with this, again is to **Name The Game**:

Hypnotherapist:

'Respectfully, I wonder if you've realised this yourself too? Each time we've looked at different possible solutions you've done something that's known in psychological literature as the 'Yes But Response'. We considered option one and you said: 'Yes but...I can't do that because...'. We considered option two and you responded by saying: 'Yes but...I can't do that because...'. And you did the same through options three to ten. Did you know sometimes, that some people have responded like this so often that it has become, for them, something of a destructive habit which holds them back often in life? I'm not saying this is that kind of problem for you. But it's worth you considering now. Let me give you an example of how it occurs.

Someone working in an office says to a colleague 'I can't think of anywhere to go on holiday this year.' The colleague tries to help by saying something like: 'Malta is nice – I went there last year and had a great time'. The 'Yes Buter' replies wistfully: 'Yes but...I don't like islands...so I can't go there'. So the colleague tries again by adding: 'How about Switzerland, that's a great place. The people are very friendly'. To which the 'Yes Buter' replies:

'Yes...but...at the time I'm planning on going it will be cold and snowy and I don't like the cold and snow'. So the colleague tries again by saying: 'How about Australia then...it will be summer there then and it's got so much variety to offer'. To which the 'Yes Buter' replies: 'Yes...but...it will be too hot for me in Australia...and anyway...I don't like the kind of variety they have in Australia. I prefer something more straight laced!'

And then a curious thing happens. The colleague says something like: 'Well I don't know what to suggest', at which point the person who has been playing something of a 'victim' role by Yes Buting, (implying they're unable to make a choice for themselves) then turns on the erstwhile 'rescuer' and says something like: 'Well you aren't much help are you!?'

My experience is that when the Yes But pattern is addressed with this kind of approach many clients have something of an 'aha! moment' and it dawns on them how self-defeating the pattern is. I then explain to them that they're now in a position of choice: 'The good thing for you is that now you're aware, which means you can choose to respond differently. Before you weren't and it just sort of used to happen, without you fully understanding what you were doing. Now you have the opportunity to really make some positive, life-affirming changes by choosing differently. My experience is that many people like you who used to do this actually catch themselves just before they're about to do it sometimes and then stop instead and respond more positively. Once you've done this a few times you'll likely find that the old unhelpful 'Yes But' response will fade away and you'll be making better choices by nature now.'

I've had clients have a laugh at themselves when a few minutes later they've been on 'automatic pilot' and have been about to respond 'Yes But' and caught themselves doing so. Saying something like: 'That was nearly a Yes But! What I mean to say is…' By telling the client that the Yes But Pattern (and Polarity Response patterns in general) are well known in the field of psychology, it 'classifies' it and 'names the game' which, because it has been brought out into the open, can no longer be 'played' as an unaddressed, self-defeating, pattern. By following up with examples that closely reflect what they're doing it brings to bear the 'weight of the field of psychology' onto their 'caught in the act' behaviour and generates tremendous leverage to help them change.

[Special note regarding Polarity Responses: Alternative points of view are valid and are what make us each the unique individuals that we are. Polarity responses are of a different order than individual points of view. They are habitual, destructive-to-communication patterns (and relationships!) that when left unaddressed reduce the possibilities of forward movement.]

Possibility To Probability

The Possibility to Probability pattern involves offering a concept to the client as being within the realm of possibility and then, due to the similarity in perceived meaning of the words, but similarly, due to their very real different meanings, transposing ('trance supposing') what's been offered as a possible suggestion to one that becomes instead a probable response based on the suggestion so offered:

The Structure:

1) 'So it's possible that you could make the changes; what do you think you will probably do first then?'

2) 'So you think it's possible to respond more effectively. How do you think you will probably begin?'

3) 'Okay. So life has many possibilities for you? [Client responds in the affirmative: 'Yes'] So which of all the many choices will you probably enjoy doing the most, soonest?'

4) 'Right. Well, you know it's possible for some people to learn to do this? [Yes] How do you think you will probably start learning it yourself?'

5) 'Okay. So you say you've got lots of possible opportunities in life. Name one that you will probably start to action then!'

Post Hypnotic Suggestion

Here's an example of how a Post Hypnotic Suggestion can be generated:

'And whenever you say the Power Words 'I feel great' to yourself, out loud or in your mind, with the intention of feeling great, your unconscious mind will respond to this suggestion by causing positive thoughts and emotions to grow stronger inside you. And the more you use your Power Words 'I feel great' the more powerful this response becomes.'

A Post Hypnotic Suggestion is a language pattern that's introduced in the process of therapy that's designed to generate desired responses in the client after the trance has concluded. Using the above example from the Power Word section of this book, you'll notice that a Post Hypnotic Suggestion has been included, which relates to the use of the words 'I feel great'. An association is generated by the therapist, so that, when the client, says the words 'I feel great', 'with the intention of feeling great' (this phrase is added so that the Post Hypnotic Suggestion is not inadvertently 'fired off' when the words 'I feel great' are used in contexts other than those being addressed) 'your unconscious will respond to this suggestion by...' (and then the desired post hypnotic response is attached to the triggering suggestion) 'causing positive thoughts and emotions to grow stronger inside you.' (Then the response is ratified and strengthened by adding...) 'And the more you use your Power Words 'I feel great' the more powerful this response becomes.' (This also encourages the client to use the post hypnotic resource.) A virtuous loop is then generated. Whereas, in the past, a vicious circle likely ensued. For instance, in business meetings, the client might have expected 'the worst', so they'd be on the lookout for 'whatever could go wrong'. As a result they'd magnify out of proportion any errors they might perceive they'd made... and then they'd feel bad. Because they felt bad, they wouldn't respond to the ongoing situation very well, so they'd then make more mistakes, and as a further result they'd feel worse... and so on. However, when a post hypnotic suggestion is included the client expects things to turn out much better. They use the trigger 'I feel great' and begin to do a Transderivational Search for thoughts and feelings <u>which support this</u>. The resultant inner sense of expectancy that they'll do well is reinforced by the belief generated by the ritual 'Affect Effect' of hypnotherapy. So, because they feel good, and because they're doing something different (from the way they have hitherto habitually responded) which helps them, their thoughts and feelings are working more positively and as a result a virtuous cycle ensues. This then becomes a self-fulfilling prophesy. The suggestion 'I feel great' helps them feel great. So because they feel great they do better, which makes them feel great.

Another version that I like which Robert Fargo uses is by suggesting a physical 'trigger' (known in NLP as an 'anchor') which acts as the catalyst to elicit the desired response. His version involves teaching the client to press a forefinger and thumb together to form the universal sign for 'okay'. It works very well. I'll often invite my client to have a conscious 'before trance' (although hypnosis is taking place) experience of doing so, as a primer, then soon afterwards, while in a 'formal' trance I'll invite them to do it again and at this point I reinforce the experience with a combination of both direct and indirect suggestion. Something like this:

'That's it. And now... aaaand in the future... whenever you use your 'Okay Trigger' it will trigger feelings of feeling okay. And as you do it here [hear] now and now notice how good you feel you understand that you are okay and your inner self can remember this feeling and let you feel okay whenever you press that forefinger and thumb together to generate the <u>universal sign for okay</u> and the more often you use your Okay [you're okay] the more powerful it becomes. So your Okay [you're okay] ... works really well... really well for you...and each time you want to feel okay you use your Okay [you're okay] and notice how better things get... and no one else will know what you're doing so it can be your special secret [many people like to have 'secret techniques' which help them] ... but they will notice the difference in how much more naturally positive you are [which causes the client to 'see themselves' from another's point of view. And as they do so, they begin anticipating seeing themselves doing well. Many people are concerned about how they will be perceived by others – which is often the cause of the problem in the first place, particularly with problems like social anxiety disorder. By subtly influencing the client's frame of reference to encompass that of 'other' and in so doing enabling them to perceive 'other' as perceiving them as 'okay' too it helps to increase the beneficial affect of the suggestion/trigger.].'

Power Words (Sutphen Style Suggestions)

<u>The Pattern</u>:

Power Words are direct suggestions. The 'New Age' Hypnotist Dick Sutphen in my opinion uses Direct Suggestion very well (you can find him on the internet). If you listen to the CDs and downloads that I recorded for Ultra Hypnosis Ltd you'll notice that in amongst the indirect hypnotherapy principles that I've employed I've also sometimes utilised Power Words/Direct Suggestion to reinforce the therapeutic work that I'm doing.

The Structure:

Here are some examples of Power Words and how they can be delivered in therapy.

1) 'You are confident!'

2) 'You feel better and better!'

3) 'Repeat this phrase in your mind after me now: 'I am confident!''

4) 'Say these words to yourself now: 'I am talented! I am talented!''

5) 'And whenever you say the Power Words 'I feel great' to yourself, out loud or in your mind, with the intention of feeling great, your unconscious mind will respond to this suggestion by causing positive thoughts and emotions to grow stronger inside you. And the more you use your Power Words 'I feel great' the more powerful this response becomes.

[See also: Post Hypnotic Suggestion]'

Predictions

The Pattern:

1)

Client:

'Things have always been hard. I'm not looking forward to the next few years. I know they'll be bad too.'

Hypnotherapist:

'I hear what you're saying. You know, the Oracle of Delphi lived hundreds of years ago and people still talk about her. You know why? Let me tell you – it's because she had a rare gift, so rare in fact that it stands out across the passage of time. The gift was the ability to predict the future, with accuracy, according to the legends. But she was, if the legends are true, one in a million. True prophesy is a rare gift. Most of us can't really predict the future. Are you telling me that you <u>are</u> gifted with real prophetic insight? Or are you just 'supposing'?'

2)

Client:

'It's all going to go wrong. I just know it.'

Hypnotherapist:

'That's a pretty strong statement. But really, how could you <u>ever truly</u> predict the future?'

3)

'I look forward with dread!'

Hypnotherapist:

'What does Dread have to say about that? Just kidding! Seriously though, how could you ever possibly really predict the future? Can anyone? However, what we can do, but it's not a good idea, is to cause 'self fulfilling prophesies' based on what we continuously tell ourselves the future is likely to be like. If we do that long enough and often enough we'll talk ourselves into living as if it was true and then go about making it true. But that's a whole different thing from it 'being written in stone' so to speak. Your statement implied that your future is predetermined. Whereas, in reality what you're really doing is determining your future by the beliefs about your future that you keep presenting to yourself. And that's good to know because it means you can change your beliefs and change the course of your future. Just think – how much better can your future start to become if you start to look at all of your potential? Don't answer that right now. Maybe just think about it. Let me tell you – I believe that you can change things radically for the better by changing the way you think to yourself. I've seen <u>others, like you</u>, do it, <u>like this</u>, and I just know you can too.'

The <u>Structure</u>:

Anthony Robbins famously stated: 'The past does not equal the future'. Sometimes clients can seem to live by the statement 'the past equals the future' and then go about predicting the worst and by doing so, they contribute, albeit, often, inadvertently, to making it happen. By challenging statements of this kind it can help clients to reconsider outmoded and unhelpful 'thought frames'. It casts doubt on the ideas which can then lead, potentially, into a needed reconsideration of them, which can then lead to change. A couple of the above examples (1 and 3) employed

Provocative Therapy style concepts. Much rapport would already have been built in order to be able to address the client in this way. The story about the Oracle of Delphi in effect says 'You're not that psychic. Maybe you're wrong about your predictions. What psychic credentials do you have to be so emphatic about that? Are you really one in a million on the PsyQ (Psychic Quotient) scale?'. And the one that starts with the 'joke' about Dread (in the sense of 'Dread' being a person) is designed to interrupt the client's negative pattern/state, by doing something out of the ordinary, with a warm and caring smile as what's said is spoken. Helpful interpretations of the behaviour patterns coupled with possible solutions are offered in the process of destabilising the unhelpful beliefs.

Pre Hypnotic Suggestion

Pre Hypnotic Suggestions are delivered linguistically before 'formal' hypnosis has taken place, to generate enhanced receptivity to Eyes-Closed Trance (and for what might occur in Eyes-Closed Trance).

The Pattern:

1) 'Now, trance is very powerful, and we're going to invite your unconscious mind to trigger a helpful feeling of calm reassurance whenever you press your thumb and forefinger together with the intention of feeling calm. Go ahead now and give it a practice run, just to get the feel of what it feels like to do it. Then when, you're in trance now, in a moment, your unconscious will add that 'extra something' which helps you to, feel good, like this.

That's it. Take a nice deep breath in and let yourself relax and as you breathe out press that forefinger and thumb together. Feel relaxed? [Which is also a suggestion to 'feel relaxed'].'

'Okay – now let's do some trancework and turn that nice calm reassurance up for you.'

2) 'You'll likely find that you'll start to notice your own physiology more after the trancework which will mean that you can choose the postures which help you feel more confident.'

3) 'After the trance I wonder if you'll notice feelings of determination or positivity first?'

4) 'During the hypnotherapy session you can experience many nice things, like allowing yourself to...take it easy...and enjoy being comfortable.'

5) 'In hypnosis your unconscious mind is listening and you might find that you begin to consciously become aware of a new solution to this situation which helps you feel more relaxed and in control, or you might notice that you start to develop a sense of awareness that...everything's going to be all right...'

The Structure:

Suggestions are offered before 'formal' Eyes-Closed Hypnosis takes place. However, they're offered in such a way as to help influence the trance that follows in desired therapeutic ways.

1) 'Now, trance is very powerful [suggestion designed to build response potential] and we're

going to invite your unconscious mind to trigger [setting an anchor linguistically] a helpful feeling of calm reassurance [describing the anchor's affect] whenever you press your thumb and forefinger together [how the anchor is generated] with the intention of feeling calm [in what context the anchor will be activated]. Go ahead now and give it a practice run [because it is only a 'practice run' that removes the pressure of 'performance anxiety' regarding the efficacy of whether or how the anchor will work for the client] just to get the feel [bringing a kinaesthetic awareness further into the picture] of what it feels like to, do it [Embedded Suggestion]. Then when, you're in trance now [suggestion that trance is taking place now] in a moment [in order for it to take place in a moment] your unconscious will add that 'extra something' [increasing the response potential] which helps you to, feel good [Embedded Suggestion] like this [Embedded Suggestion]. That's it. Take a nice deep breath in [introducing relaxed breathing to engender relaxation in order to link the relaxed feeling, implicitly, with the triggering of the anchor] and let yourself relax [Embedded Suggestion] and as you breathe out press that forefinger and thumb together [triggering of the process timed on the relaxing out-breath to generate the anchor]. Feel relaxed? [Which is also a suggestion to 'feel relaxed'].

Okay – now let's do some trancework and turn that nice calm reassurance up for you [which implies that they already have some in order for it to be 'turned up].'

2) 'You'll likely find that you'll start to notice your own physiology more [this implies that they have

already begun to notice their habitual physiological patterns] after the trancework which will mean that you can choose the postures which help you feel more confident [you will be feeling more confident after the trance because you will naturally be adopting physiological structures which generate feelings related to confidence].'

3) 'After the trance I wonder if you'll notice feelings of determination or positivity first [you will notice feelings – which will likely be in the range of positivity and determination]?'

4) 'During the hypnotherapy session you can experience many nice things [which is a suggestion designed to generate reassurance in the client about the nature of their ensuing trance experience – it will be nice] like allowing yourself to... take it [Embedded Suggestion] easy... and enjoy being comfortable [Embedded Suggestion].'

5) 'In hypnosis your unconscious mind is listening and you might find that you begin to consciously become aware of a new solution [you will become aware of a solution at some level which will likely also include conscious awareness] to this situation which helps you feel more relaxed [you will gain assistance to feel more relaxed] and in control, [and you will gain assistance to feel more in control] or you might notice that you start to develop a sense of awareness that... everything's going to be all right... [Embedded Suggestion].'

Pre Hypnotic suggestions can also be employed to begin setting in motion a nested loop sequence as a prelude to further loops that will be added during 'formal' trance, the results of which will manifest for the client after the therapy session has concluded. Here's an example: 'I once knew someone who was in pretty much the same situation as you it seems and what she started to do was think of <u>all the nice things</u> that have happened too...and that helped her a lot...now as you gently close your eyes... that's right... isn't it <u>nice</u> to know that it is possible to... [further loops are added and therapy takes place...at which point the client is guided back to full awareness...] ...that's right...welcome back... oh...by the way...I asked the client I told you about who began to think of the <u>nice things</u> that have happened to give me a call in about a week to let me know what <u>nice things</u> she had already begun to notice... would you be kind enough to do the same too? Here's my number. Thanks.'

Prescribing The Behaviour

I once worked with a client who was referred to me by another therapist whose presenting problem was that she said she was possessed by a demon. The other therapist had been faced with the spectacle of the woman walking into his treatment room, jumping onto his therapy coach, curling up into a foetal position and then laying on the couch shaking violently and being unresponsive to any kind of therapy. Eventually he managed to end the session by telling her that he'd phoned me and had arranged an appointment for her with me. Not knowing quite what to expect (but being forewarned about what had happened) I arrived at the clinic early and immediately began to change the layout of the room in order to eliminate the client's ability to take control of the situation, as she had during the previous session with the other therapist. I did so by putting my coat and a portable CD player/tape recorder onto the couch (which I plugged into a socket nearby) along with some other items. I then placed two wooden hardback, upright chairs at a 45% angle to each other. When the woman arrived, I found her sitting in the waiting room in what can best be described as a 'demure' posture with a summer floral dress on, looking like she wouldn't say boo to a goose. However, as she walked up the stairs and crossed the threshold of the treatment room a glazed, fixed, stare took hold in her eyes and a morose look appeared on her face. We both became seated on the hard chairs and I began to take some case notes along with a signed disclaimer from her in which was included a record of the fact that I'd suggested to her that she should probably visit her GP about her 'problem'. As I was doing so her demeanour continued to worsen until eventually she started to make guttural groaning noises (like you'd hear in a horror film). As I write now I remember then thinking to myself something like 'Oh shit!', and then I 'heard myself' spontaneously say to her (which in hindsight makes me wonder who was the most possessed person in the room out of the two of us! ☺): **'Was that an in breath or an out breath?'** in a very authoritative voice. She was stunned by the question and said in a shocked and annoyed tone. **'I don't know!'**. (Notice: in order to answer the question a major state change had taken place). So I replied: **'Well next time it happens** (I had begun to prescribe the behaviour. In effect I was telling her that there would likely be a next time and that, in effect, I was allowing it to happen. This meant that she was no longer in control of her power game) **let me know, because it could be important!'** Once more I said this in a very unfazed and authoritative manner. A few moments later she started again. So I said quickly, as soon as she began: **'In breath or out breath?'**. She replied in an even more irritated voice: **'I don't know!'**. This happened a few more times until she said - in a slightly exasperated and unsure manner: **'I think it was an in breath'**. To which I replied: **'Good!' If it changes let me know.'**.

And then she stopped playing that particular control drama and instead <u>switched</u> instead to another tactic. As we were talking, she suddenly started to slant her body to an odd angle (almost as if she were going to fall off of the chair) while fluttering her eyelids, as if some 'demon' were taking control of her again. So, this time, I spontaneously clapped my hands together loudly and shouted **'You're flaking out on me here!'**. Immediately she stopped. Only to try another tactic...

She told me that the demon had warned her not to keep her appointment with me. And then she began to tell me that sometimes the demon would possess her in such a way that she would start to jump around the room. So I said **'SHOW ME!'**. I stood up and said: **'Is it a little jump like this?'** And I took a small jump across the treatment room myself. **'Or a big jump like this'**: and I took an even bigger jump across the treatment room. She then got up and joined in (following my instructions to enact the behaviour – thereby turning the behaviour pattern from one of control, on her part, in which she had hitherto exercised power over others, due to their fear and uncertainty about how to respond to her and her 'demon', to one of compliance, in which I first enacted the behaviour and then <u>instructed</u> her to join me).

From this point our conversation proceeded in an almost 'normal' manner. She no longer tried any control games. The demon appeared to have disappeared.

At one point I even looked at her and said: **'I think we both know that someone's playing a game here. Don't we?'** As I said it, I smiled. And she said **'Yes!'**

It turned out that she was able to get a lot of attention from others by acting out similar behaviours to those detailed above around them. However, when I utilised surprise and the principle of Prescribing The Behaviour it resulted in her extinguishing her power game (also known as a 'control drama') and gaining an admission from her that it was all just a 'game'.

Towards the end of the session she paid me a 'compliment', of sorts, by telling me: **'You're crazier than I am!'**. Which, interestingly, I think meant that, in effect, she'd had to review and alter her perceptions about her own supposed 'craziness', in order to be able to make such a statement to me! She needed to look at herself in relation to our interaction from a <u>meta position</u> in order to conclude that actually she was less 'crazy' than the therapist. And it was as a result of me responding with this, seemingly unfazed, authoritative–in-the-face-of-'possession' behaviour and by prescribing her own control patterns to her that we rapidly reached a point at which she confirmed that it was just a game that she used (and probably half believed to be true) in order to get attention from those around her in the very 'humdrum' life she appeared to be living.

Some people are addicted to adrenalin. And her game kept giving her the 'fix' she needed.

For the reader's reference, as a precaution, having been forewarned of what I suspected could be an attention seeking pattern (of a massive order) at the outset of the therapy I told her that everything would be recorded – which it was, from start to finish, on the tape recorder that I'd placed on the couch. This was an indirect way of saying that I'd have a record of everything we both did and said - and I still have the tape.

Presuppositional Language (1)

Time

The Pattern:

1) 'You know – you know – that as you become aware that already something good is taking place within...'

2) 'And after you notice you are smiling again...'

3) 'I don't know whether you'll make that change right now as you continue to take action which manifests your chosen vocation into your life...'

4) 'Before today you might have wondered whether you could do it but now, and in your future as you

continue to see solutions presenting themselves to you, you just naturally do it now...'

5) 'Every time you dwell on that positive idea it reinforces itself for you...'

6) 'Each time you do this starting from tomorrow...'

7) 'Beginning today...that special something which is good for you...'

8) 'Even up until yesterday when you used to think XYZ ...that part of you which knew you could think ABC was just waiting to help you understand this now.'

9) 'Time and time again you'll notice while you're life is improving that...'

10) 'During the next opportunity that arises, between each boost of energy that you notice... before you do it really well... you'll know that every time you do it like this... you feel good...and afterwards...you feel good too because the positive experience joins your inner records of positive experiences so that they grow stronger... and before you know it... but you will know it before too long...you sense a continuing sense of positivity growing stronger every day... so as you have learned from the past you can look forward to the future too... today... knowing that the temporary setbacks that have occurred have been replaced by an enduring source of inner-peace and self-esteem...'

<u>The Structure</u>:

1) 'You know – you know – that as you <u>become</u> [time element] aware that <u>already</u> [time element] **something good is taking place within** [presupposition that something good is taking place]...'

2) 'And <u>after</u> [time element] you notice **you are smiling again** [presupposition that the client will be smiling again]...'

3) 'I don't know whether you'll **make that change** [presupposition of change] <u>right</u> <u>now</u> [time element] as you <u>continue</u> [time element] to **take action** [presupposition that the client will be taking action] which **manifests your chosen vocation** [presupposition that the action will manifest their chosen vocation] into your life...'

4) '<u>Before</u> [time element] <u>today</u> [time element] you might have wondered whether you could do it [presupposition relating to potential capability] but <u>now</u> [time element] and in your <u>future</u> [time element] as you <u>continue</u> [time element] to **see solutions presenting themselves to you**, [presupposition that solutions will present themselves] you just naturally do it <u>now</u> [time element and Embedded Suggestion that the client will do it naturally]...'

5) '<u>Every</u> <u>time</u> [time element] you **dwell on that positive idea** [presupposition that the client will dwell on that positive idea] it reinforces itself for you...'

6) 'Each time [time element] you do this [presupposition that the client will do this] starting from tomorrow [time element]...'

7) 'Beginning today [time element]... that special something [presupposition that there is a special something] which is good for you...'

8) 'Even up until yesterday [time element] when you used to [time element] think XYZ [presupposes that the client used to think XYZ – in the past]...**that part of you which knew you could think ABC** [presupposes that there is a part which can think ABC] was just waiting [time element] to help **you understand this now** [Embedded Suggestion and time element].'

9) 'Time and time [time element] again you'll notice while [time element] you're life is improving [presupposition that the client's life will be improving] that...'

10) 'During [time element] the next [time element] **opportunity that arises** [presupposition that an opportunity will arise], between [time element] each boost of energy that you notice [presupposition that there will be boosts of energy which the client will notice] ...before [time element] you do it really well [presupposition that the client will do it really well]...you'll know that every time [time element] **you do it like this** [presupposition that the client will do it like this] ...you feel good...and afterwards [time element]...you feel good too [Embedded Suggestion] **because the positive experience** [presupposition that it is a positive experience] joins **your inner records** [presupposition that the client has inner records] of

positive experiences [presupposition that the inner records contain positive experiences] so that they grow stronger...and <u>before</u> [time element] **you know it** [presupposition that the client will know it] ...but you will know [Embedded Suggestion] it <u>before</u> [time element] <u>too</u> <u>long</u> [time element]...you sense a [Embedded Suggestion] <u>continuing</u> [time element] sense of positivity growing [Embedded Suggestion] stronger <u>every</u> <u>day</u> [time element]...so as **you have learned** [presupposition that learning has taken place] from the <u>past</u> [time element] you can look <u>forward</u> [time element and Embedded Suggestion] to the <u>future</u> [time element] **too** ['too' presupposes learning from the past in conjunction with looking forward to the future]...<u>today</u>...[time element] knowing that the <u>temporary</u> [time element] **setbacks** [presupposes that there were setbacks – but that they were only temporary] that <u>have</u> <u>occurred</u> <u>have</u> <u>been</u> [time element] replaced by an <u>enduring</u> [time element] **source of inner-peace and self-esteem** [presupposition that there is a source of inner-peace and self-esteem with which to replace the previous experience].'

[See also Change of Time Verbs and Adverbs]

Presuppositional Language (2)

<u>Space</u>

<u>The Pattern</u>:

1) 'When you go to Royan and notice the different fashion...'

2) 'While you're moving over there...'

3) 'Each time you sit down and take it easy...'

4) 'So as you step forward and...'

5) 'Leaving what you don't want behind and moving into what you like...'

6) 'Stepping into those good feelings...'

7) 'When moving forward in that positive way that you know how...'

8) 'Each time you move from here to here ...'

9) 'And as you let your thoughts rise above the situation...'

10) 'Moving that energy around your body and sensing a certain flow beginning to occur... more... travelling to the place inside that it needs to go to inspire you to step back from how you used to think about it all and decide to change direction and begin to move forwards to a better place. And I wonder... I'm curious... as you move into these new resources ...what will you sense is happening that tells you there is more good around than you used to realise?...but now that you make it a habit to move forward into the good... taking a stand... stepping up to another better level of life and enjoying looking down from this higher place and understanding how small those problems really always were and how big the opportunities really are... and here... it feels good... but then you already really knew it would...'

<u>The Structure</u>:

1) 'When you go to Royan [change of place element] and **notice the different fashion** [presupposition of different fashion that the client will notice]...'

2) 'While you're moving [change of place element] over there...'

3) 'Each time you sit down [change of place element] and take it easy...'

4) 'So as you step forward [change of place element] and...'

5) 'Leaving what you don't want behind [change of place element] and moving into [change of place element] what you like...'

6) 'Stepping into [change of place element] those good feelings...'

7) 'When moving forward [change of place element] in that positive way that you know how...'

8) 'Each time you move [change of place element] from here to here [change of place element] ...'
9) 'And as you let your thoughts rise above [change of place element] the situation...'

10) 'Moving [change of place element] that energy around [change of place element] your body and sensing a certain flow beginning to occur... more... travelling [change of place element] to the place inside [change of place element] that it needs to go to inspire you to step back [change of place

element] from how you used to think about it all and decide to change direction [change of place element] and begin to move forwards [change of place element] to a better place [change of place element]. And I wonder... I'm curious... as you move into [change of place element] these new resources... what will you sense is happening that tells you there is more good around than you used to realise?...but now that you make it a habit to move forward [change of place element] into [change of place element] the good... taking a stand [change of place element]... stepping up to [change of place element] another better level [change of place element] of life and enjoying looking down [change of place element] from this higher place and understanding how small those problems really always were and how big the opportunities really are... and here [change of place element]... it feels good...but then you already really knew it would...'

Presuppositional Language (3)

<u>Temporariness and Permanence</u>

<u>The Pattern</u>:

1) 'Nothing lasts for ever...that's true enough...even great empires rise and fall...so think how impermanent an unwanted feeling is...and let that disappear now too...'

2) 'Sensing a certain lasting happiness that remains with you...in a special way...'

3) 'That momentary doubt is replaced by a fixed commitment to follow through...'

4) 'Now and in the long-term life is getting better and better...'

5) 'I know you're clever enough to realise that any of the so-called short-term 'benefits' of smoking that you just mentioned bear no relation to the frighteningly possible, long term, shall we say, perhaps, even permanent, consequences...'

6) 'So, you say you've gotten a brief 'chilled out' kind of feeling when you were drinking...but in the long term you know you could damage your brain, your heart, your liver and your kidneys. There's no comparison really when you look at it like this, is there? So, tell me, what else don't you like about drinking?'

7) 'Restructuring those unwanted up-until-now long-lasting emotional responses and making them fleeting, temporary, transient, unstable...until they just totally disappear and replacing them with uplifting, long lasting, enduring, permanent, stable thoughts, feelings and emotions... and it seems to me that... permanently speaking... now... things are getting better...'

8) 'Briefly, for a moment, consider what you'd rather be doing... tell you what!... take a few moments to think about it for a while longer... why not even let those good thoughts begin to take on a degree of permanence... becoming...for you... an enduring sense of inspiring reality that remains always with you... continuing to make things better and better... and that's nice to know...'

9) 'I remember a client who decided that she was no longer prepared to let a temporary emotion like

fear permanently hold her back... so she invited her inner self to make the time-span of the old fear emotion shrink... so that it became shorter and shorter...more and more fleeting... until it's temporary nature became so temporary that it just disappeared all together to be replaced by this beautiful sense of expectancy that something good, something which totally, permanently in an amazingly enduring way lets confidence start to always be there when it's needed... I wouldn't be surprised at all if you quietly ask your unconscious mind to do something like this for you now you also notice a change for the better too...'

10) 'Taking a hitherto temporary idea and making it a permanent part of your reality...'

The Structure:

1) 'Nothing lasts for ever [temporariness element] ...that's true enough... even great empires rise and fall...so think how impermanent [temporariness element] an unwanted feeling is... and let that disappear [temporariness element] now too...'

2) 'Sensing certain lasting [permanence element] happiness that remains [permanence element] with you...in a special way...'

3) 'That momentary [temporariness element] doubt is replaced by a fixed [permanence element] commitment to follow through...'

4) 'Now and in the long-term [permanence element] life is getting better and better...'

5) 'I know you're clever enough to realise that any of the so-called short-term [temporariness element] 'benefits' of smoking that you just mentioned bear no relation to the frighteningly possible, long term [permanence element], shall we say, perhaps, even permanent [permanence element], consequences…'

6) 'So, you say you have gotten a brief [temporariness element] 'chilled out' kind of feeling when you were drinking… but in the long term [permanence element] you know you could damage your brain, your heart, your liver and your kidneys. There's no comparison really when you look at it like this, is there. So, tell me, what else don't you like about drinking?'

7) 'Restructuring those unwanted up-until-now long-lasting [temporariness element] emotional responses and making them fleeting [temporariness element] temporary [temporariness element] transient [temporariness element] unstable [temporariness element]… until they just totally disappear [temporariness element] and replacing them with uplifting, long lasting [permanence element], enduring [permanence element], permanent [permanence element], stable [permanence element] thoughts, feelings and emotions…and it seems to me that… permanently speaking [permanence element]… now…things are getting better…'

8) 'Briefly, [temporariness element] for a moment, consider what you'd rather be doing… tell you what!… take a few moments [temporariness element] to think about it for a while longer [permanence element]… why not even let those

good thoughts begin to take on a degree of permanence [permanence element]... becoming... for you... an enduring [permanence element] sense of inspiring reality that remains [permanence element] always with you... continuing [permanence element] to make things better and better... and that's nice to know...'

9) 'I remember a client who decided that she was no longer [temporariness element] prepared to let a temporary emotion like fear permanently hold her back [temporariness element]... so she invited her inner self to make the time-span of the old [temporariness element] fear emotion shrink... so that it became shorter and shorter... more and more fleeting [temporariness element]... until it's temporary [temporariness element] nature became so temporary [temporariness element] that it just disappeared [temporariness element] all together to be replaced by this beautiful sense of expectancy that something good, something which totally, permanently [permanence element] in an amazingly enduring [permanence element] way let confidence start to always [permanence element] be there when it's needed... I wouldn't be surprised at all if you quietly ask your unconscious mind to do something like this for you now, you also notice a change for the better too....

10) 'Taking a hitherto temporary [temporariness element] idea and making it a permanent [permanence element] part of your reality...'

Presuppositional Language (4)

<u>Change</u>

<u>The Pattern</u>:

1) 'The thing about the transforming nature of experiencing hypnotherapy is...'

2) 'And when something starts to feel different...'

3) 'And as you sense that your inner you is converting all of that energy into something more useful...'

4) 'The alteration of perspective...'

5) 'More and more the way you adapt...'

6) 'It's like you can translate the desire to think in more uplifting ways into uplifting thoughts...'

7) 'And the restructuring of your perceptions lets you notice a different way of looking at the world – one which helps you two feel free. Whenever you say One to Free with the intention of feeling free like this. And the transformational effect is quite noticeable in a certain kind of way.'

8) 'As you reform your habitual responses you notice that this reformation results in a new you – the real you.'

9) 'How will you know that this realignment of your deep core values has shifted?"

10) 'It's all about realigning yourself with your true ideals – the things that are really important to you.'

11) 'You don't not have to totally experience the subtle variation in your mood right away – although you can – I think it's nice to curiously wonder expectantly how it is beginning to shift right now and how as it changes you become more aware of a transformational awareness that something is beginning to radically alter within, without you really having to do much to translate these new, better, thoughts, feelings and emotions so that you continue to be and become the fullest positive expression of yourself in every good and wonderful way and while you are experiencing this and while you gently yet powerfully improve what needs changing things naturally get better and you sense the signs of your recovery let you enhance your increasing sense of expanded positivity...and this helps you to help yourself advance as you further enrich your life.'

The Structure:

1) 'The thing about the <u>transforming</u> nature of experiencing hypnotherapy is...'

2) 'And when something <u>starts</u> to feel different...'

3) 'And as you sense that your inner you is <u>converting</u> all of that energy into something more useful...'

4) 'The <u>alteration</u> of perspective...'

5) 'More and more the way you <u>adapt</u>...'

6) 'It's like you can <u>translate</u> the desire to think in more uplifting ways into uplifting thoughts...'

7) 'And the <u>restructuring</u> of your perceptions lets you notice a <u>different</u> way of looking at the world – <u>one</u> which helps you <u>two</u> feel <u>free</u>. Whenever you say One to Free with the intention of feeling free like this. And the <u>transformational</u> effect is quite noticeable in a certain kind of way.' [My thanks to Nick Othen for the 'One to Free' language pattern.]

8) 'As you <u>reform</u> your habitual responses you notice that this <u>reformation</u> results in a new you – the real you.'

9) 'How will you know that this <u>realignment</u> of your deep core values has shifted?'

10) 'It's all about <u>realigning</u> yourself with your true ideals – the things that are really important to you.'

11) 'You don't not have to totally experience the subtle <u>variation</u> in your mood right away – although you can – I think it's nice to curiously wonder expectantly how it is beginning to <u>shift</u> right now and how as it <u>changes</u> you become more aware of a <u>transformational</u> awareness that something is beginning to radically <u>alter</u> within, without you really having to do much to <u>translate</u> these new, better, thoughts, feelings and emotions so that you continue to be and <u>become</u> the fullest positive expression of yourself in every good and wonderful way and while you are <u>experiencing</u> this and while you gently yet powerfully <u>improve</u> what needs <u>changing</u> things naturally <u>get</u> <u>better</u> and you sense the signs of your <u>recovery</u> let you <u>enhance</u> your <u>increasing</u> sense of <u>expanded</u> positivity...and this

helps you to help yourself <u>advance</u> as you <u>further</u> <u>enrich</u> your life.'

Prior Cause

<u>The Pattern</u>:

Client statement:

'I'm feeling worried so I won't be able to do it.'

A)

'Feeling worried just means you haven't discovered how to feel calm yet.'

B)

'You only think you won't be able to do it because no one has shown you yet.'

A/B)

'Feeling like that is telling you that you need to change your approach so that doing it is natural.'

<u>The Structure</u>:

The client's statement is a 'Cause And Effect' statement. In effect it reads: 'I'm feeling worried [Cause And Effect] so I won't be able to do it. The Prior Cause pattern enables the therapist to deal with the issue by referring to 'Prior Cause'. The Prior Cause can be addressed to the first part of the client's statement (as in example 'a'), the second part of the client's statement (as in example 'b') or to both elements (as in example 'a/b'). It's designed to help the client to disengage the 'Cause And Effect' thinking that they're involved in, in order to help them reframe the situation to one of a better perspective.

A)

'<u>Feeling</u> <u>worried</u> just means you haven't **discovered how to feel calm yet**.'

B)

'You only think you won't be able to <u>do</u> <u>it</u> **because no one has shown you yet**.'

A/B)

'<u>Feeling</u> like that **is telling you that you need to change your approach** so that <u>doing</u> <u>it</u> **is natural**.'

Pronouns

<u>The Pattern</u>:

1) 'You know it can help you.'

2) 'She's going to be a real asset.'

3) 'They don't need to know what you're thinking...just show them what you can do.'

4) 'And when you smile at her...'

5) 'Of course you can tell him...'

6) 'You can put that in the past.'

7) 'This is no longer necessary. Maybe even never was?'

8) 'You don't need those any more. Maybe even never did?'

9) 'That can fade away and this can replace it.'

10) 'Who knows how much better you will feel around him and around her? You will respond resourcefully when he is around. And around her too.'

The Structure:

We use pronouns regularly in our day-to-day conversations. Being aware of them gives us the opportunity to choose to use them strategically. If for instance, the mention of someone's name (or the name of a condition) is likely to be detrimental at some stage in the process of therapy, the hypnotherapist can instead use pronouns to refer to them (there's another example of a pronoun), or it (and another pronoun) without needing to specifically use a name. Similarly, it (there's another example of a pronoun) can be used to avoid overuse of a particular source of resource being addressed. And they (another example) can be employed to suggest resources which are not specifically named in order that the client can unconsciously generate them (and another) without excessive guidance on the part of the therapist as to how they (and another) will manifest..

1) 'You know <u>it</u> can help you. (There is an 'it' that exists. In this case 'it' is the unconscious mind).'

2) '<u>She</u>'s going to be a real asset. (There is a female in existence).'

3) '<u>They</u> don't need to know what you're thinking...just show <u>them</u> what you can do. (There is a group in existence).'

4) 'And when you smile at <u>her</u>...(There is a female in existence).'

5) 'Of course you can tell <u>him</u>...(There is a male in existence).'

6) 'You can put <u>that</u> in the past. (Something exists).'

7) '<u>This</u> is no longer necessary. Maybe even never was? (Something exists).'

8) 'You don't need <u>those</u> any more. Maybe even never did? (Some things exist).'

9) '<u>That</u> can fade away and <u>this</u> can replace it. (Some things exist)."

10) 'Who knows how much better you will feel around <u>him</u> and around <u>her</u>? (There is a female and a male in existence) You will respond resourcefully when <u>he</u> is around. (There is a male in existence) And around <u>her</u> too. (There is a female in existence)'

Proper Names

The Pattern:

Proper Names is, as the term suggests simply the use of a person's (or other subject's) name. You can use them to be very specific.

1) 'Did you see <u>Gill</u> <u>Webb</u> when she was last on TV? She's certainly highly skilled. She likes to help people learn how to use hypnosis to improve their lives. The <u>Sunday</u> <u>Times</u> did an article with her too you know!'

2) 'Listening to <u>Andrea</u> <u>Lindsay</u> on <u>2CR</u> <u>Radio</u> successfully demonstrating hypnotherapy is exciting isn't it? They've featured her a lot recently.'

3) 'Can you consciously unpack everything <u>Kerin</u> says? All of the time? Can you be sure that you can? Or can't you be sure that you can't? Or can't you be sure that you can?... that's right... and when I say the word 'awake' you'll remember reading these words and learning more and return to full conscious awareness... ready to enrol on the next <u>Eos Seminars</u> <u>Ltd</u> training course in professional hypnotherapy. Awake!' (☺ Just kidding!)

4) '<u>Peter</u> and <u>Pam</u> are cool dudes. If you go to <u>Royan</u> you might even see them there. <u>France</u> is such a great place.'

5) '<u>Rose</u> was with <u>Max</u> the other day in <u>Winchester</u>. They'd just been to see <u>Richard</u> and <u>Gladys</u> <u>Williams</u> in <u>Swindon</u>. <u>Mabel Chiswick</u>, <u>Queenie</u> and <u>Ernie</u> <u>Webb</u> dropped by too after they'd been to <u>Southampton</u>.'

6) 'Liza and Steve really epitomise the 'Jet Set'. Where will their next holiday be? Will it be America, South Africa, Australia or Thailand? Who knows?'

7) 'Alice and Fleur are going to do really well in life. You can just tell. I wonder if they will use NLP in some capacity?'

8) 'Ele and Melissa are very clever – opportunity is coming their way. Bournemouth is full of opportunity.'

9) 'Rob likes going in and out of trance. It's now a natural part of his life. He knows more about Indirect Hypnosis than he knows he knows!'

Pseudo Cleft Sentence

The Pattern:

1) 'What you're learning about indirect hypnosis is going to be very helpful.'

2) 'What you can do to change is begin by taking it easy.'

3) 'What will help you most is slowing down for a moment.'

4) 'What you can do to improve things is to ask your inner self.'

5) 'What happens as you change is that you start to feel better.'

<u>The Structure</u>:

The Pseudo Cleft Sentence method is used for offering subtle suggestions through the form of the special word structure being employed, which causes the recipient to consciously 'lock onto' the latter part of the phrase while the opening part of the suggestion is absorbed at a deeper level. The pattern is characterised by a 'What...is' framework.

1) '**What** <u>you're</u> <u>learning</u> <u>about</u> <u>indirect</u> <u>hypnosis</u> [absorbed by unconscious mind] **is** going to be very helpful [conscious level element of the pattern].'

2) '**What** <u>you</u> <u>can</u> <u>do</u> <u>to</u> <u>change</u> [absorbed by unconscious mind] **is** begin by taking it easy [conscious level element of the pattern].'

3) '**What** <u>will</u> <u>help</u> <u>you</u> <u>most</u> [absorbed by unconscious mind] **is** slowing down for a moment [conscious level element of the pattern].'

4) '**What** <u>you</u> <u>can</u> <u>do</u> <u>to</u> <u>improve</u> <u>things</u> [absorbed by unconscious mind] **is** to ask your inner self [conscious level element of the pattern].'

5) '**What** happens <u>as</u> <u>you</u> <u>change</u> [absorbed by unconscious mind] **is** that you start to feel better [conscious level element of the pattern].'

Punctuation Ambiguity

<u>The Pattern</u>:

1) 'The wonderful thing about going into trance is good for you.'

2) 'Feeling happier each day by day you get better.'

3) 'And this suggestion is absorbed powerfully by your unconscious mind knows what to do to help you.'

4) 'Are you ready to feel good feelings are coming your way?'

5) 'And you can listen to my voice influences you inside which makes you feel good ideas are coming to you know what to do now as things get better respond sooner because it means things get better quicker and quicker good things become a part of your life is improving right now you understand this deep inside that's it go deep inside now.'

The Structure:

This is one of my favourite hypnotic / techniques are useful for helping clients to change. Two well-formed statements are combined in such a way that they form a statement which is not grammatically correct (also known as 'ill formed') but which is very 'well-formed' so to speak, for use in a therapeutic context, and which results in the facility to offer a number of suggestions which become increasingly hard to decipher at a conscious level, but which are readily absorbed at an unconscious level. I incorporate this method often and find that it helps to generate some very deep trance responses. The client, often, in effect, 'switches off' at a conscious level (because what's being said is so hard to unpack, consciously) and this allows the client's unconscious mind to work without any critical, conscious, interference.

1) 'The wonderful thing about going into trance / is good for you.'

2) 'Feeling happier each day / by day you get better.'

3) 'And this suggestion is absorbed powerfully by your unconscious mind / knows what to do to help you.'

4) 'Are you ready to feel good / feelings are coming your way.'

5) 'And you can listen to my voice / influences you inside which makes you feel good / ideas are coming to you / know what to do now as things get better / respond sooner because it means things get better / quicker and quicker good things become a part of your life / is improving right now you understand this / deep inside / that's it go deep inside now.'

Q

Questions (Closed)

Briefly, because this subject has been covered extensively many times by other writers, 'closed questions' are designed (when knowingly used) to facilitate short replies. Questions like:

Will you?
Can you?
Did you?
Have you?
Are you?

...are more likely to receive 'yes' or 'no' answers. They're called 'closed' because they have the effect of drawing limited responses which can sometimes 'close' or end a communication cycle.

Questions Facilitating A Therapeutic Response

The Pattern:

1) 'I wonder when you will first become aware that you are feeling different.'

2) 'How do you think you will begin to sense that something good is happening?'
3) 'What do you think will be most nice for you after you are experiencing more confidence?'

4) 'How good are things going to be after you've solved this?'

5) 'Which of the many new options which your inner self is generating for you here [hear] now do you think you will become aware of first?'

<u>The Structure</u>:

A question is asked which has implicit within it a presupposition that implies that in order to be able to answer what is posed the client will be doing so from a perspective that acknowledges that a therapeutic response will be experienced by the client (even if the client's 'answer' is just to wonder how the presupposed situation will occur, which is itself a form of having accepted the suggestion that it likely will).

1) 'I wonder <u>when</u> you will first become aware that <u>you are feeling different</u>.'

2) '<u>How</u> do you think you will begin to sense that <u>something good is happening</u>?'

3) '<u>What</u> do you think will be <u>most nice for you</u> after you are experiencing more confidence?'

4) '<u>How good are things going to be</u> after you've solved this?'

5) '<u>Which</u> of the many <u>new options</u> which your inner self is generating for you here [hear] now do you think you will become aware of first?'

Questions Facilitating New Response Potentials

The Pattern:

A)

Induction Questions:

1) 'Have you noticed how easy it is for you to go into trance?'

2) 'Are you aware of your changing awareness?'

3) 'What level of trance are you going to choose to experience do you think?'

4) 'Can you listen to the sound of the clock as you go inside now?'

5) 'Are you listening more to me consciously or more to me unconsciously as your perceptions continue to shift and your experience changes again?'

The Structure:

You'll notice that the above questions are posed in such a way that for the receiver to even just consider answering them it will, in all likelihood, generate more trance.

B)

Questions To Direct Associations:

1) 'When you consider this relaxed feeling in place of that old unwanted tension you said you used to have – how much better is it to feel relaxed like this?'

2) 'When you consider the difference between being out of trance and being in trance now what do you remember, consciously, about your trance experience.'

The Structure:

This category of Questions That Facilitate New Response Potentials is designed to direct the receiver's attention to a desired outcome.

1) 'When you consider this relaxed feeling [focus of attention] in place of [as a replacement of] that old [in the past] unwanted [relinquish 'ownership' of it] tension [naming issue] you said you used to have [which is now in the past] – how much better [comparison] is it to feel relaxed [desired response] like this [as a present phenomenon]?'

2) 'When you consider the difference [invites a comparison] between being out of trance [one state of being] and being in trance [desired focus] now [a present experience] what do you remember, consciously, about your trance experience [refocus on the experience of trance].'

Questions (Hypnotic)

'How did you know / How do you do that?'

Hypnotic Questions are designed to elicit further hypnotic reasoning and hypnotic affect. By rhetorically asking clients questions like 'How did you know that?', and… 'How did you do that?' it causes them to 'go inside' to search for an answer to the question.

For instance:

1) 'And there's a part of <u>you</u> which knows what the next thought is going to be before <u>you</u> know that you're going to think it. How do <u>you</u> do that?'

2) 'Think about this for a moment. Your <u>inner self</u> knows how to tie your shoelaces for <u>you</u> – but you'd have to consciously think about it first in order to be able to explain how <u>you</u> do it. But <u>another</u> part of <u>you</u> can do it without thinking. How do <u>you</u> know how to do that – without having to consciously think about how <u>you</u> do it? And <u>you</u> can wonder how much more that part of <u>you</u> knows which can help <u>you</u> which <u>you</u> don't yet know that <u>you</u> know.'

3) 'And the rhythm of your breathing has altered quite nicely now. But <u>you</u> didn't have to think about it in order for it to happen. <u>You</u> probably didn't even notice when it started. How do you do that?'

4) 'That's right…how did you know…that you could go into trance just as easily as this? Maybe ^{you} didn't while _{you} knew _{you} did.'

(That's right…how did you know…that you could go into trance just as easily as this? Maybe ^{you} [voice lifts to address the conscious mind] didn't while _{you}

[voice deepens to address the unconscious mind] knew you [voice deepens again to address the unconscious mind] did.)

The therapist can also ask questions and utilise the client's answer:

'Hypnotherapist: How do you do that?'

Client: 'I don't know.'

Hypnotherapist: 'That's right – You don't know!'

Questions (Open)

Just as the subject of Closed Questions (covered above) has been addressed extensively in other works by other writers so to has the topic of Open Questions. Therefore this example will take the form of a brief reference. Open Questions are, as the title suggests, designed (when used intentionally) to elicit detailed answers. Words like:

How
What
Why
When
with Whom

Are all more likely to receive a response with some depth to it:

'**How** can you begin to change things?'

'**What** option is best in the present moment?'

'**Why** do you prefer this option over this option?'

'**When** can you start to do this?'

'**With whom** do you think this will be most appreciated?'

Quotes

The Quotes method offers a useful way to relay information to a client, in an indirect manner. Milton often used to say things like: '**Well my friend John said that he was dealing with a situation like this the other day and he found that the more he relaxed the more easy it became...',** as a means of suggesting something important to his client(s), in this case the possibility of employing relaxation - without it seeming to be too obvious, direct or 'demanding' a suggestion. By 'quoting' someone else's experience it helps to convey a potential solution – but without the client feeling under duress to respond in the same way as did the subject of the story – as they might if they were told for example 'what you should do is...'. The client can instead freely receive the message (example) that's embedded within the story being told and then apply an appropriate response, as befits their own situation. Sometimes if a person is told directly that they 'should' respond in a certain way to a given situation they will reject the suggestion feeling that by so doing they are asserting their independence (or, instead, in some cases unknowingly exhibiting a Polarity Response). Naturally it would be considered inappropriate for a hypnotherapist to seek to compel a client to respond in any particular manner. Offering examples in this form however allows for the hypnotherapist to sidestep any possible resistance while respecting the client's ability to choose. It's often been said that many of Milton's clients did not consciously perceive the embedded messages that he presented to them and as a result they felt that he'd simply chatted with them about things that appeared unrelated to their presenting problems, so deeply embedded were the solutions he conveyed. Nevertheless, oftentimes the suggestions took root and began to manifest in beneficial ways in the clients' thoughts and behaviour patterns. Anthony Robbins, in my opinion, uses this principle often in the form of the little anecdotal stories he tells about his clients as he's conveying pertinent messages to his large audiences.

The hypnotherapist can embed suggestions by using quotes in the following manner too:

'My friend John was dealing with a situation like this and [2nd Position:]....he said 'How should I feel?'....and [1$^{st\ position}$] I said '<u>You can feel relaxed</u>'.'

This turns the quote into a medium for offering quite a direct suggestion to the client without it seeming to be such:

'I said '<u>You can feel relaxed</u>.'

R

Rapid Suggestions

<u>The Pattern</u>:

'Those amazingly, powerful, life-changing, resources that you will find yourself experiencing for all the best, most helpful, most life-affirming, reasons...'

<u>The Structure</u>:

A number of helpful suggestions are offered rapidly, often in a sequence, which may appear to be purely descriptive (but which are equally suggestive of desired outcomes) to create an environment for desired change.

'Those <u>amazingly</u>, <u>powerful</u>, <u>life-changing</u>, <u>resources</u> that you will find yourself experiencing for all the <u>best</u>, <u>most helpful</u>, <u>most life-affirming</u>, reasons...'

<u>Another example</u>:

'Maybe you will <u>change now</u>, <u>change easily</u>, <u>change quickly</u>, <u>change directly</u>...or maybe you will gently <u>change for the better</u>, <u>change how you feel</u>, <u>become a new person</u>, <u>become the real you</u>...I wonder?'

Reality Strategy (Sleight Of Mouth)

Sleight of Mouth principles were first delineated by Robert Dilts as he himself modelled Richard Bandler's language patterns. Additional contributions have been made by Steve and Connirae Andreas. A number of Sleight of Mouth patterns now exist, which are covered in this book. Sleight of Mouth patterns are utilised to unravel and in the process depotentiate adverse Complex Equivalence and/or Cause and Effect statements made by the client. [See: Analogy, Another Outcome, Apply To Self, Challenge, Change Of Reference Frame Size, Chunk Size, Consequences, Counter Example, Hierarchy Of Criteria, Intention, Meta Frame, Model Of The World, Reality Strategy, Redefine, Switch Referential Index.] In this example the principle of Reality Strategy is employed.

The Context:

Client statement: 'Being stupid makes me feel worthless.'

The Pattern:

A)

'How do you know you're stupid? [opens up the first part of the statement for reappraisal]'

B)

'How do you know that you feel worthless? [opens up the second part of the statement for reappraisal]'

C)

'How do you know that you think you're stupid and that that makes you feel worthless? [opens up both elements of the statement for reappraisal].'

Rear Loaded Suggestions:

<u>The Pattern</u>:

1) 'Wouldn't it be better to change sooner... think about it?'

2) 'There are other alternatives you know... think about that!'

3) 'You're cleverer than that... consider that for a moment!'

4) 'It's going to improve... expect it.'

5) 'Other people change and so can you... get ready.'

<u>The Structure</u>:

In essence, a suggestion is presented and then intensified by 'rear loading' it with a statement designed to enhance the prior suggestion.

1) 'Wouldn't it be better to <u>change</u> sooner... <u>think about it</u>!'

2) 'There are <u>other alternatives</u> you know... <u>think about that</u>!'

3) 'You're <u>cleverer</u> than that... <u>consider that for a moment</u>!'

4) 'It's going to <u>improve</u>... <u>expect it</u>!'

5) 'Other people <u>change</u> and so can you... <u>get ready</u>!'

Recapping Questions

<u>The Pattern</u>:

1) 'So you want to do this because... it will help improve the quality of your life?'

2) 'So you chose hypnotherapy because your friend got a good result with it?'

3) 'The reason you've decided to do this is?'

4) 'So, let's recap, you want to become a non-smoker because?'

5) 'Right! So, what I understand you're saying is...?'

<u>The Structure</u>:

The examples provided above show that Recapping Questions can be used to <u>review</u> what has already been covered, while at the same time allowing for any <u>clarification</u> to occur, which may be necessary. If no clarification is necessary then the Recapping Question can serve to further <u>confirm</u> the nature of what the client has said up to the point at which the Recapping Question is asked. In a sense, then, the question acts in much the same manner as a sales person's 'closing' technique. This is to say that, what has been previously covered in the process of therapy has been 'ratified' by the client as being correct and therefore, does not need to be clarified to any further degree. This means that the process of therapy can proceed in a prioritised solution-focussed manner, in order to clarify and ratify each element of the process. This procedure produces a firm foundation, ensuring that both the client and therapist are in accord with each other and working in a unified way towards a desired outcome.

Redefine (Sleight Of Mouth)

Sleight of Mouth principles were first delineated by Robert Dilts as he himself modelled Richard Bandler's language patterns. Additional contributions have been made by Steve and Connirae Andreas. A number of Sleight of Mouth patterns now exist, which are covered in this book. Sleight of Mouth patterns are utilised to unravel and in the process depotentiate adverse Complex Equivalence and/or Cause and Effect statements made by the client. [See: Analogy, Another Outcome, Apply To Self, Challenge, Change Of Reference Frame Size, Chunk Size, Consequences, Counter Example, Hierarchy Of Criteria, Intention, Meta Frame, Model Of The World, Reality Strategy, Redefine, Switch Referential Index.] In this example the principle of Redefine is employed.

(A not equal to B)

<u>The Pattern</u>:

Client Statement: 'Being stupid makes me feel worthless.'

A)

'<u>Being</u> anything is a lot more than how you feel you are in any snapshot moment of time.   Being is about who you are – and you are a lot more than how you think you feel at the moment.'

B)

'<u>Worthless</u> is what you would say about something like a used train ticket.'

A/B)

'To make such a statement means that you desire more <u>wisdom</u> and more <u>worth</u> in your life. All truly <u>wise</u> and <u>worthwhile</u> people start by first noticing how they feel about where they are and that motivates them to do and become more.   Well done!'

Referential Shifting

<u>The Pattern</u>:

I remember hearing Stephen Brooks employ this principle. He said to a client: **'That's what you think – it's not what he thinks'**. This artfully translated the client's, internal, associated thoughts and feelings relating to a prior experience from an emotionally charged first position perspective, into a dissociated (once removed) second position, simply by asking the client to consider another person's point of view in the given scenario. All in the space of just nine words. In NLP terms it was like causing the client to go through an 'instant meta mirror' re-evaluation of the situation (meaning rapidly experiencing a third position point of view and an instant integration of the new perspective). Sometimes it can be useful to employ Referential Shifting therefore to help distance a client from emotionally charged elements that have been evoked by recalling a given situation.

Here are a couple of examples:

1) 'You say it's bothering you – how do you think they're feeling?'

2) 'No. It wouldn't feel good to you. How do you think she/he would feel about it though? What does that tell you?'

Reframing

Meaning Reframing

Client statement: 'I'm afraid!'

1) Hypnotherapist: 'That fear just means that you're being cautious. And that's a good thing.'

2) Hypnotherapist: 'There's a thin line between fear and excitement.'

The Structure:

A meaning reframe offers an alternative meaning to the situation being experienced.

1) Hypnotherapist: 'That fear just means that you're being cautious. And that's a good thing. [This means that the feeling of fear was 'being helpful'. What's more, the client is being applauded for demonstrating sufficient caution.]'

2) Hypnotherapist: 'There's a thin line between fear and excitement. [This means that maybe the experience isn't fear after all. Maybe the meaning of the feeling is excitement?]'

Context reframing:

The Pattern:

Client Statement: 'I'm afraid.'

1) 'And how could that be useful now?'

2) 'I find that when I've experienced that feeling myself, in the past, that that fear was usually just a message to tell me to take care over something – or to deal with a situation that required some attention. What message do you think that feeling of fear you told me you were having was telling you?'

The Structure:

The structure is self-evident. In the above examples questions are asked which look for a context in which the client can offer a <u>positive</u> <u>interpretation</u> to their experience.

1) 'And how could that be useful now [in what context could the fear be helpful]?'

2) 'I find that when I've experienced that feeling myself, in the past, that that fear was usually just a message to tell me to take care over something – or to deal with a situation that required some attention. [The therapist offers his/her own reframed interpretation of the experience of fear.] What message do you think that feeling of fear you told me you were having was telling you [in what context could the feeling be helpful]?'

<u>Content Reframe</u>:

Client statement: 'I'm boiling over with rage about her behaviour.'

1) Hypnotherapist: 'I understand. But anger can be very helpful in situations like this because you can constructively channel that high energy emotion to help you generate the determination to solve this amicably and within the law.'

2) Hypnotherapist: 'Angry for sure. I know. I can see alright that you're pretty het up and bothered about this. I'd probably be annoyed and feel naffed off in that situation too. It must be quite frustrating too - or something?'

<u>The Structure</u>:

In these examples the content of the message has been reframed, for instance, from rage to anger, to naffed off. It's met at a similar level (rage and anger are almost synonymous) and then scaled down, through words which have similar but lesser meanings each time. Finally, in the second of the two content reframes, the emotional charge is then changed from anger to frustration.

1) Hypnotherapist: 'I understand. But <u>anger</u> can be very helpful in situations like this because you can constructively channel that <u>high</u> <u>energy</u> <u>emotion</u> to help you generate the <u>determination</u> to solve this amicably and within the law.'

2) Hypnotherapist: '<u>Angry</u> for sure. I know. I can see alright that you're pretty <u>het</u> <u>up</u> and <u>bothered</u> about this. I'd probably be <u>annoyed</u> and feel <u>naffed</u> <u>off</u> in that situation too. It must be quite <u>frustrating</u> too - or <u>something</u>?'

<u>Specifics Reframing</u>:

<u>The Pattern</u>:

1)

Client Statement: 'Studying physics is really difficult.'

Hypnotherapist: 'Which part have you been finding difficult?'

2)

Client statement: 'I hate being in large groups.'

Hypnotherapist: 'What specifically don't you like about being in large groups?'

<u>The Structure</u>:

When a client says, for example, that something is difficult the hypnotherapist can reframe what's been said by chunking down to specifics by saying: 'Which part was difficult?'.   This implies that 'everything else' isn't difficult, and it makes the difficulty seem smaller because it now occupies just a 'part' of the whole situation (most of which isn't difficult).

1) Hypnotherapist: 'Which <u>part</u> have you been finding difficult?'

2) Hypnotherapist: 'What <u>specifically</u> don't you like about being in large groups?'

Relative Clauses

<u>The Pattern</u>:

1) 'Hypnotherapists who utilise indirect approaches have a wide range of methods to help people...'

2) 'The thing about NLP that I like is its flexibility.'

3) 'What some people who live in Bournemouth do that you might like to consider too, is drive into the New Forest for a walk.   It's quite peaceful in the New Forest.'

4) 'The amazing thing about your Inner Self that I think is helpful to know, is that the thoughts which you are not yet aware of that are helping you make changes show that it's you, Sally, who knows what is best for you!'

5) 'It's nice to know that because you are moving forward and enlisting your Protective Self... which continues to take care of you... and your Creative Self... who can help you to find new ways to be safe... while also allowing you to enter into life more again... is because it takes place inside that means that it is influential.'

<u>The Structure</u>:

Relative Clauses use complex noun arguments (a noun being descriptive of a person, place or thing). This takes place in the form of a statement, which has a noun, immediately followed by the words, who, which or what. Complex Noun arguments help to lend gravitas (in the sense of authority) to the statement being made. The relative clause modifies the noun which has preceded it. It therefore changes the scope; from being purely a descriptive noun, to one which introduces something (a clause), which, in relation to the noun (relative), modifies the statement.

1) '**Hypnotherapists** [noun] <u>who</u> [relative clause - modifies] utilise indirect approaches have a wide range of methods to help people...'

2) 'The thing about **NLP** [noun] <u>that</u> [relative clause - modifies] I like is its flexibility.'

3) 'What some people who live in **Bournemouth** [noun] do <u>that</u> [relative clause - modifies] you might like to consider too, is drive into the New Forest for a walk. It's quite peaceful in the New Forest.'

4) 'The amazing thing about your **Inner Self** [noun] <u>that</u> [relative clause - modifies] I think is helpful to know, is that the **thoughts** [noun] <u>which</u> [relative clause - modifies] you are not yet aware of that are helping you make changes show that it's you, **Sally** [noun], <u>who</u> [relative clause - modifies] knows what is best for you!'

5) 'It's nice to know that because you are moving forward and enlisting your **Protective Self**... [noun] <u>which</u> [relative clause - modifies] continues to take care of you... and your **Creative Self**... [noun] <u>who</u> [relative clause - modifies] can help you to find new ways to be safe... while also allowing you to enter into life more again... is because it takes place **inside** [noun] <u>that</u> [relative clause - modifies] means that it is influential.'

Relaxing The Changes To Happen

<u>The Pattern</u>:

1) 'And while you're taking it easy here, today, isn't it nice to know that you can relax the changes to happen like this?'

2) 'Relaxing the changes to happen in trance is a nice way to change, many people think.'

3) 'And whenever you start relaxing the changes to happen like this again in the future they will become more and more effective.'

4) 'That's right. And you don't have to try to force this to happen. In trance it's all about relaxing the

changes to happen. And that seems to me like a nice way to change.'

5) 'I remember one person who found that relaxing the changes to happen, like you're doing now, was such a nice experience and that things began to improve so much, that now, she often uses the process of trance to relax even more positive things into her life.'

The Structure:

This pattern helps to diffuse 'performance anxiety' on the part of the client. If a client has worries about whether or not they or 'the hypnosis' will be able to help them (as some clients do), the use of this pattern can help to reframe the issue from being one of perceived (by the client) effort and stress to one of 'relaxing the changes to happen'. This generally results in the client becoming comfortable about participating in the process. And as performance anxiety is depotentiated the client can begin to positively explore the opportunities of therapy.

Repeated Words

The Pattern:

Two Word Repeats

'So, with each breath you … you… can… can… go… …go… inside… inside… so… so… your… your… unconscious… unconscious… can…'

Two And Three Word Repeats

'So, with each breath you ... you... can... can... go... go... inside... inside... so... so... your... your... unconscious... unconscious... can... can ... help... help... you... you... you...'

The Structure:

These patterns are wonderful for inducing trance. Spoken in a rhythmic way they naturally 'flow' and create a very trancey mood. [Specific examples of these patterns can be found on the Ultra Hypnosis CDs and downloads titled 'Positively Positive', 'Confidently Confident' and 'Mind-Body Healing'.] By leaving gaps of increased duration, every now and again, this too, I suspect, causes the client to begin to expectantly await the next word to be spoken...while...the rhythm... generates more... ... ... trance... trance... as it... all... all... ... happens.... happens... ... . happens.

Repetitive Cue Words

The Pattern:

1) 'Okay – and you can do this too.'

2) 'And as you also find new solutions...'

3) 'Let's refer back to that feeling that you said you want to experience more often.'

4) 'So, when you do this again...'

5) 'That's right. And you no longer think that you need to do this either.'

<u>The Structure</u>:

Repetitive Cue Words refer to words which, by their nature, imply a repetition (revisiting) of the context being considered.

1) 'Okay – and you can do this <u>too</u>.'

2) 'And as you <u>also</u> find new solutions...'

3) 'Let's refer <u>back</u> to that feeling that you said you want to experience more often.'

4) 'So, when you do this <u>again</u>...'

5) 'That's right. And you no longer think that you need to do this <u>either</u>.'

Repetitive Verbs And Adverbs

<u>The Pattern</u>:

1) 'As you realign your conscious mind with your inner talents think how much better things can become.'

2) 'As you remember to remember solutions...'

3) 'That's right. And you can reconfirm to yourself that you are a talented person.'

4) 'Every time you recall what it was that motivated you to do this you can take pride in reaffirming to yourself that you are a good person.'

5) 'It's like restoring your sense of self worth while at the same time renewing your sense of optimism. But then, I expect, deep inside, just like I know, you know, you deserve to return to your true ideals and repay yourself with some positive feelings for all the progress you've made and repeat those good feelings often. It's all about replacing unwanted feelings with ones that you'd rather re-experience and replenish them as often as you want to. Remember it's as simple as reminding your inner self that you want a total renewal of your most positive attributes. You know, making profound change like this can be a bit like having something of a rebirth. Changing from how you were, to who you are. And when you reconsider things from this enhanced perspective and notice all that you've achieved it might be nice to allow yourself to allow your process of personal regeneration to continue trusting in the wisdom of your inner mind to let everything work out as best it should.'

<u>The Structure</u>:

The Repetitive Verbs and Adverbs pattern uses words beginning with 're' to convey a sense of additional emphasis to the subject being addressed. For instance, rather than 'consider', the hypnotherapist could say 'reconsider' which implies a certain amount of consideration has already taken place. Rather than 'think about' the hypnotherapist could say 'remember', or 'recall' which also implies that the thoughts to be considered already existed. The word 'invigorate' could become 'reinvigorate', which similarly suggests referral to an already existent resource.

1) 'As you <u>realign</u> your conscious mind with your inner talents think how much better things can become.'

2) 'As you <u>remember</u> to remember solutions...'

3) 'That's right. And you can <u>reconfirm</u> to yourself that you are a talented person.'

4) 'Every time you <u>recall</u> what it was that motivated you to do this you can take pride in reaffirming to yourself that you are a good person.'

5) 'It's like <u>restoring</u> your sense of self worth while at the same time <u>renewing</u> your sense of optimism. But then, I expect, deep inside, just like I know, you know, you deserve to <u>return</u> to your true ideals and <u>repay</u> yourself with some positive feelings for all the progress you've made and <u>repeat</u> those good feelings often. It's all about <u>replacing</u> unwanted feelings with ones that you'd rather <u>re-experience</u> and <u>replenish</u> them as often as you want to. <u>Remember</u> it's as simple as <u>reminding</u> your inner self that you want a total <u>renewal</u> of your most positive attributes. You know, making profound change like this can be a bit like having something of a <u>rebirth</u>. Changing from how you were, to who you are. And when you <u>reconsider</u> things from this enhanced perspective and notice all that you've achieved it might be nice to allow yourself to allow your process of personal <u>regeneration</u> to continue trusting in the wisdom of your inner mind to let everything work out as best it should.'

Replaying

<u>The Pattern</u>:

1) 'And every time you replay that positive feeling it will continue to become a deep and significant part of your developing emotional range. Which means that things can continue to improve.'

2) 'Your inner self knows how to replay a good thought and turn it into a good feeling and each time you replay this good thought and each time it becomes a good feeling you can remember that you have the ability to replay it whenever and wherever you need to.'

3) 'How often do you think your inner self will replay these suggestions to you on a deeper than conscious level in order for the changes to powerfully integrate inside?'

4) 'I'd like to invite your inner self to replay these suggestions - and new and better feelings for you as and when appropriate in order that you consciously notice that things are now shifting in your favour.'

5) 'The thing that I like about making changes in hypnosis is that each time you find your unconscious replays a nice thought or a nice feeling for you in the future – along with that sense of optimism that accompanies them - so that each time it happens it helps improve the present moment is that it can be like replaying giving yourself the present of a good thought and good feeling in the present moment. So each replay of something good helps you presently live in the

present and present yourself with a better and new perspective each time you replay them like this.'

The Structure:

The Replaying pattern offers a way for the therapist to introduce the concept of ongoing, continual change, which draws on resources that are already in existence (such as positive thoughts and emotions, and post hypnotic suggestions) within the client and suggests that they can be replayed (which means re-experienced) in the future in the context of whatever situation the client requires the replayed resources to occur.

Resist And Yield

The Pattern:

1) 'There's nothing to stop you closing your eyes now.'

2) 'That relaxed state is developing rather nicely... but don't go into a hypnotic trance until it's your turn.'

3) 'Now I know that there is something that you want to tell me, but let's agree to hold it back until you know the time is right.'

The Structure:

In essence, the therapist offers a suggestion that either removes a prohibition which has been implied (example 1) or which includes a prohibition against its immediate enactment (example 2). A 'quirk' in our collective human nature (speaking very generally now) is our desire to possess things that we can't easily have. The Resist And Yield pattern makes use of this. As a result, the client is likely to follow the suggestions offered. Example 2 will also work well with clients who demonstrate a polarity response.

Example 3 is a bit different. I was working with a woman who was referred to me by her mother – because she (the mother's daughter – my client) had been repeatedly sexually abused. The client, so to speak, kept wandering around the issue, without directly addressing it. I knew we needed to deal with the issue - and I sensed that this avoidance pattern on her part might take a long time to work its way out. I also felt that it was important for the woman in question to raise the issue with me – rather than me 'steam rollering in' to address it. So by using the phrase above, I acknowledged that I had an understanding of her reason for being with me, but I also conveyed my respect for her and the sense that we could work at a measured pace – while respectfully suggesting that she would start to deal with the issue when the time was right. As a result, within a relatively short period of time of me saying: **'Now I know that there's something you want to tell me, but let's agree to hold it back until you know the time is right.'** ...the client started to talk to me about the relevant issues. [For example 2 see also Reverse Set Double Bind.]

Resistant Clients

Despite the unrealistic phrases that you sometimes hear (for instance: 'There's no such thing as a resistant client – only an un-resourceful therapist'), every now and again most psychotherapists will encounter a client, who, for a myriad number of reasons, appears to be unresponsive, difficult or even resistant to the process of therapy. In the supervision sessions I've offered to various therapists I've found that it's a phenomenon that's (sometimes) part of the working life of each psychotherapist. It can, therefore, be useful to have some 'prepared responses' to, where possible, melt the resistance in order to help the client begin to deal with his/her issues constructively.

Here are a couple of phrases that could be employed to help a client begin to fully participate in trancework.

1) 'Of course, you could resist but that's not why you're here. [As mentioned elsewhere in this book, I learned this phrase from reading a script by **Marshall Sylver**.]'

2) 'Everyone can go into trance when they want to. And I respect you and I know that you also know that you are in charge and that the responsible and mature thing to do to assist your trance experience so that you will fully benefit too is to relax and ….let it happen. And I know that: You could resist – but why would you? [The last sentence is one that I've borrowed from Andrea Lindsay. She employs it on the Ultra Hypnosis CDs and downloads called 'Stop Smoking – Start Living'.] You would only be resisting yourself because it's you who is choosing

to make this change today. Which tells me that you are in alignment with your goals and outcomes by coming here today to make this change – and what a wonderful thing it can be to let your life improve and start to experience more of the good that is available because you have demonstrated by your actions that this is what you want - really deep inside!

I once used an approach where I included the first example above and one very similar to the second example too in a smoking cessation session several years ago. I'd helped one client with hypnotherapy to become a non-smoker. Soon afterwards she met an 'old friend' and when her 'old friend' learned that my client was now a non-smoker she chided her for doing it without telling her. It turned out that, at some time in the past, they'd made an agreement with each other that if ever one was going to stop the other would do so too. However, they'd drifted apart, hence my client visiting me independently. My client's 'friend' insisted that she give her my phone number so that she could book an appointment with me too. However, before the 'friend' could call me, my original client phoned to apologise to me <u>in</u> <u>advance</u> for referring her 'friend' to me. In the process she gave me some feedback about her 'friend's' temperament. Soon afterwards the 'friend' did indeed phone to book a session herself. There was an undercurrent of aggression in her manner and a polarity response. So I utilised the above mentioned principles with help her. Soon afterwards my original client phoned me to tell me that her friend had also stopped smoking after the hypnotherapy session but (demonstrating an ongoing polarity response – despite a positive result) that she had dismissively said that 'it was nothing to do with that hypnotherapist!'. ☺

Resource Double Binds

The Pattern:

1) 'Your conscious mind can wonder what resources you have while your unconscious activates them for you.'

2) 'As you consciously consider what resources would be most helpful, your inner self is even now creating them.'

3) 'As you inwardly create your new resources, outwardly you can experience them.'

4) 'Outside you sense new resources are happening while inside you choose which ones to experience.'

5) 'It doesn't matter if you are not yet consciously sure what resources you will experience, because unconsciously you already know.'

The Structure:

Resource Double Binds are basically Double Binds which have as their 'Bind focus' the suggestion of implied resources. The Bind is offered in such a way that whatever conclusion the client draws it will (at all levels) be one that involves an improvement in their condition because of the resources being triggered by the Resource Double Bind's presupposition that what is suggested is in the process of taking place.

1) 'Your <u>conscious</u> mind can wonder what <u>resources</u> you have while your <u>unconscious</u> activates them for you.'

2) 'As you <u>consciously</u> consider what <u>resources</u> would be most helpful, your <u>inner self</u> is even now creating them.'

3) 'As you <u>inwardly</u> create your new <u>resources</u>, <u>outwardly</u> you can experience them.'

4) '<u>Outside</u> you sense new <u>resources</u> are happening while <u>inside</u> you choose which ones to experience.'

5) 'It doesn't matter if you are not yet <u>consciously</u> sure what <u>resources</u> you will experience, because <u>unconsciously</u> you already know.   [For more examples of the structure of Binds of this nature see: Double Binds].'

Respect Phrases

<u>The Pattern</u>:

1) 'And you can make these changes in the exact appropriate, helpful, healthful ways that are right for you.'

2) 'You will accept the suggestions which are right for you and use them in ways that suit your unique circumstances.'

3) 'You will make these changes in normal, balanced and harmonious ways.'

4) 'Remembering that you can be true to yourself. As you continue to be and become the fullest positive expression of yourself, in every good and every wonderful way.'

5) 'And remember, you can awaken at any time you choose, fully able to deal with whatever requires your attention by saying to yourself, out loud or in your mind, the word 'awake' and you'll awaken feeling at ease in every good way.'

<u>The Structure</u>:

I include various Respect Phrases often during hypnotherapy sessions so that my clients understand (consciously and unconsciously) that only changes which are for <u>their</u> <u>highest</u> good will manifest. A 'safety switch' anchor is also included, in the form of suggesting to the clients, at the outset, that they can end the trance ('awaken') <u>at</u> <u>any time</u> by using the cue word 'awake' to do so. In so doing the hypnotherapist demonstrates consideration for the client by ensuring that all of the work that occurs is done in the context of the client's desired outcome and overall well-being, and in the agreed knowledge that the client can end the session at any time or choose whether or not to respond to any and all suggestions offered. I remember Richard Bandler incorporating a similar principle in a group hypnosis session in which he suggested that we (those of us in the group) would never accept a suggestion which wasn't for our highest good (meaning in any situation, hypnotic or otherwise)...including from <u>himself</u>! (Which I thought was very professional of him.)

1) 'And you can make these changes in the exact <u>appropriate</u>, <u>helpful</u>, <u>healthful</u> ways that are <u>right for</u> <u>you</u>.'

2) 'You will accept the suggestions <u>which</u> <u>are</u> <u>right for</u> <u>you</u> and use them in <u>ways</u> <u>that</u> <u>suit</u> <u>your</u> <u>unique circumstances</u>.'

3) 'You will make these changes in <u>normal</u>, <u>balanced</u> and <u>harmonious</u> <u>ways</u>.'

4) 'Remembering that you can <u>be</u> <u>true</u> <u>to</u> <u>yourself</u>. As you continue to <u>be</u> <u>and</u> <u>become</u> the <u>fullest positive</u> <u>expression</u> <u>of</u> <u>yourself</u>, in <u>every</u> <u>good</u> and <u>every</u> <u>wonderful</u> <u>way</u>.'

5) 'And remember, you can awaken at any time you choose, <u>fully able to deal with whatever requires your attention</u> by saying to yourself, out loud or in your mind, the word '<u>awake</u>' and <u>you'll awaken feeling at ease in every good way</u>.'

Response Contingent Bind Double Bind

<u>The Pattern</u>:

1) 'Can you relax into trance with your eyes closed as well as with your eyes open?'

2) 'Can you visualise this with your eyes open as well as with your eyes closed.'

3) 'Can you go into trance sitting down as well as laying down?'

4) 'Can you go into hypnosis while sitting back in the chair as well as sitting forward in it?'

5) 'Can you count yourself down into trance as well as relaxing your body into trance?'

The Structure:

A Response Contingent Bind Double Bind manifests depending upon the response that the recipient gives to the question. If the client responds with an affirmative 'yes' answer then it's manifested as a Bind. However, if they have to 'try out' both options to <u>discover</u> the answer, it's a Double Bind. Binds can be decided at a conscious level, whereas Double Binds are manifested at an unconscious level. The answer to a Double Bind is always revealed in the process of its manifestation. It's outside of conscious choice and therefore inside unconscious control.

Notice this pattern exhibits the: 'Can you...as well as...' structure. This means that a question is posed with an either/or both possibility as an answer.

1) '**Can you** relax into trance with your eyes closed <u>as well as</u> with your eyes open?'

2) '**Can you** visualise this with your eyes open <u>as well as</u> with your eyes closed?'

3) '**Can you** go into trance sitting down <u>as well as</u> laying down?'

4) '**Can you** go into hypnosis while sitting back in the chair <u>as well as</u> sitting forward in it?'

5) '**Can you** count yourself down into trance <u>as well as</u> relaxing your body into trance?'

Reversed Coué's Law

<u>The Pattern</u>:

1) 'Curiously, you can even try not to think about feeling different, and you'll still feel different. This change is that powerful for you that it even works when you try not to think about it happening. So just think how good it is going to be when you are just getting on with your life and letting it happen.'

2) 'Don't think about feeling good. It's not necessary right now. You can just let it happen in its own good way.'

3) 'Here's a pleasant experiment that you might like to try. See if you can resist thinking about feeling good for the next five days and notice what happens. This change is that powerful that it even works when you try and resist thinking about it! Which means that it's really going to be wonderful for you – is it not – when you're not resisting and allowing it to happen as you want it to.'

4) 'Now your inner self will make this happen in the best way for you. And if you want to prove to yourself how wonderfully powerful this is – you can even try and resist thinking about the changes tomorrow – and you'll find that you think about them anyway.'

5) 'Even people who, for whatever unknown reason, try and resist the positive changes, and that might

sound curious to you, but sometimes people do, they find that even when they try and resist the changes, if they are the right changes for them, if their inner wisdom chooses them, then they will happen anyway. Actually, sometimes I like to try to not think about the hypnotic changes I've made in my own life, and I notice too that, for instance, even when I try not to think about a hypnotic suggestion, say, to do with feeling positive, like: 'You will feel positive', I still think about feeling positive. Try it now. Try not to remember the suggestion: 'You will feel positive'. Try really hard and notice that you will think about it, at some level, in some way, even if it's just to think about thinking about it in order to not think about it. Which means that you've been thinking about it and the change is continuing to work for you. **You will feel positive!** And that is nice to know!'

The Structure:

Emile Coué's famous dictum: 'Whatever you resist persists' explains the principle that Richard Bandler often expounds when he reminds us that we cannot process negation. That's to say that in order to not think about something, we first have to think about it in order to not think about it. Someone says to you for instance 'Don't think of Winston Churchill'... and instantly thoughts of Winston Churchill pop into your mind. This principle is useful for hypnotherapists to remember because it can be utilised to help clients to stop trying to 'stop thinking about' their psycho-emotional problems, because, in so doing they're actually manifesting the very things they're trying to overcome! By trying to not think about a problem the client creates the problem. However by suggesting resistance to the suggested solution instead in the manner illustrated here the opposite effect is encouraged in the sense that the client is actually induced (paradoxically) to consider the beneficial suggestion being offered.

1) 'Curiously, you can even <u>try not to think about</u> feeling different, and you'll still feel different. This change is that powerful for you that it even works when you <u>try not to think about</u> it happening. So just think how good it is going to be when you are just getting on with your life and letting it happen.'

2) <u>'Don't think about</u> feeling good. It's not necessary right now. You can just let it happen in its own good way.'

3) 'Here's a pleasant experiment that you might like to try. <u>See if you can resist thinking about</u> feeling good for the next five days and notice what happens. This change is that powerful that it even works when you <u>try and resist thinking</u> about it! Which means that it's really going to be wonderful for you – is it not – when you're not resisting and allowing it to happen as you want it to.'

4) 'Now your inner self will make this happen in the best way for you. And if you want to prove to yourself how wonderfully powerful this is – you can <u>even try and resist thinking about the changes</u> tomorrow – and you'll find that you think about them anyway.'

5) '<u>Even</u> people who, for whatever unknown reason, <u>try and resist</u> the positive changes, and that might sound curious to you, but sometimes people do, they find that even when they <u>try and resist</u> the

changes, if they are the right changes for them, if their inner wisdom chooses them, then they will happen anyway. Actually, sometimes <u>I like to try to not think about the hypnotic changes</u> I've made in my own life, and I notice too that, for instance, <u>even</u> when I <u>try not to think about</u> a hypnotic suggestion, say, to do with feeling positive, like: 'You will feel positive', I still think about feeling positive. <u>Try</u> it now. <u>Try not to remember</u> the suggestion: 'You will feel positive'. <u>Try</u> really hard and notice that you will think about it, at some level, in some way, even if it's just to think about thinking about it in order to not think about it. **Which means that you've been thinking about it** and the change is continuing to work for you. **You will feel positive!** And that is nice to know!'

Reverse Set Double Bind

<u>The Pattern</u>:

1) 'Now. I understand that it's taken some time for you to choose to enter therapy. And I respect that. And there are obviously things that you want to deal with in your own time. So let's agree that you will introduce them when you are good and ready. Okay.'

2) 'Now – you've mentioned that there is a deeper issue. I also understand that you need to address it in the right way. So, how about we specifically agree that you hold it back until you're ready to let me know what it is?'

3) 'I understand that there are many things you'd like to share with me. But I'd like you to hold some

of it back for now. Only tell me when you're good and ready.'

4) 'You mentioned some secrets that you want to share but you are not sure when and how? Well, let's both understand now that you only need to let me know what they are at the right time.'

5) 'And there are certain concerns which have been bothering you – I understand that. And don't even tell me about them just yet. Only at the right time. Okay!'

The Structure:

The Reverse Set Double Bind is a form of Bind that can be employed when a client indicates that they want to discuss something, but are hesitant, for whatever reason, about getting started. A suggestion is offered, in the form of a Bind, which has as its outcome the presupposition that the client will address the issue in question. However, an element within the Bind suggests that, although the issue will be raised, it will take place only after a certain criterion is met. [Obviously, patterns like this should be used with integrity and with the highest respect for the client. If it's clear that a client does not want to discuss something, which from a therapist's perspective, appears to need to be discussed, on an ethical level, it is, I suggest, better to reach that point by raising the issue in other ways. Perhaps by explaining, overtly, why, as a therapist, you might consider that the subject in question would benefit by being explored. The examples of the Reverse Set Double Bind here are offered in the context of a client expressing the desire to explore some issues, but demonstrating some uncertainty as to exactly when and how. Not, 'whether' or 'if'.]

1) 'Now. I understand that it's taken some time for you to choose to enter therapy. And I respect that. And there are obviously <u>things that you want to deal with</u> in your own time. So let's agree that <u>you will introduce them when you are good and ready</u>. Okay.'

2) 'Now – you've mentioned that there is <u>a deeper issue</u>. I also understand that you need to address it in the right way. So, how about we specifically agree that <u>you hold it back until</u> you're ready to let me know what it is?'

3) 'I understand that there are <u>many things you'd like to share</u> with me. But I'd like you to <u>hold some of it back for now</u>. Only <u>tell me when you're good and ready</u>.'

4) 'You mentioned some <u>secrets that you want to share</u> but you are not sure when and how? Well, let's both understand now that <u>you only need to let me know what they are at the right time</u>.'

5) 'And there are <u>certain concerns</u> which have been bothering you – I understand that. And <u>don't even tell me about them just yet</u>. <u>Only at the right time</u>. Okay!'

Reverse Yes Set

<u>The Pattern</u>:

1) 'You wouldn't expect to know how the changes will take place before you go into trance would you?'

2) 'You wouldn't expect the changes to happen before the trance has happened would you?'

3) 'You wouldn't expect the trance to take place before you relax would you?'

4) 'You wouldn't expect to feel different before the changes have taken place would you?'

5) 'You wouldn't expect this problem to fade away before we have entered trance would you?'

<u>The Structure</u>:

The Reverse Yes Set pattern involves the asking of a question, which is designed to elicit a 'no' answer, but, paradoxically, the 'no' answer is actually, by implication a 'yes' answer, because it is in agreement with the premise of the questioner's question. It sounds a bit unusual – but then you can't be expected to understand it until you've first learned about it. Can you? So, in essence, a Reverse Yes Set occurs when a question is asked which elicits a 'no' answer, BUT, the 'no' answer is actually in agreement with the questioner's stance.

Here's another example of how this might take place conversationally:

Client: 'I found you okay. The directions you sent me were very helpful.'

Hypnotherapist: 'So they weren't difficult after all?'

Client: 'No (Yes by agreement)'

Hypnotherapist: 'Now you didn't just arrive to talk about my directions?'

Client: 'No (Yes by agreement)'

Hypnotherapist: 'So what you want to look at then isn't unrelated to what we talked about on the phone?'

Client: 'No – it is related (Yes by agreement).'

Reversing Presuppositions

The Pattern:

Student's Statement:

'I didn't train directly with Milton Erickson so I'll never be a good hypnotherapist.'

1) 'How could not training directly with Milton Erickson actually help you be a good hypnotherapist?'

2) 'In what way can not training with Milton Erickson actually make you a good hypnotherapist?'

3) 'How is not training with Milton Erickson actually the same as becoming a good hypnotherapist?'

4) 'In what way would not training directly with Milton Erickson actually equal becoming a good hypnotherapist?'

5) 'How has not training directly with Milton Erickson actually meant that you are becoming a good hypnotherapist?'

6) 'In what way does not having trained directly with Milton Erickson actually mean that you can become a good hypnotherapist?'

7) 'How would not training directly with Milton Erickson actually cause you to become a good hypnotherapist?'

8) 'In what way is not training directly with Milton Erickson actually useful for making you a good hypnotherapist?'

9) 'How might not training directly with Milton Erickson actually be helpful in causing you to become a good hypnotherapist?'

10) 'What do you think there might be about not training directly with Milton Erickson that might actually contribute to you becoming a good hypnotherapist?'

The Structure:

The Student's Statement: 'I didn't train directly with Milton Erickson so I'll never be a good hypnotherapist', presupposes that in order to be a 'good hypnotherapist' it is imperative that direct training with Milton Erickson takes place. Obviously that's not true (although of course it would be helpful).   The   Reversing   Presuppositions   pattern (developed   by   Connirae   Andreas)   is   geared   to reverse such limiting presuppositions, in order to help the client expand their paradigm of what is and what isn't (supposedly) possible.   You'll notice that the word 'actually' acts as pivot of sorts.   The therapist asks a question (which sets the frame) because the client has made a statement in which, from their 'model of the world' (NLP-speak for their perspective), there is no other conclusion that could be drawn than that which they've stated.   It is (the client   is   suggesting)   a   fact.   So,   in   asking   a question, it immediately, with subtlety, begins to suggest that 'it ain't necessarily so?'.   The pivotal word <u>actually</u> is a very powerful word when used in this   context   because   it   implies   that   the presupposition (the veracity of which has just been questioned)   might   not   actually   be   as   solid   as suggested.   The   therapist   then   follows   with   a counter – which is still in the form of a question, which suggests that there are other alternatives to the client's hitherto fixed point of view which might actually   help   them   to   achieve   whatever   they thought   they   couldn't.   The   Reversing Presuppositions Pattern offers an alternative, in the form   of   a   question,   that   it   might   actually   be possible that the opposite of the client's statement is true.

1) '<u>How could</u> not training directly with Milton Erickson   <u>actually</u>   help   you   <u>be   a   good hypnotherapist</u>?'

2) '<u>In what way</u> can not training with Milton Erickson <u>actually</u> make you <u>a good hypnotherapist</u>?'

3) 'How is not training with Milton Erickson actually the same as becoming a good hypnotherapist?'

4) 'In what way would not training directly with Milton Erickson actually equal becoming a good hypnotherapist?'

5) 'How has not training directly with Milton Erickson actually meant that you are becoming a good hypnotherapist?'

6) 'In what way does not having trained directly with Milton Erickson actually mean that you can become a good hypnotherapist?'

7) 'How would not training directly with Milton Erickson actually cause you to become a good hypnotherapist?'

8) 'In what way is not training directly with Milton Erickson actually useful for making you a good hypnotherapist?'

9) 'How might not training directly with Milton Erickson actually be helpful in causing you to become a good hypnotherapist?'

10) 'What do you think there might be about not training directly with Milton Erickson that might actually contribute to you becoming a good hypnotherapist?'

Revivification

<u>The Pattern</u>:

'That's right...and you may choose to remember a relaxing trance that you've enjoyed before or perhaps even a time when you've been pleasantly daydreaming...letting your imagination wander and I wonder where you can let your imagination wander to again today?'

<u>The Structure</u>:

Revivification is about helping the client to re-experience (revivify) a therapeutically desired outcome. Whether it's recalling a previous trance, as they go into trance, to facilitate the present trance, or, perhaps remembering a positive emotion, or thought, in order to draw on it again, as a resource in the now, or maybe recalling an event from the past, in order to use the associations to that event in some therapeutic context.

'That's right...and you may choose to <u>remember a relaxing trance</u> [revivification of context] that you've <u>enjoyed before</u> [revivification of context] or perhaps <u>even a time</u> [revivification of context] when you've been <u>pleasantly daydreaming</u> [revivification of process] ...letting your <u>imagination wander</u> [revivification of process] and I wonder where you can let your <u>imagination wander</u> [suggestion that a similar experience to that which has been elicited, which involved the client allowing their imagination to wander will take place again in the present moment] to again today?'

Reward

<u>The Pattern</u>:

1) 'And just think how rewarding it's going to be to live like this now.'

2) 'That's right – congratulate yourself for deciding to make these changes.'

3) 'We both know that it hasn't been easy. But you did it anyway. So you can give yourself a pat on the back and recognise all of your achievements. Remember, you are allowed to feel good like this.'

4) 'You know, you merit a good sense of self approval for the good things you've done with this situation. It's been a good endeavour on your part and you deserve to acknowledge that.'

5) 'What's more, every time you follow through and do XYZ you will notice that your inner self rewards you with a nice boost of positivity. So being true to your ideals will make you feel good in more ways than one.'

<u>The Structure</u>:

A number of useful things can occur for the client when the Reward principle is employed:

A) The client can gain a sense of 'reward' for their achievement, on a personal level (after all – many clients will have been dealing with some pretty difficult issues, so a reward acts as a nice counter balance to the problematic experiences that they will likely have encountered) and...

B) On a subtle level the method implies that a line has been drawn underneath the problematic events that have taken place, suggesting, implicitly that things are improving. And...

C) The therapist can also introduce Post Hypnotic Suggestions of a 'reward factor', which are in effect anchors that are designed to occur, when required, to help reinforce the desired new cognitive behavioural pattern (as in example 5).

Rhetorical Questions

The Pattern:

1) 'My God, my God, why hast thou forsaken me?'

2) 'What does it matter if you leave?'

3) 'Who's bothered about it anyway?'

4) 'I don't suppose it matters. And I wonder if anyone else does either?'

5) 'What difference will it make if we continue anyway?'

The Structure:

I remember, about 20 years ago, asking a Christian minister a question. The question was about why, if Jesus Christ was the Divine Son of God, and, therefore fully aware of his mission on Earth, why did he ask the very famous question that I quoted in the example above. The minister explained to me that the question was a Rhetorical Question.

Jesus did know the answer. He posed it, out loud, in order that it would be recorded and passed down through history, to make people of his (and future) generation(s) consider what a great price he'd paid in order to liberate people from the results of their (our) collective and individual sins that occur when we all, from time to time, 'miss the mark' (the original meaning of the word 'sin'). That's how I learned about Rhetorical Questions. I learned that a Rhetorical Question is not 'really', so to speak, a question for information, made by the questioner, but rather a statement, made in the form of a question, which is designed to cause the receiver(s) of the question to think about what's being posed.

Rhythm

A useful 'rule of thumb' to remember when delivering hypnotherapy is that a good tempo to aim for is about one third of 'normal' conversational pace. Of course, it's good to 'up tempo' sometimes and to speak slower at other times (as well as raising the tone, or whispering, from time to time, etc). In my opinion, Paul McKenna has an excellent 'hypnotic voice' and he maintains good rhythm and tonality.

Rhythming And Rhyming

The Pattern:

'And each day now you sense that you are,
beginning to develop your talents by far,
so in all the best places and in all the right ways,
you continue to find that you wonderfully amaze,

yourself now with how well you do,
as you begin to feel really good about you.'

The Structure:

Rhythming and Rhyming is a name I've given to a method that I learned from Richard Bandler (I never heard him give a 'label' to it). You can hear it employed on the Ultra Hypnosis CDs and downloads called: 'Positively Positive', 'Confidently Confident' and 'Mind Body Healing'. Accelerated Learning research has demonstrated that rhythm and rhyme are excellent tools for being employed in the context of helping people to learn. They're equally useful in the therapeutic context too. We all remember: 'Red sky at night, Shepherd's delight. Red sky in the morning, Shepherd's warning'; which teaches us, from a very early age, about a meteorological phenomenon that we can look to, to indicate the up-coming weather patterns. Why is it so easy to remember? Because there's an intrinsic rhythm in the structure of the proverb, which is also coupled with rhyme.

'And each day now you sense that you **are**,
beginning to develop your talents by **far**,
so in all the best places and in all the right **ways**,
you continue to find that you wonderfully **amaze**,
yourself now with how well you **do**,
as you begin to feel really good about **you**.'

S

Scope Ambiguity

The Pattern:

1) 'And I wonder whether it will be those amazing thoughts and feelings which let you know that things are different?'

2) 'You can notice pleasant calm and relaxation.'

3) 'Isn't it nice to know that those happy feelings and emotions are becoming more and more a part of your life?'

4) 'Can you notice those positive emotions and thoughts?'

5) 'And a most amazing thing about those uplifting experiences and emotions is that...'

The Structure:

The Scope Ambiguity introduces a sense of indistinctness into the meaning of words that follow a modifying word. A modifying word means a word that introduces a quality to a word or words (which I call 'context words') which follow its use. For instance: Those <u>amazing</u> indirect hypnotherapists. The word 'amazing' modifies the following (context) words 'indirect hypnotherapists' to give them a modified meaning (they are amazing). Without the modifier 'Those indirect hypnotherapists' is quite a different statement. However, the effect of the Scope Ambiguity introduces an ambiguous modification, in as much as it's not possible to discern (without clarification) whether the modifying word applies to just one following point of reference or two (or more). The ambiguity is introduced by the use of the word 'and'. As you'll notice in the highlighted examples which follow below, the modifying word is then followed by a context word, plus the word 'and' and another context word. However, <u>does the modifier apply to the first context word or both</u>? Of course, without clarification it's not possible to tell. Hypnotically speaking, it's a very useful pattern for the delivery of therapy.

1) 'And I wonder whether it will be those <u>amazing thoughts</u> **and** <u>feelings</u> which let you know that things are different?'

2) 'You can notice <u>pleasant</u> <u>calm</u> **and** <u>relaxation</u>.'

3) 'Isn't it nice to know that those <u>happy feelings</u> **and** <u>emotions</u> are becoming more and more a part of your life?'

4) 'Can you notice those <u>positive</u> emotions **and** <u>thoughts</u>?'

5) 'And a most amazing thing about those <u>uplifting experiences</u> **and** <u>emotions</u> is that...'

The therapist can 'hitch-hike' the second context word, which is implicitly modified, for therapeutic affect. Considering example number 5 (directly above); a client could recently have enjoyed some 'uplifting experiences', the fact of which they've shared with the therapist, to which (by implication) 'uplifting emotions' (which will likely have been a part of the 'uplifting experiences' and, importantly, therefore a **Truism**) are suggested and 'hitch-hiked' onto the statement. By 'hitch-hiking' words in this way it depotentiates conscious questioning about whether or not it's possible or not for the client to access uplifting emotions, because, they've been elicited for the client in an indirect way.

Seeding

The Pattern:

1) 'I know people have wondered about how it is that by simply deepening their breathing, so that as they go within, so inner wisdom can become available, inside, below the level of your conscious awareness, just beneath the threshold, the place where you... understand... how good it is to find insights... which help you... as you begin to let yourself go inside now...'

2) 'Your higher nature knows how best to let you experience an uplifting sense of inner change and you can hand it to yourself, so to speak, so that from this new and elevated potential you can sense a higher purpose beginning to evolve and I wonder if you will sense it happening before one of those hands gently begins to lift up from your lap, will it be the left or will it be the right... that's right... you'll find out which one it is when your unconscious raises your awareness as you start to sense it is happening... now...'

3) 'Isn't it nice to say 'hi' to your unconscious? Knowing that at all the times you want to you can remember that it's high time to feel good and you can do this by standing up positively and noticing how much better things are when you naturally choose a positive upright posture like this.'

4) 'Sometimes I like to think about things in different ways. And many clients tell me that they like to consider things from new and different perspectives. And it can be good to reflect on the principle that it's nice to start to believe something that's helpful. I wonder, what do you imagine will be the first experience that lets you know that things are different and better? Think about this for a moment.'

5) 'That's right and as you adjust your posture, you know you can alter your position at any time, just as you can switch or amend your thoughts, beliefs and ideas... and while you do this your unconscious can start to change XYZ so that it becomes transformed into ABC.'

The Structure:

Seeding is a method (that's similar to Embedded Suggestions) in which a theme can be introduced, in order to help the client gently move in the direction of the, soon to be suggested, desired outcome. Words which convey the same, or similar, meaning to the intended desired outcome are 'seeded' into the overall message being offered so that the client becomes 'acclimatised' albeit, indirectly, to the concept that is to be introduced.

1)

Desired outcome: going into trance.

'I know people have wondered about how it is that by simply <u>deepening</u> their breathing, so that as they go <u>within</u>, so <u>inner</u> wisdom can become available, <u>inside</u>, <u>below</u> the level of your conscious awareness, just beneath the threshold, the place where you...<u>under</u>... stand... how good it is to find <u>in</u>...sights... which help you... as you begin to let yourself **go inside now**...'

2)

Desired outcome: arm levitation.

'Your <u>higher</u> nature knows how best to let you experience an <u>uplifting</u> sense of inner change and you can <u>hand</u> <u>it</u> <u>to</u> <u>yourself</u>, so to speak, so that from this new and <u>elevated</u> potential you can sense a <u>higher</u> purpose beginning to evolve and I wonder if you will sense it happening before one of those hands gently begins to **lift up from your lap**, will it be the left or will it be the right... that's right...you'll find out which one it is when your unconscious <u>raises</u> your awareness as you start to sense **it is happening... now**...'

3)

Desired outcome: development of upright posture.

'Isn't it nice to say 'hi' to your unconscious? Knowing that a <u>tall</u> (at all) the times you want to you can remember that it's <u>high</u> time to feel good and you can do this by **standing up positively** and noticing how much better things are when you naturally **choose a positive upright posture** like this.'

4)

Desired outcome: think about the positive outcome.

'Sometimes I like to <u>think</u> about things in different ways. And many clients tell me that they like to <u>consider</u> things from new and different perspectives. And it can be good to <u>reflect</u> on the principle that it's nice to start to <u>believe</u> something that's helpful. I wonder what do you <u>imagine</u> will be the first experience that lets you know that things are different and better? **Think about this** for a moment.'

5)

Desired outcome: prepare to make some cognitive behavioural changes.

'That's right and as you <u>adjust</u> your posture, you know you can <u>alter</u> your position at any time, just as you can <u>switch</u> or <u>amend</u> your thoughts, beliefs and ideas...and while you do this your unconscious can start to **change XYZ so that it becomes transformed into ABC**.'

Selectional Restriction Violation

<u>The Pattern</u>:

1) 'And as you picture your new office and notice how it welcomes you.'

2) 'It's like the mountain is sharing the knowledge it's gained over its many years of watching.'

3) 'Time is telling you to get on with it and take action.'

4) 'As you step into your inner temple and notice the energy it's sending you.'

5) 'That's it. I can almost hear your computer calling you myself. It's saying: 'Write the book. Write the book'.'

The Structure:

The Selectional Restriction Violation attributes high order qualities to animals, objects or concepts (like the concept of time, for instance), which are usually deemed to be only within the realm of the human experience (for example, consider: 'those dancing people' with 'those dancing flowers'. People consciously choose to dance. As far as we know, flowers don't. Do they?).

1) 'And as you picture your new <u>office</u> and notice how it <u>welcomes you</u>.'

2) 'It's like the <u>mountain</u> is <u>sharing the knowledge</u> <u>it's gained</u> over its many years of watching.'

3) '<u>Time</u> is <u>telling you</u> to get on with it and take action.'

4) 'As you step into your <u>inner temple</u> and notice the energy <u>it's sending you</u>.'

5) 'That's it. I can almost hear your <u>computer calling you</u> myself. <u>It's saying</u>: 'Write the book. Write the book'. [This is a bit of a border-line example, which falls within the spirit of the law, in as much as the speaker has said: 'I can almost hear...', which implies that it is a metaphorical expression. Of course, all the other examples are really metaphors too.]'

Semantically Charged Words

<u>The Pattern</u>:

1) 'Something good has happened. Something has changed. And you fully comprehend it.'

2) 'And as you deservedly experience these feelings of peace and tranquillity...'

3) 'That's right.   And you can totally notice the difference.'

4) 'Okay. Truthfully now – you're ready to change?'

5) 'Being a therapist means that you're working compassionately to help others and that's a good place to be.'

<u>The Structure</u>:

Semantically Charged Words amplify the strength of the sentences of which they form part. They turn the intensity of the meaning which is being conveyed up several levels. Rather than 'she is caring'; it becomes; 'she is <u>totally</u> caring', or 'she is <u>extremely</u> caring', or 'she is <u>fervently</u> caring', or 'she is <u>passionately</u> caring'. (How many readers recall Tony Robbins using an expression like, for example: 'She was <u>totally</u> jazzed...'?)

<u>The Pattern</u>:

1) 'Something good has happened. Something has changed. And you <u>fully</u> comprehend it.'

2) 'And as you <u>deservedly</u> experience these feelings of peace and tranquillity...'

3) 'That's right. And you can <u>totally</u> notice the difference.'

4) 'Okay. <u>Truthfully</u> now – you're ready to change?'

5) 'Being a therapist means that you're working <u>compassionately</u> to help others and that is a good place to be.'

The semantic element of a conversation relates to the <u>meaning</u> being conveyed. So, Semantically Charged Words are words which convey <u>a charged meaning</u> to the context in which they appear.

Sensation Double Binds

<u>The Pattern</u>:

1) 'And I wonder if you will become aware of new feelings of positivity or inspiration?'

2) 'And the inner you knows how to do this. And it can help you feel better by feeling more confident.

And by feeling more calm. And I wonder, what will you feel, more confident or more calm?'

3) 'How is it going to happen? How are you going to notice the changes? Will they appear as a sense of relief or freedom?'

4) 'Happiness is a curious thing. For some people it begins to take root as a feeling of liberating indifference around inconsequential things that used to unnecessarily bother them, but which never really needed to. For others it starts as a feeling that there is a lot of good in the world – if you only just choose to notice it. How will your happiness start: As a feeling of liberating indifference or a feeling of good in the world?'

5) 'Improvements can take place at any time. A wave of relaxation or a sense of peacefulness? Both are possible. But what will your unconscious start to let you notice first?'

The Structure:

This pattern is basically a Double Bind – but with an emphasis on sensation. Because therapists are generally working with issues relating to cognition (thinking) and emotion (feelings/sensation) it can be useful to become adept at introducing emotional options (choice) to clients in order to help them to shift from 'stuck states' to other available ranges of emotional experience. Remember Simple Binds ('would you like the red one or the blue one?') can be chosen at a conscious level ('I'd like the blue one thanks!'), whereas Double Binds can only be chosen unconsciously, which means that we have to wait and see what the answer is. We have to wait for the answer to manifest (as a behaviour, thought process, etc) in order to know what it is. (Hypnotherapist: 'Will you feel calmer or more relaxed as your eyes close? What do you notice as your eyes are closing? Client: 'Umm. I'm starting to feel calmer'.)

1) 'And I wonder if you will become aware of new feelings [new feelings are the focus of the Bind] of positivity [possibility one] or inspiration [possibility two]?'

2) 'And the inner you knows how to do this. And it can help you feel better [feeling better is the focus of the Bind] by feeling more confident. And by feeling more calm. And I wonder, what will you feel, more confident [possibility one] or more calm [possibility two]?'

3) 'How is it going to happen? How are you going to notice the changes [changes are the focus of the Bind]? Will they appear as a sense of relief [possibility one] or freedom [possibility two]?'

4) 'Happiness [the focus of the Bind] is a curious thing. For some people it begins to take root as a feeling of liberating indifference around inconsequential things that used to unnecessarily bother them, but which never really needed to. For others it starts as a feeling that there is a lot of good in the world – if you only just choose to notice it. How will your happiness [the focus of the Bind] start: As a feeling of liberating indifference [possibility one] or a feeling of good in the world [possibility two]?'

5) 'Improvements [the focus of the Bind] can take place at any time. A wave of relaxation [possibility one] or a sense of peacefulness [possibility two]? Both are possible. But what will your unconscious start to let you notice first?'

Sensing [See also Mind Reading]

The Pattern:

1) 'You know that I sense you are getting ready to change.'

2) 'I sense that something good is taking place within you.'

3) 'I sense that you are ready to start to do something different.'

4) 'I sense you do know what the answer is.'

5) 'I sense you know what you must do next.'

The Structure:

This is a form of 'Mind Reading'. By using the expression 'I sense' the therapist has, by implication, an insight into the client's thoughts and emotions. Hypnotically, when used appropriately, this can enhance rapport. It often adds a sense of authority to the statement being made. Sensing, along with other forms of Mind Reading, when used in conjunction with each other, offer a greater range of opportunities to utilise 'Mind Reading' principles to help clients, without what is occurring becoming too obvious, due to repetition of form.

(For example: I <u>sense</u> that the changes are going to pleasantly surprise you. I <u>know</u> you will enjoy them and I <u>think</u> they are going to take place sooner than you expected. Because I <u>understand</u> that you are ready to change now...)

1) 'You know that <u>I sense</u> **you are getting ready to change**.'

2) '<u>I sense</u> that **something good is taking place within you**.'

3) '<u>I sense</u> that **you are ready to start to do something different**.'

4) '<u>I sense</u> **you do know what the answer is**.'

5) '<u>I sense</u> **you know what you must do next**.'

Sensory Overload

<u>The Pattern</u>:

'And you don't have to not think about your left foot left there right now or when trance is going to happening right now you sense that that's right you sense that that trance is happening but you don't not never have to go right inside right now you can listen to what you hear here or hear here what you are listening too as a part of you can hear the rhythm of the clock while not focusing on the sensations of the chair which are gently supporting you and every time you listen to the sound of my voice a part of you can count backwards from 100 to 1 thinking or not thinking about those hands resting in your lap...or that left foot left resting right here right now...as you continue to take it easy.'

The <u>Structure</u>:

As the name suggests, the senses (inner and outer) are overloaded (at a conscious level) so that the client will find it difficult to over-analyse what's taking place and instead just relax and let the unconscious mind come to the fore and help. As in the previous example of the Confusion Technique (covered above) the final element of the communication, however, is very clear, because, after a state of confusion, such as that which is generated by Sensory Overload, the mind looks for a way out of the uncertainty, and it will hone in on the first obvious statement/suggestion that follows the Sensory Overload/Confusion state.

'And you don't have to not... think about your left foot... left... there... right... now... or when trance is going to... happening right now... you sense... that... that's right... you sense that... that trance... is happening... but you don't... not never... have to... go right inside... right now... you can listen to what you hear... here... or hear... here... what you are listening too... as a part of you can.... hear the rhythm of the clock... while not focusing on... the sensations of the chair... which are gently... supporting... you... and every time you listen to the sound of my voice.... a part of you can... count backwards from 100 to 1... thinking or not thinking about those hands... resting in your lap...or that left foot... left resting... right here... right now...as you continue to **take it easy**.'

Sensory Specific Language

Sensory Specific Language is a term used in NLP to denote communication which purposefully does not allow for personal interpretation of an observed event to colour the therapist's communication. In 'strict' NLP-speak rather than saying 'you're looking upset' you'd say, perhaps, 'I notice you're frowning', or instead of: 'he was livid', you'd say, 'he thumped his fist on the table, his face turned red and the veins on his neck stood out'. (Maybe adding: 'I think he may have been livid.') In reality, an understanding of the difference between personal interpretation of an observed event and the reality of the event is useful because it can help therapists exercise caution around introducing their own ideas into what's being observed and/or commented on. (Maurice Chevalier's song 'I Remember It Well' is a wonderful example of how an interpretation, or memory, of an event can be peculiar to the observer, and not necessarily a factual interpretation, or recollection, of what actually occurred.) As with the use of 'clinical' Clean Language, however, in real life, a middle ground is usually found, in which the therapist is careful to ensure that they do not 'jump to conclusions' and colour things with their own interpretation, while, at the same time, the language does not become so analytical that the rapport element within a natural human interaction becomes 'lost' in the 'technique'.

Serial Suggestions

The Pattern:

'And you can send a relaxing feeling into those feet, and then allow it to let those legs relax too, those knees, upper legs and then that upper body unwinding, and those shoulders, arms, neck and head all just feeling very comfortable now.'

The Structure:

Serial Suggestions are suggestions which are offered in a <u>sequential</u> fashion. They can act to compound each other so that the focus of the message (which in the above example is about relaxing into trance) is reinforced by all the other components of the sequence.

Here's another example:

'And as you begin to write, you can notice a sense of creativity and as your fingers begin to work on the keyboard that sense of inspiration can increase and as you continue to type the words that you find easily appear...your creativity can increase... as you continue to write your book... and with every word you type...you notice a sense of inspiration and the knowledge that things are moving forward.'

Shifting

The Pattern:

'How do you feel about feeling angry?'

<u>The Structure</u>:

Shifting is useful for helping a client to move beyond a 'stuck state' and to consider another point of reference to the one they've been 'trapped' in or habituated to. By asking 'How do you feel about feeling...?', the client will usually shift to another emotional frame of reference (metaphorically 'taking a step away' from the named emotion, so that they can 'see the wood' and not just 'the trees').

Another approach, which is in the form of a suggestion that's designed to help a client shift from one limiting belief into another (helpful belief) is one that I learned from Neil French who delivered hypno-analysis training courses for many years. It is a nice suggestion which I've used many times since first being introduced to it. Here it is: 'Something that you thought would be difficult turns out to be ridiculously easy'.

Shock

Milton Erickson, Richard Bandler, Anthony Robbins and, the founder of Provocative Therapy, Frank Farrelly all use 'shock' to help people 'snap out of' habituated self-defeating attitudes.

Farrelly is a master of the art and I recommend seeing him live (along with reading his must-have book called Provocative Therapy, co-written with Jeff Brandsma). The 'shock' can be introduced through the use of precision directed 'profanity', unexpected behaviour, humour and whatever else is appropriate in any given moment. For instance:

1)

<u>Shock</u>:

Client:

'You can spot evil people a mile off. Good people are polite - and evil people aren't!'

Therapist:

'Damn it, you're right! I totally agree with you.'

2)

<u>Unexpected Behaviour</u>:

Client:

'I must tell you before we go any further that I have three degrees and I'm a Fellow of the Fellowship of Top Business Managers.'

Therapist:

Looking disinterested: 'So you're that important huh!'

3)

<u>Humour</u>:

Client:

'I'm not sure you can fully understand what I'm telling you?'

Therapist:

'Hold up! Wait I minute! I <u>do</u> understand what you're saying. And I'm not surprised. You're English! People expect that kind of opinion from English people!'

[See also: The Wizard of Wisconsin appendix below which is a detailed article about Frank Farrelly's approach to psychiatric work. Frank was trained directly by Carl Rogers, the developer of Person Centred Counselling and he was himself (Frank) extensively modelled by Richard Bandler and John Grinder, the developers of NLP.]

Shoelace Tying

This is a useful point of reference in order to begin to 'play down the conscious mind' by 'playing up' the unconscious mind. Many clients will have wrestled with their problems, at a conscious level, for some considerable time before seeking hypnotherapy. This, axiomatically suggests that its resolution lies outside of the conscious mind's lone ability to resolve. So, by appealing to another element of the person's Greater Self it can act to create a sense of expectancy and hope (which is itself therapeutic) while also shifting the balance in the direction of eliciting unconscious intervention.

How does shoelace tying fit into this? Well, for most people this is a form of universal experience. We all tie our shoelaces, without having to think very much about how we do it. In fact if we did have to think about it, in order to explain it to someone else, it would probably become harder than expected. However, most everyone can do it without thinking about <u>how</u> they're doing it, on cue. So, by using this example of unconscious learning a distinction can be made between a person's conscious and unconscious resources, with the emphasis placed upon the greater resources which are available to the unconscious mind.

<u>Here's an example</u>:

'I hear what you're saying. I empathise with how you're feeling and how difficult this has been. And it seems to me that what you've learned from all of this is that you want to change – after all you've tried lots of ways to do so – but you just haven't consciously discovered how. And that's okay, because sometimes it's better to let your unconscious show you how. After all – you can tie your shoelaces can't you? And you don't have to think about how you do it. That's because you just naturally let your unconscious knowledge of how to do it translate itself into all of those movements that are necessary in taking the laces in each hand, and threading them in a certain way to make a bow. Without really having to give it much thought! Just like you don't have to consciously think about doing the breathing you're doing for yourself. Your unconscious does that for you too. Just like it governs all of the other miracles within that help your body to work so well. And it even knows where the next thought is coming from before you've consciously thought it. So, how about you stop trying too hard to consciously sort this out? Give yourself a bit of a rest. Quit wrestling with it and let your unconscious mind – the part of you which ties your shoelaces for you without you really having to think very much about it – help you out instead now.'

Silence

<u>The Pattern</u>:

The use of <u>strategic</u> silence can be very useful.

<u>The Structure</u>:

Silence is a useful tool. It can be employed for example to allow moments of quiet during the delivery of hypnotherapy in order to give clients time to sort, evaluate, make sense of and explore their thoughts and experiences. It can also be utilised to generate a sense of <u>expectancy</u> as the listener waits for the next word to be spoken:

'The use of strategic ………………………………………… silence …can be very ………………………………………… useful.'

Simple Binds

[See Bind.]

Simple Deletion

The Pattern:

1) 'And as you sense things are developing...'

2) 'And that specific idea...'

3) 'Those feelings continue...'

4) 'Certain thoughts are thought....'

5) 'How nice it is to relax into a pleasant state of hypnosis and become aware of changes. Lots of people do this you know, every day around the world and they enjoy those changes too...'

The Structure:

1) 'And as you sense things... [What things specifically?] are developing...'

2) 'And that specific idea... [What specific idea specifically?]'

3) 'Those feelings... [What feelings specifically?]'

4) 'Certain thoughts... [What thoughts specifically?] are thought.'

5) 'How nice it is to relax into a pleasant state of hypnosis and become aware of changes [What changes specifically?]. Lots of people do this you know, every day around the world and they enjoy those changes [What changes specifically?] too.'

Something that is referred to, but is not specified has been, in these examples, in effect, 'deleted' from each sentence and is therefore left up to the unconscious mind to conclude. Non specific phrases like this can generate a very 'trancey' atmosphere and, in the context of the supportive and directed-at-the-best-possible-outcome context in which such suggestions are set they can therefore help to elicit good levels of trance and overall high levels of receptivity to the entire therapy process. The client becomes accustomed to the indirect approach of the therapy and tends to 'go with the flow' of the indirectness and implied suggestions (along with the direct suggestions which usually form a part of most hypnotherapy sessions) which maximises the opportunity of positive unconscious intervention and support.

Simple Generalisation

The Pattern:

1) 'And as those resources become available to you.'

2) 'So those talents which you have.'

3) 'Making those old problems fade away.'

4) 'Discovering ideas which help you.'

5) 'Letting go of problems and taking hold of solutions.'

<u>The Structure</u>:

This language pattern introduces generalised concepts (which are also Simple Deletions) in the form of Nominalisations in order to introduce a 'universal classification' into what's being addressed (thereby making it generalised) in order that by extending the reference frame from specific to general the therapist can maximise the positive impact of the emphasis being offered. For instance in Example 5, immediately above, rather than a 'problem' being referred to 'problems' are addressed in the context of a therapeutic intervention (which implies a wider healing event) as 'solutions' (not a 'solution') are introduced.

1) 'And as those <u>resources</u> become available to you.'

2) 'So those <u>talents</u> which you have.'

3) 'Making those old <u>problems</u> fade away.'

4) 'Discovering <u>ideas</u> which help you.'

5) 'Letting go of <u>problems</u> and taking hold of <u>solutions</u>.'

Simple Time Bind

<u>The Pattern</u>:

1) 'Would you like to start on this today or tomorrow?'

2) 'Would you prefer to do this now or in a few moments?'

3) 'What would work best for you? Doing this this evening or tomorrow morning?'

4) 'Okay. So you're going to write out an action plan. Shall we do this now or after this meeting?'

5) 'Are you going to go into a nice trance right now or in a moment or two?'

The Structure:

This is a nice language pattern which can be introduced to presuppose that something will take place. The only question (seemingly) is when?

1) 'Would you like to start on this <u>today</u> or <u>tomorrow</u>?'

2) 'Would you prefer to do this <u>now</u> or <u>in a few moments</u>?'

3) 'What would work best for you? Doing this <u>this evening</u> or <u>tomorrow morning</u>?'

4) 'Okay. So you're going to write out an action plan. Shall we do this <u>now</u> or <u>after</u> this meeting?'

5) 'Are you going to go into a nice trance right <u>now</u> or <u>in a moment or two</u>?'

Some People...

The Pattern:

1) 'Some people find the changes happen within hours and some people notice them instantly.'

2) 'Some people like to allow the changes to gently happen in their own good time.'

3) 'Some people find that it's good to reconsider things, from a different perspective.'

4) 'Some people like to go into trance to experience its benefits often.'

5) 'Some people find that things just seem to gently work themselves out almost 'all by themselves'.'

The Structure:

I recall hearing hypnotherapist Robert Farago use the 'some people' pattern very well. It's basically a form of metaphor, of the type used by Milton Erickson in his, now famous, 'My Friend John' approach. By using the expression 'some people' and then explaining what the 'some people' being referred to do, in a given situation, it allows the therapist the opportunity to offer suggestions which are less likely to be consciously challenged, criticised or over analysed by the client, because the therapist is not giving the client direct instructions, he/she is, instead, simply letting the client know about what 'some people' do in similar situations. This will generally create a 'follow response' in the sense that the client will begin to do the same thing as the 'some people' being referred to.

Sorting Patterns:

<u>The Pattern</u>:

1)

A)

'That's right – and the further away you push that image the smaller it becomes.'

B)

'So...as all these good things are drawing closer, right into your life...you will become aware of how improved things are.'

C)

'Good! Well done! That's it. Just move right away from that old way you used to think about it as you now move closer...and closer...and closer towards that positive feeling...until it becomes a part of you.'

2)

A)

'So, let's specifically consider what exactly do you need to do next, first?'

2)

'Let's do something.'

C)

'Let's specifically reframe that particular picture of you in the school playground and then replace it with something better.'

3)

A)

'Just think, how many others will this project that you've started benefit?'

B)

'Consider how much better your life is going to be when you do this.'

C)

'I agree with you. It's a good idea and it seems to me that this is a really 'win-win' situation too. You benefit and so does everyone else too!'

4)

A)

'So, what's good about this?'

B)

'So, what don't you like about smoking?'

C)

'So, first, tell me what don't you like about smoking? And then tell me what is good about being a non-smoker?'

5)

A)

'What do you think is best?'

B)

'What do you think everyone else will think is best?'

C)

'So, it seems to me that everyone else will be in agreement. That's what you think?'

6)

A)

'So, you want a better job. What can you do to begin to find one?'

B)

'So, you're in debt by about £100,000. What must you first do to begin to clear it?'

C)

'So, the good news is, you know you can get a better job and that will help you start to clear those debts that you need to deal with.'

7)

A)

'Yes. If you've practised self-hypnosis before you'll find that hypnotherapy is very similar.'

B)

'Of course, hypnotherapy is different from self-hypnosis. The difference is that in hypnotherapy someone else is guiding you through the process.'

C)

'Because self-hypnosis and hypnotherapy are very similar you already know pretty much what to experience, the only difference being is that I'll be joining in with you.'

8)

A)

'Okay. So what can you do now?'

B)

'Right. Tell me about what needs to take place next?'

C)

'Okay. So tell me first, what do you need to do now? And then what?'

<u>The Structure</u>:

Sorting Patterns language draws on the distinctions made in NLP about how people/groups of people categorise the world and their experiences in it. They are (Sorting Patterns) quite polar (it's 'this' <u>or</u> 'that'). The hypnotherapist who understands this principle can use the skill to ascertain which natural Sorting Patterns the client is using and as a result choose his/her language to fit, therefore being more influential because of the natural rapport which will be taking place. Sometimes the hypnotherapist may choose to make reference to both polar extremes of the pattern being employed in order to highlight the contrast – and sometimes the mutually beneficial elements of both.

1)

<u>Moving Away From</u>

A)

'That's right – and the <u>further away you push that image</u> the smaller it becomes.'

<u>Moving Towards</u>

B)

'So...as all these good things are <u>drawing closer</u>, right into your life...you will become aware of how improved things are.'

<u>Moving Away From and Towards</u>

C)

'Good! Well done! That's it. Just <u>move right away from</u> that old way you used to think about it as you now <u>move closer</u>...and <u>closer</u>...and <u>closer</u> towards that positive feeling...until it becomes a part of you.'

2)

<u>Specificity</u>

A)

'So, let's <u>specifically</u> consider what <u>exactly</u> do you need to do <u>next</u>, <u>first</u>?'

<u>Generality</u>

2)

'Let's do <u>something</u>.'

Specificity and Generality

C)

'Let's <u>specifically</u> reframe that <u>particular</u> picture of <u>you in the school playground</u> and then replace it with <u>something better</u>.'

3)

Sorting For Others

A)

'Just think, how many <u>others</u> will this project that you've started benefit?'

Sorting For Self

B)

'Consider how much better <u>your life</u> is going to be when you do this.'

Sorting For Others and For Self

C)

'I agree with you. It's a good idea and it seems to me that this is a really 'win-win' situation too. <u>You benefit</u> and so does <u>everyone else</u> too!'

4)

A)

Sorting For Good

'So, what's <u>good</u> about this?'

B)

<u>Sorting For Bad</u>

'So, what <u>don't you like</u> about smoking?'

C)

<u>Sorting For Good And Bad</u>

'So, first, tell me <u>what don't you like about smoking</u>?   And then tell me <u>what is good about being a non-smoker?</u>'

5)

A)

<u>Internal Frame Of Reference</u>

'What do <u>you think</u> is best?'

B)

<u>External Frame of Reference</u>

'What do you think <u>everyone else will think</u> is best?'

C)

<u>Internal And External Frames of Reference</u>

'So, it seems to me that <u>everyone else</u> will be in agreement. That's what <u>you think</u>?'

6)

Possibility

A)

'So, you want a better job. What <u>can</u> you do to begin to find one?'

Necessity

B)

'So, you're in debt by about £100,000. What <u>must</u> you first do to begin to clear it?'

Possibility And Necessity

C)

'So, the good news is, you know <u>you can</u> get a better job and that will help you start to clear those debts that <u>you need</u> to deal with.'

7)

Similarity

A)

'Yes. If you've practised self-hypnosis before you'll find that hypnotherapy is very <u>similar</u>.'

Difference

B)

'Of course, hypnotherapy is <u>different</u> from self-hypnosis. The difference is that in hypnotherapy someone else is guiding you through the process.'

Similarity And Difference

C)

'Because self-hypnosis and hypnotherapy are very <u>similar</u> you already know pretty much what to experience, the only <u>difference</u> being is that I'll be joining in with you.'

8)

A)

In Time

'Okay. So what can you do <u>now</u>?'

B)

Through Time

'Right. Tell me about what needs to take place <u>next</u>?'

C)

In Time And Through Time

'Okay. So tell me first, what do you need to do now? And then what?'

[The terms 'In Time' and 'Through Time' are not as obvious in their meaning as are the other divisions of Sorting Patterns covered above. Simply put, generally speaking, people who are deemed to be 'In Time' tend to live in (are associated to) the present moment (if you were to ask an In Time person to spatially locate the past and the present in relation to where they were standing, there's a pretty good chance that the past would be behind them and the future in front of them) whereas people who are 'Through Time' (tending to be dissociated from the present) have an awareness of time as something of a linear continuum stretching out in front of them (in which they have a perception, in their minds, of the past, present and future laid out before them 'over there' from right to left; they 'see' the expanse of time, in a panoramic sort of way, whereas an In Time person tends to be located 'in the moment' with time situated behind and ahead of them].

So, What Does This Tell You? Let Me Tell You...

The Pattern:

'So, what does this tell you...let me tell you...it means that you can now do ABC with a greater sense of flexibility...and...'

The Structure:

The 'So, what does this tell you, let me tell you…' pattern allows the hypnotherapist to raise a question in the client's mind and then quickly suggest a therapeutic answer that by implication is 'owned' by the client because the premise is based on the phrase/question 'so what does this tell you'. To arrive at an answer which is accepted by the client it means that that's what it 'tells' them.

For Example:

'So, <u>what does this tell you</u>…**let me tell you**…<u>it means that</u> you can now do ABC with a greater sense of flexibility…and…'

[Obviously the 'let me tell you' suggestion that follows must be within the realm of the client's stated desired outcome and ability to attain.]

Specific Deletions

The Pattern:

1) 'That thing that you've been thinking about in detail which you've told me that you want to change…let's begin to change it now.'

2) 'You've wanted to reconsider the way you do this for a long time now. You've been looking for ways to increase your choices. You told me that up until now you only had that one option, but now we are going to create more for you…'

3) 'You specifically want to experience more of this better emotion. You know what it is, why you want it and when you want to experience it...so let's start to make it happen now.'

The Structure:

In this pattern, something(s) has been deleted, but it is referred to so specifically, that its meaning is understood.

1) 'That thing that you've been thinking about in detail which you've told me that you want to change [the deleted element will be quite clear to the client, due to the specificity surrounding the context in which it's being referred to]...let's begin to change it now.'

2) 'You've wanted to reconsider the way you do this for a long time now [in this example, what is deleted is something that the client has talked with the therapist about – so it's obvious what is meant]. You've been looking for ways to increase your choices [This too, refers, in this example, to something that has been discussed and understood by the client and the therapist, so the meaning is quite specific]. You told me that up until now you only had that one option, but now we are going to create more for you...'

3) 'You specifically want to experience more of this better emotion [The words 'this better emotion', clearly relate to a particular emotion, already understood by both the client and the therapist.] You know what it is [This, in this context is a Truism, while the 'what it is', while specifically referred to is deleted – and this theme continues in

the words that follow], why you want it [it is specifically understood, if not specifically 'labelled'] and when you want to experience it [and again, 'it' is understood, while not called by 'its' name]...so let's start to make it happen now.'

Spelling The Suggestion

<u>The Pattern</u>:

Spelling suggestions can enhance the positive impact of the meaning of the word being spelt out to the client.

<u>The Structure</u>:

1) 'I wonder when you will first notice feelings of **C...A...L...M**...?'

2) 'You can begin to feel...**G...O...O...D**...!'

3) 'The wonderful thing about beginning to ... **R... E... L... A... X**... is...'

4) 'Now is the time to introduce some...**F... U... N**... into your life.'

5) 'You've been very busy but now is a good time to take it easy... **S... L... O... W**... down and relax.'

Spurious Not

<u>The Pattern</u>:

1) 'Consider.   Are you not already noticing the difference?'

2) 'And is it not nice to know that you're improving already?'

3) 'And I'm curious about whether you might not already know more about this than you think?'

4) 'And I wonder are you not already thinking about things differently?'

5) 'Could you not already be improving?'

<u>The Structure</u>:

The use of the word not is actually used in such a way that it elicits agreement.

1) 'Consider.   Are you <u>not</u> **already noticing the difference**?'

2) 'And is it <u>not</u> nice to know that **you're improving already**?'

3) 'And I'm curious about whether you might <u>not</u> **already know more about this than you think**?'

4) 'And I wonder are you <u>not</u> already **thinking about things differently**?'

5) 'Could you <u>not</u> already **be improving**?'

Stacking

<u>The Pattern</u>:

1) 'Consider. If you do this today, how much better are things going to be already by tomorrow and then how much better are they going to be for the future?'

2) 'Think about what improvements you're going to notice and then imagine how this is going to positively impact your life.'

3) 'Suppose you did say 'yes' to this opportunity. Just think about how much better things are going to be. What will you notice changes in your life?'

4) 'Maybe! Just maybe? If you started this today and then did this next, things would begin to improve so much that you'd achieve both of these goals by next week and the cumulative effect would be so helpful that everything else would get easier as a result?'

5) 'Take a moment to marvel about how simple it would be to fill in that application form and as a result you'd be enrolled and that means that your life will be changing massively for the better. How great is that!'

<u>The Structure</u>:

Stacking involves helping the client to build an internal representation of an outcome that's very compelling. The hypnotherapist can do this by Stacking concept upon concept.

1) 'Consider. If you <u>do this today</u>, how <u>much better</u> are <u>things</u> going to be <u>already</u> by <u>tomorrow</u> and then <u>how much better</u> are they <u>going to be</u> for the <u>future</u>?'

2) 'Think about what <u>improvements</u> you're going to <u>notice</u> and then <u>imagine</u> how <u>this is going to positively impact your life</u>.'

3) '<u>Suppose</u> you did say 'yes' to this <u>opportunity</u>. Just <u>think</u> about how <u>much better</u> <u>things</u> are going to be. What will you notice <u>changes</u> in <u>your life</u>?'

4) '<u>Maybe</u>! Just <u>maybe</u>? If <u>you started this today</u> and then did <u>this next</u>, <u>things</u> would begin to <u>improve</u> <u>so much</u> that you'd <u>achieve</u> both of these <u>goals</u> by <u>next week</u> and the <u>cumulative effect</u> would be <u>so helpful</u> that <u>everything else</u> would get <u>easier as a result</u>?'

5) 'Take a moment to <u>marvel</u> about how <u>simple</u> it would be to <u>fill in that application form</u> and as a <u>result</u> you'd be <u>enrolled</u> and that means that your <u>life will be changing massively</u> for the <u>better</u>. <u>How great is that</u>!'

Static Words

<u>The Pattern</u>:

1) 'NLP teaches us that all problems can be solved instantly.'

2) 'Psychotherapy says that the roots of psychological problems can be traced back to childhood.'

3) 'Everyone knows that hypnotherapy causes people to go instantly into a trance.'

4) 'Hypnosis will never put me under.'

5) 'History shows us that you can't trust Martians.'

The Structure:

The term Static Words refers to words that are used as if they have a fixed meaning. The static word appears to represent an entire class. However, by honing in on the specifics and recovering the edited information alternative interpretations can be drawn.

1) 'NLP teaches us that all problems can be solved instantly.'

All forms of NLP? Is the field of NLP represented by one body which speaks for everyone?

2) 'Psychotherapy says that the roots of psychological problems can be traced back to childhood.'

All forms of Psychotherapy? Do any schools of psychotherapy teach otherwise?

3) 'Everyone knows that hypnotherapy causes people to go instantly into a trance.'

All hypnotherapy? Is there any hypnotherapy which doesn't cause people to go instantly into a trance?

4) 'Hypnosis will never put me under.'

What hypnosis? Is there only one kind of hypnosis? Is there a hypnosis that could put you under?

5) 'History shows us that you can't trust Martians.'

All history? Is there any history which shows that Martians can be trusted? Is there only one interpretation of history?

Stop

The Pattern:

1) 'Stop and think for a moment...'

2) 'Stop and consider how things might be if...'

3) 'Stop and notice exactly what takes place as...'

4) 'Stop and let yourself take it easy...'

5) 'Okay. Let yourself stop and slow down for a moment.'

The Structure:

We're all conditioned to respond to the word 'stop' at an early stage in life. This conditioning can be utilised to introduce a pause in a client's train of thought in order to suggest something helpful. 'Stop ...and ABC'.

Style Of No Style

This is not so much a language pattern but the embodiment of an ideal. Bruce Lee the revolutionary developer and exponent of various martial arts principles also stated that the highest form of martial prowess was a form without form. Rather than rigid, fixed models of behaviour he favoured a 'style of no style'. This was based on his concept of 'Learn the rules then dissolve the rules'. Which is to say, that to become proficient you must first learn your art by 'the rules' until you reach a point that you no longer need a fixed structure but are instead fluid and natural and able work spontaneously. This is the mark of a good hypnotherapist/NLP practitioner. The habitual use of fixed scripts or rote, step-by-step NLP techniques, is by its very nature a limited way of working. Whereas, starting with scripts, and techniques can be useful, but excellence comes from learning the principles and then being fluid enough to use them in wider ways. The same is true of Indirect Hypnotherapy language patterns. First there is the learning of the patterns, often in a rote way. That helps to 'get the feel' of what's being learned. In fact, that's how I myself learned many of them, at first. I repeated the various language patterns to myself over and over until they became committed to memory, then I disassembled each pattern – much like many of them have been detailed in this book and then I reassembled them again. I repeated this until I understood the operating principles behind the rote patterns that I'd learned. At that point, I like to believe, I began to move beyond fixed examples and into more fluid indirect language.

Submodality Language

<u>The Pattern</u>:

1) 'Listen up to what your unconscious is telling you.'

2) 'If you don't start to do something it could turn into a bitter experience.'

3) 'Get in touch with your own sense of what is right.'

4) 'You'll begin to notice the sweet smell of success.'

5) 'Move yourself closer to making your dreams your reality.'

6) 'Never let yourself forget it.'

7) 'You can make your future brighter starting right now.'

<u>The Structure</u>:

Submodality Language is used to influence the client's submodality experience. This can add importance and deeper meaning to what's being said.

1)

<u>Auditory</u>

'<u>Listen up</u> to what your unconscious is telling you.'

There are many other words that can influence auditory submodalities. Some of them include: hear, loud, noisy, quiet, sounds.

2)

Gustatory / Taste

'If you don't start to do something it could turn into a <u>bitter</u> experience.'

There are many other words that can influence gustatory submodalities. Some of them include: sharp, sour, sweet, tangy, and tasteful.

3)

Kinaesthetic / Feeling

'Get <u>in touch</u> with your own sense of what is right.'

There are many other words that can influence kinaesthetic submodalities. Some of them include: comfortable, feeling, heavy, light, warmth.

4)

Olfactory / Smell

'You'll begin to notice the <u>sweet</u> smell of success.'

There are many other words that can influence olfactory submodalities. Some of them include: aroma, fragrance, perfume, scent, smell.

5)

<u>Space</u>

'Move yourself <u>closer</u> to making your dreams your reality.'

There are many other words that can influence spatial submodalities. Some of them include: area, break, closeness, expanse, distance.

6)

<u>Time</u>

'<u>Never</u> let yourself forget it.'

There are many other words that can influence temporal submodalities. Some of them include: future, historically, now, past, then.

7)

<u>Visual</u>

'You can make your future <u>brighter</u> starting right now.'

There are many other words that can influence visual submodalities. Some of them include: Brilliant, clear, dark, intense, vivid.

Subordinate Clause Of Time

<u>The Pattern</u>:

1) 'As you go into trance...'

2) 'Prior to making the changes you might notice...'

3) 'After your unconscious has improved things...'

4) 'During the hypnosis you will...'

5) 'Since you've decided to shift a couple of stone...'

6) 'When you do this you will notice that...'

7) 'While this happens this can happen too...'

8) 'Before you go into trance remember...expect the best...because the best is the best to expect...'

<u>The Structure</u>:

The Subordinate Clause of Time works on the level of temporal perception and presupposition. Each of the above examples includes a presupposition, which is generated by the part which refers to time.

1) '<u>As</u> you go into trance... [Going into trance is presupposed]'

2) '<u>Prior</u> to making the changes you might notice... [Making changes is presupposed]'

3) '<u>After</u> your unconscious has improved things [Improvement is presupposed]'

4) 'During the hypnosis you will... [Hypnosis is presupposed]'

5) 'Since you've decided to shift a couple of stone... [A decision that has been made is presupposed]'

6) 'When you do this you will notice that... [Doing 'this' is presupposed]'

7) 'While this happens this can happen too... [Something happening is presupposed]'

8) 'Before you go into trance remember...expect the best...because the best is the best to expect... [Going into trance is presupposed]'

Suggestion Of Unconscious Learning / Behaviour

The Pattern:

'And while you may have consciously not been aware of all of those things you have just learned.... didn't you(?)... your unconscious can remember for you... didn't it? After all... how many times have you remembered something from long ago which you'd thought you'd forgotten but which your unconscious has remembered?'

The Structure:

This is another example (of the same category as the one covered above called Shoelace Tying) in which emphasis is placed upon unconscious learning, which can help to 'play down' the conscious mind's involvement and 'play up' the unconscious mind's resources and involvement.

'And while you may have <u>consciously</u> not been aware of all of those things <u>you have just learned</u>…. didn't you(?)… your <u>unconscious can remember for you</u>… didn't it?   After all… <u>how many times have you remembered something from long ago</u> which you'd thought you'd forgotten <u>but which your unconscious has remembered</u>? [This example is based on a language pattern that I learned from Alan Jones, a hypnotherapist and NLP trainer.   It also includes an emphasis on recovering memory.]'

Suggestions To Generate Arm Levitation

<u>The Pattern</u>:

'I don't know whether you will discover your right arm lifting by itself or your left arm moving before you notice it.'

<u>The Structure</u>:

'I don't know [this statement is a Truism, because only the client can know] whether you will discover your right arm lifting [this is an Embedded Command to suggest the lifting of the arm] by itself [this is a Conscious Unconscious Double Bind] or your left arm moving before you notice it [this is a Double Dissociated Double Bind].'

Contingent Suggestion Addition (to the above):

'…**As** you discover something NOW. Some people find that their arm begins to lift spontaneously in trance. **And** what's that happening to that arm now?'

If Arm Doesn't Levitate:

'Isn't that curious about how maybe you wondered about that heaviness that you may not have noticed until now.'

[This example is based on my observations of Stephen Brooks' approach to achieving arm levitation. I've employed it myself in practice, amongst other approaches, and found that it works well. One of my favourite approaches is one I learned from Richard Bandler. Basically you say something like: 'Okay! Lift your arm up to here. That's right. And now close your eyes and go allll the way dowwwwn'. You're guaranteed a levitation with this approach, <u>because you begin with one</u>!]

Switch Referential Index (Sleight of Mouth)

Sleight of Mouth principles were first delineated by Robert Dilts as he himself modelled Richard Bandler's language patterns. Additional contributions have been made by Steve and Connirae Andreas. A number of Sleight of Mouth patterns now exist, which are covered in this book. Sleight of Mouth patterns are utilised to unravel and in the process depotentiate adverse Complex Equivalence and/or Cause and Effect statements made by the client. [See: Analogy, Another Outcome, Apply To Self, Challenge, Change Of Reference Frame Size, Chunk Size, Consequences, Counter Example, Hierarchy Of Criteria, Intention, Meta Frame, Model Of The World, Reality Strategy,

Redefine, Switch Referential Index.] In this example the principle of Switch Referential Index is employed.

The Pattern:

Client statement:

'Always wondering makes me feel inadequate.'

'(A) Always wondering (B) makes me feel inadequate.'

The Structure:

A)

'I wonder as well.'

'Others wonder too.'

B)

'I wonder what else you could feel other than inadequate?'

A/B)

'I wonder and I don't feel inadequate.'

'Wouldn't it be weird if whenever we wondered about anything we all felt inadequate?'

'Sylver Method'

I remember learning a language pattern which was attributed to the American stage hypnotist, Marshall Sylver, which I think is useful for generating a solution-focussed state with clients, while affirming their ability to make choices. It also helps to depotentiate 'resistance' or polarity responses. Here it is:

'Of course you could resist but that's not why you're here [hear].'

Symptom Prescription

[See 'Prescribing the Behaviour']

Syntactic Ambiguity

The Pattern:

1) 'While I'm talking to you in trance...now...'

2) 'Helping helpers can be helpful...'

3) 'Amazing hypnotherapists can be nice...'

4) 'Training people can be nice...'

5) 'As you are listening to me in trance now...'

The Structure:

The Syntactic Ambiguity occurs when the role of a word cannot be ascertained due to the context in which it appears.

1) 'While I'm talking to you in trance...now... [Who is in trance? The speaker or the hearer?]'

2) 'Helping helpers can be helpful... [Is there a group of people called 'helping helpers' who are helpful? Or does this mean that helping people who are 'helpers' is helpful?]'

3) 'Amazing hypnotherapists can be nice... [Is there a group of people who are 'amazing hypnotherapists' who are also nice? Or does it mean that it can be nice to amaze hypnotherapists?]'

4) 'Training people can be nice... [Is there a class of people called 'training people' who are also nice? Or does it means that it is nice to train people?]'

5) 'As you are listening to me in trance now... [Who is in trance? The speaker of the hearer?]'

T

Tag Questions

<u>The Pattern</u>:

1) 'You can do this, can you not?'

2) 'You want to make a change, do you not?'

3) 'It's easy, is it not?'

<u>The Structure</u>:

Tag questions make it difficult to say no. They depotentiate resistance and can help to overcome a polarity response. They're called 'Tag Questions' because the question is tagged onto the end of a statement, in such a way that it sounds like it is purely a question, when, at a deeper level, it's an embedded statement that's designed to evoke agreement. Some people suggest that one of the reasons it can be useful to employ Taq Questions with people who exhibit a polarity response is, because they habitually respond in a polarised way to what's said to them, by ending with a question like 'can you <u>not</u>?' they'll naturally respond in the opposite direction of 'can you <u>not</u>' which equals (=) 'you can', which in turn helps the process of therapy to move in the right direction.

1) 'You can do this, <u>can you not</u>?'

2) 'You want to make a change, <u>do you not</u>?'

3) 'It's easy, <u>is it not</u>?'

Taking It To Threshold

<u>The Pattern</u>:

The Taking it to Threshold approach involves stretching a belief so much that it becomes impossible for the client to maintain and is, as a result, undone. Frank Farrelly is a master of doing this with his Provocative Therapy approach.

<u>The Structure</u>:

1) 'So, let me see if I'm understanding this right. You've got to sort out your best friend's money problems, then there's the situation with your brother, that <u>you</u> feel <u>you</u> need to deal with, in order to help him, plus you're trying to save up enough money, yourself, to fix the local church roof? Hold up a minute. I've got a good idea. I know a good tailor. I'm sure we could do a deal with DC Comics and arrange some kind of licensing agreement for you, so that you can officially start wearing a bright red and blue costume with a big red 'S' displayed proudly on your chest. Up, up and away! You know what I mean [smile].'

2) 'So you need cigarettes because they're your 'daily life savers'? Boy. They even improve your health? Wow! That just goes to show that you can't believe everything you read in the papers or on the front of a cigarette packet [smile].'

3) 'So, let me recap what you just said. You'll never get anywhere because you're incapable of doing anything right? Geez! So you mum still ties your shoelaces for you? Your dad zips your anorak up. And, with great respect... and maybe this is a bit rude to ask, but are you really saying that someone still has to help you go to the toilet too? That you never got by that potty training stuff because you're supposedly soooo incapable of doing <u>anything</u> right? I don't think so! [smile]. I think you're more capable than you're giving yourself credit for. You've been learning how to do things right for longer than you've been considering. What you've been doing though is focusing on what you think you didn't do right – and not noticing how many millions of things you've been doing right for the past 40 years of your life. It's just a matter of perspective and it sound to me like you are in need of a helpful perspective readjustment. Right!'

Tautology

<u>The Pattern</u>:

1) 'And as you make these changes which are more than adequate enough for you to do...'

2) 'And as you quickly speed up...'

3) 'While you are altering and changing...'

4) 'Think and consider deeply just how good this is going to become now...'

5) 'Feel these nice good feelings...'

The Structure:

A tautology involves the use of a word which repeats a meaning already conveyed by another word which has been used to describe something. It can be used to add emphasis to a conveyed idea.

1) 'And as you make these changes which are more than <u>adequate</u> <u>enough</u> for you to do...'

2) 'And as you <u>quickly</u> <u>speed</u> up...'

3) 'While you are <u>altering</u> and <u>changing</u>...'

4) '<u>Think</u> and <u>consider</u> deeply just how good this is going to become now...'

5) '**Feel** these <u>nice</u> <u>good</u> **feelings**...'

Teasing

The Pattern:

1) 'You can't go into a trance can you?'

2) 'What – you mean you could do this – reeeelllyyy?'

3) 'No, no, don't start feeling too positive about things too quickly. Come on. Talk about wanting it all in one go. Phew! When you get started there's no stopping you is there?'

4) 'Ohhh! So you do know how to ABC then?'

5) 'Now, this isn't a competition or anything. But I once worked with a client who used to leave her hypnotherapy sessions really enthusiastic to see how soon afterwards she could make the changes.'

The Structure:

Teasing can be used to 'make light' of an issue in order to help a client elicit a desired response. By introducing humour in a respectful and appropriate way it often enables a client to 'loosen up' and as this happens things can seem to become more manageable.

Tell You

The Pattern:

1) 'In a moment I'm going to tell you something very important...'

2) 'I'm now going to say something that will help you...'

3) 'I'm going to share something vital with you now...'

4) 'Listen, I'm going to explain something to you...'

5) 'I'm going to tell you something that I think you want to know...'

The Structure:

We don't usually say 'I'm going to tell you something' before telling a person something. By doing so therefore it adds importance to whatever follows the 'I'm going to tell you' part.

Tempo

<u>The Pattern</u>:

'And… as… you… s l o w   r   i   g   h   t … dooooown…   noticehowfastthingsstarttochange! And… that… feeeeelllllssss g   o   o   d.'

<u>The Structure</u>:

Good use of Tempo is an important element of trancework. In the above example you'll notice that the speaker is talking in a slow measured way and proceeds to slow things down by drawing the words out until he/she reaches a certain point at which moment she/he speeds up, in the process of which, he/she introduces the suggestion that change is starting to take place, fast. At which point the speaker slows down again. Having embedded the up-tempo suggestions within the gentle Tempo structure.

Temporal Predicates

<u>The Pattern</u>:

1) 'How often now do you think you will be able to look back and notice now when things started to improve today…'

2) 'Now, yesterday you were considering making changes tomorrow which is now today which means that as you start to change now...'

3) 'Isn't it nice to know that at this moment something good is happening which will positively influence all of your tomorrows...'

4) 'Today a new course has been set so that now and tomorrow things are different and as your tomorrows become your now you'll be able to enjoy this experience in its full splendour...'

5) 'Now change!'

The Structure:

1) 'How <u>often</u> now do you think you will be able to <u>look back</u> and notice <u>now</u> <u>when</u> things started to improve <u>today</u>...'

2) '<u>Now</u>, <u>yesterday</u> you were considering making changes <u>tomorrow</u> which is <u>now</u> <u>today</u> which means that as you <u>start</u> to change <u>now</u>...'

3) 'Isn't it nice to know that at this <u>moment</u> something good is happening which will positively influence all of your <u>tomorrows</u>...'

4) '<u>Today</u> a new course has been set so that <u>now</u> and <u>tomorrow</u> things are different and as your <u>tomorrows</u> become your <u>now</u> you'll be able to enjoy this experience in its full splendour...'

5) '<u>Now</u> change!'

I especially like Andrea Lindsay's use of this pattern in her promotional material which reads: '**Changing your tomorrows today...**' ™. [Used with permission]. [www.halohypnotherapy.com]

That's A Very Good Question...

The Pattern:

Client:

'Will the hypnosis mean that I'm totally confident always in every situation?'

Hypnotherapist:

'That's a very good question. And I'm sure you've got a very good reason for asking me it. [pause] Would you like to tell me what it is?'

Client:

'Yeah. Well. I need to know that I'll feel more confident so that I can give a speech at my brother's wedding.'

The Structure:

This is a pattern that I learned from my dad (Peter Webb) which he himself learned from his time in the world of Direct Sales. One of the things he taught his sales teams is that an unanswered question could remain an objection (albeit, if unanswered, a hidden objection). However, just as in the field of hypnotherapy, where therapists are sometimes presented with presenting problems which are actually something of a 'cover' for more 'real' issues, so too, some questions can also hide deeper, more specific needs. So, a good way of offering the question back to the client in order to get to the (potentially) deeper issues is to acknowledge the client's question ['That's a very good question'], acknowledge the client's need to ask it ['and I'm sure you've got a very good reason for asking me it']...and then elicit what that deeper need is ['would you like to tell me what it is?']. This pattern is very effective for removing objections and getting to deeper issues, which the therapist can then respond to from a proactive position rather than a 'defensive' one.

That's Right

<u>The Pattern</u>:

1) 'That's right. You're doing really well.'

2) 'That's right! How did you know how to do that?'

3) 'That's right! You can do it that way too.'

4) 'And as you take it easy. [Client moves in trance] That's right. You can adjust your posture to move in the right direction all the time.'

5) '[Client moves their head] That's right. You've got it. You're moving <u>a</u> <u>head</u> now. Thing are starting to change. That's right.'

<u>The Structure</u>:

This pattern can be used in a Tony Robbins style 'up-time' conversational hypnosis way and/or in a 'downtime' Milton Erickson trancey kind of way. It can be used to reassure a client that they're doing things in the 'right' way, without explicitly commenting on what they're doing. For example; I've heard Anthony use it with a sense of exclamation in his voice ('That's right!') in order to introduce to his 'client' (a delegate at the fire-walk seminar) a pleasant feeling of surprise that 'they've got it'. The well-known 'That's Right Trance' that's covered in the wonderful book called 'Training Trances' by Julie Silverthorne and John Overdurf details a very good method for generating a minimalist trance simply by using the words 'That's right' as a bio-feed back commentary on the client's trance experience. This 'loop' (the client does something indicative of trance, so the therapist acknowledges it by saying 'that's right', which causes the client to go deeper into trance and exhibit further trance phenomena, which the therapist then acknowledges, which causes the client to generate more trance phenomena, and so on) is a very powerful induction process.

1) 'That's right. You're doing really well. [Milton style]'

2) 'That's right! How did you know how to do that!? [Tony style]'

3) 'That's right! You can do it that way too! [Tony style]'

4) 'And as you take it easy. [Client moves in trance] That's right. You can adjust your posture to move in the right direction all the time. [Milton style]'

5) '[Client moves their head] That's right. You've got it. You're moving a head now. Things are starting to change. That's right. [Milton style]'

Think About It...

The Pattern:

1) 'Think about it. How good will it be to do this soon?'

2) 'Think about it. Won't it be great to be free of this?'

3) 'Think about it. Isn't it better when you look at it from this perspective?'

The Structure:

A comment is made which suggests that the person will think about what follows at a deeper level because the suggestion has been 'front loaded' with the words 'Think about it...'.

Think About That... Then Think About This...

The Pattern:

'Hypnosis is a great way to improve the quality of your life.

Think about that. Then think about this.

Because you can improve the quality of your life with hypnosis and because you are entering hypnosis now, then that means things are already changing.

Think about that. Then think about this.

And with each moment you are in hypnosis now things have already started to get better.

Think about that. Then think about this.

And because you've already entered hypnosis and the benefits have started to grow then this means that you can look forward to an improvement very soon.

Think about that. Then think about this.

If you are able to look forward to improvements already then things must have started to get better.

And that's really nice to know...'

The Structure:

As you followed the example given above you'll have noticed that a reasoning <u>process</u> or 'theme' occurs within the overall pattern which is emphasised by the suggestions to 'think about that' and 'think about this'. As the client becomes drawn into the reasoning process the therapist can gently yet powerfully help them to shift from one frame of reference to another quite quickly, due to the inherent process of the pattern. You can hear an example of this method in the Ultra Hypnosis CD/download called 'Saying Goodbye To Anxiety', in which a similar instance is utilised. [www.ultrahypnosis.co.uk].

You'll notice that the Complex Equivalence Pattern and the Magical Because Pattern have also been included, to provide a linguistic thread - and leverage components to what's occurring. You'll also notice temporal language is employed in order to shift from a current to a past state which implicitly suggests that the desired changes have <u>already</u> taken place (through the shift to the past tense) and that means that the improvements are therefore <u>already</u> (current and ongoing state) a part of the client's repertoire.

Think About This...

1) 'Think about this. How good will it be to do this soon?'

2) 'Think about this. Won't it be great to be free of this?'

3) 'Think about this. Isn't it better when you look at it from this perspective?'

A comment is made which suggests that the client will think about what follows at a deeper level because the suggestion has been 'front loaded' with the words 'Think about this...'.

Thinking / Thought Binds

The Pattern:

1) 'Which thoughts will you think that start to make a difference?'

2) 'Now, let yourself develop an idea but don't consciously notice what it is until your unconscious is ready to let you become aware of it and help you.'

3) 'Now consider what you are becoming aware of without considering what it is until you are ready to consider integrating it now into your life.'

4) 'And you can think thoughts without having to think them and notice ideas without having to notice them.'

5) 'There's a part of you which is thinking about letting you start to think differently. And when do you think you'll notice that you're thinking differently?'

The Structure:

Thinking Binds and Thought Bind are basically, Double Binds, Conscious Unconscious Binds, Double Dissociated Double Binds and Conscious Unconscious Double Dissociated Double Binds which have as an integral part of their structure the concept of thinking and/or thought. This can be a useful focal point for suggestions because much of the work that takes place in the field of Indirect Hypnotherapy is directed at the process of the client's rumination.

Time Binds

<u>The Pattern</u>:

1) 'I wonder whether you'll find yourself using this resource on the first opportunity or will it be the second?'

2) 'Do you think that you will decide to apply for that new job by Tuesday or will it be by Thursday?'

<u>The Structure</u>:

A desired outcome is 'bound' to happen by the use of temporal language. In the first example (which is a Time Double Bind, by way of contrast with the second example) time is used to suggest that imminent use of a 'resource' by the client is a given. All that needs to be ascertained is <u>when</u> it will happen. And this response will be an unconscious process because the client will have to 'wait and see' when the resource is applied because they're waiting to discover when they will 'find yourself' using it (which means that it's outside of conscious influence). The second example (which is a basic Time Bind - because the person can exercise conscious choice over the matter) while being more available to conscious consideration and evaluation nevertheless generates a certain amount of influence to (in this example) apply for a job within a certain time frame. However the **critical difference** between a **Time Bind** and a **Time Double Bind** is that with a Time Bind an element of conscious choice will remain to be exercised, whereas with a Time Double Bind it's more likely that an unconscious response to the suggestion will occur. [See also: Ordinal Number, Temporal Language and Time Double Binds.]

Time Distortion

The Pattern:

1) 'A minute of trance time can seem like an hour and an hour of normal time can seem like a minute.'

2) 'In trance, time can go faster or slower or slower or faster and it may seem faster than it is or slower than it isn't but it will happen one way, or the other.'

3) 'You may feel that time is slowing down in trance or that normal time is happening at a different rate. That all depends on how your unconscious wants you to notice what's different about time for you at the moment you need to notice it.'

4) 'You may feel that you've been in trance for just a few minutes while in normal time it's been for longer than you thought or it may seem as if normal time has happened normally but that it all seems different in trance.'

The Structure:

Time Distortion suggestions are (as the above examples demonstrate) designed to influence the possibility (likelihood) that the client will alter their perception of the flow of time. This in itself is a very hypnotic experience. It also helps to generate something of an Affect Effect. [See Affect Effect]

Time Double Binds

The Pattern:

1) 'I wonder whether you will start to notice the change today or tomorrow?'

2) 'I wonder whether you will notice that you use this resource on the first occasion or whether you'll find that it starts to happen from the second?'

3) 'I wonder if you will notice that your unconscious lets you know the time is right to apply for that new job by Tuesday or will it be Thursday?'

The Structure:

In example 1 above a change is suggested – all that remains is to ascertain when it will occur. This implies that it is to be an unconscious response which is 'bound' to occur. It is therefore a Time Double Bind. Example 2 suggests that a resource will be utilised, but that the client will 'notice' it occurring, almost as if they're observing themselves using it, which suggests that it will be an unconscious manifestation of the trait. Another Time Double Bind. Example 2 similarly poses a question (which is more of a suggestion) that the client will 'notice' that their unconscious 'lets them know' the outcome. This powerfully suggests that it will be an unconscious response – which is 'bound' to take place because they will become aware that a part of them is letting them know the answer to the Bind, thereby making it a Time Double Bind.

[See also Time Binds.]

Time Released Suggestions

<u>The Pattern</u>:

1)

Hypnotherapist:

'Skilled Indirect Hypnotherapists like to help their clients continue to make changes even after they've opened their eyes by saying 'get ready to feel good."

[Allow some time to elapse]

'Now open your eyes as you return to the room. And get ready to feel good.'

2)

'People who get good results at helping people to change invariably utilise Indirect Hypnosis to help them do so.'

[Allow some time to elapse]

'Okay. Let's use some Indirect Hypnosis now and go into trance to make some changes.'

3)

'Empathic therapists are always interested in knowing that their clients are doing okay.'

[Allow some time to elapse]

'Okay. How are you doing... okay?'

4)

'People who are really skilled at helping others overcome addictions are so skilled because they've had to overcome an addiction themselves. They've lived it. It's more than just a theory.'

[Allow some time to elapse]

'When I myself beat cigarettes/drink/over-eating I found that the first thing that I noticed was that my self-esteem improved quickly.'

5)

'Gifted healers are by their very nature honest.'

[Allow some time to elapse]

'...I can honestly say it was the best demonstration of healing I've seen in a while. Would you like me to show you how it works?'

The Structure:

A Time Released Suggestion is designed to work at an unconscious level. First the therapist makes a statement which includes within it a deeply Embedded Suggestion, which will be released to the receiver's unconscious mind at a later time. After an appropriate time has elapsed the therapist triggers the fulfilment of the suggestion by activating it.

1)

Hypnotherapist:

'**Skilled Indirect Hypnotherapists** [this is the deeply Embedded Suggestion] like to help their clients continue to make changes even after they've opened their eyes by saying 'get ready to feel good.''

[Allow some time to elapse]

'Now open your eyes as you return to the room. And get ready to feel good. [This is the activation of the suggestion]'

2)

'**People who get good results at helping people to change** [this is the deeply Embedded Suggestion] invariably utilise Indirect Hypnosis to help them do so.'

[Allow some time to elapse]

'Okay. Let's use some Indirect Hypnosis now [this is the activation of the suggestion] and go into trance to make some changes.'

3)

'**Empathic therapists** [this is the deeply Embedded Suggestion] are always interested in knowing that their clients are doing okay.'

[Allow some time to elapse]

'Okay. How are you doing... okay? [This is the activation of the suggestion.]'

4)

'People who are really skilled at helping others overcome addictions [this is the deeply Embedded Suggestion] are so skilled because they've had to overcome an addiction themselves. They've lived it. It's more than just a theory.'

[Allow some time to elapse]

'When I myself beat cigarettes/drink/over-eating [this is the activation of the suggestion] I found that the first thing that I noticed was that my self-esteem improved quickly.'

5)

'Gifted healers [this is the deeply Embedded Suggestion] are by their very nature honest.'

[Allow some time to elapse]

'...I can honestly [this is the activation of the suggestion] say it was the best demonstration of healing I've seen in a while. Would you like me to show you how it works?'

Tonal Dissociation

The Pattern:

'Sometimes I'll talk to you and sometimes I'll talk to you. Now I know that you know how to make changes while you may be wondering how the changes will occur. But you don't have to know because you know which means that you can relax while you make the changes for you.'

The Structure:

'Sometimes I'll talk to ^{you} and sometimes I'll talk to $_{you}$. Now I know that $_{you}$ know how to make changes while ^{you} may be wondering how the changes will occur. But ^{you} don't have to know because $_{you}$ know which means that ^{you} can relax while $_{you}$ make the changes for ^{you}.'

The hypnotherapist can generate dissociation between the conscious and unconscious mind by projecting his/her voice to different spatial locations as he/she addresses each 'part'. This can be very therapeutic because often clients will have consciously struggled with a problem for a long time before seeking therapy. In the above example the conscious mind is addressed by the raising of the voice and the lifting of the head, while the unconscious mind is addressed by the deepening of the voice and the lowering of the head. By utilising Tonal Dissociation to 'play down the conscious mind' this method can act as a significant source of relief for the client, because it suggests that they no longer have to consciously wrestle with the problem like they have been doing, because the unconscious part of them, which is being addressed, is being addressed in such a way as to suggest that the therapy can now take place at an unconscious level.

[The Ultra Hypnosis CDs/downloads, 'Mind Body Healing', 'Positively Positive' and 'Saying Goodbye to Anxiety' contain examples of this principle. URL: www.ultrahypnosis.co.uk.]

Tonality

The Pattern:

1) 'You can do this?'

2) 'You can do this!'

3) 'YOU CAN DO THIS.'

4) 'Youuu caaaan doooo this.'

The Structure:

Effective use of Tonality is an important element to the application of good hypnotherapy. Paul McKenna, Richard Bandler, Robert Farago and Dick Sutphen all make good use of tonality in their trancework (have a listen to some of their CDs). Ultra Hypnosis CDs and downloads make particular use of varying tonality styles to enhance the therapeutic components of the trances being presented. [URL: www.ultrahypnosis.co.uk]

Transderivational Search

The Pattern:

1) 'And there's a part of you which knows how you'd prefer to feel and I know that that part of you can begin to make you aware of this now.'

2) 'I wonder what kind of resource you'd need and how you'd start to use it?'

3) 'Go inside and consider, if you were going to do it differently how would you do it?'

4) 'Maybe a certain memory can begin to remind you of what you need to know? Or a certain feeling reveal something helpful? Think about this for a moment and just let yourself notice what you notice.'

5) 'You can gently recall what you need to know and allow yourself time to consider what that is now. You might sense a certain thought. Perhaps an idea? Maybe even a feeling, or a memory, or an idea for a solution will start to come to mind. Just invite your inner-self to appropriately reveal to you something which is helpful and then relax and wait and notice what it is.'

The Structure:

A Transderivational Search (TDS) is a term that's used in NLP to indicate the process of 'going inside' and searching for relevant information, which might manifest in the form of a feeling, thought, sensation or memory, etc. The language patterns provided here as examples have been designed to elicit such searches in very indirect ways, thereby making it more likely that in each instance a helpful result will occur. TDS then is NLP-speak <u>for the process of accessing and searching through acquired experiences and understandings</u> in order <u>to locate a fitting response</u>. For example: If I were to ask someone: 'When did you last see a rose?'... the person would in turn be required to do a search of their memory-banks in order to access the answer. Similarly, if I were to ask someone: 'What do you think the best outcome could be?' the respondent will be required to draw upon his/her past experiences, common sense and reasoning ability (which are developed through experience) in order to calculate the odds of the 'best outcome' based on the information recovered from 'within'. You can loosely liken the process of a TDS to using the Find facility in the Edit menu of a Microsoft Word program. A required word (or experience, etc, in the case of a human TDS search) is entered into the Find feature (equating, for instance, to a question being posed) and then 'Find Next' is selected, causing the program to search through the entire document in order to locate all relevant instances of the required text (which parallels the natural process that human beings exhibit in order to locate relevant information from the unconscious).

1) 'And there's <u>a part of you which knows how you'd prefer to feel</u> and I know that that part of you can <u>begin to make you aware of this now</u>.'

2) '<u>I wonder what kind of resource you'd need</u> and how <u>you'd start to use it</u>?'

3) '<u>Go inside and consider</u>, if you were going to do it differently <u>how would you do it</u>?'

4) 'Maybe <u>a certain memory</u> can begin to <u>remind you</u> of what <u>you need to know</u>? Or a <u>certain feeling reveal something</u> helpful? Think about this for a moment and just <u>let yourself notice what you notice</u>.'

5) 'You can <u>gently recall</u> what <u>you need to know</u> and allow yourself time to <u>consider what that is now</u>. You might <u>sense a certain thought</u>. Perhaps an idea? <u>Maybe even a feeling</u>, or <u>a memory</u>, <u>or an idea for a solution will start to come to mind</u>. Just invite <u>your inner-self to appropriately reveal</u> to you something which is helpful and then relax and wait <u>and notice what it is</u>.'

Triggers

[See Anchoring]

Trinity Phrases

<u>The Pattern</u>:

'Now you know... that you are... ready to do... this right now... this means that... changes are happening... which help you... go right inside...'

<u>The Structure</u>:

This pattern is very similar to Coupled Words except that a trinity of words (in this case meaning a group of three) is used instead. The effect is the same; rhythmic, unusual and quite hypnotic.

Truisms

<u>The Pattern</u>:

'As you sit in that chair breathing, noticing the sound of the music that's playing.'

<u>The Structure</u>:

A Truism is a comment on something that's factual:

'As you sit in that chair breathing, noticing the sound of the music that's playing.'

When a therapist comments on several Truisms in succession it becomes possible to add a suggestion to the preceding Truisms which will more readily be accepted by the client because, in effect, the therapist will have created what's known as a '**Yes Set'** sequence. This consists of the delivery of several statements with which the client will likely agree. Once a person has entered into agreement several times they are more likely to agree with other things that are said:

'As you sit in that chair breathing, noticing the sound of the music that's playing...and as you're hearing the sound of the clock and becoming aware of the warmth of the sun upon your face a certain part of your deeper mind can let your natural creativity continue to release itself so that you can use it when you want to now...'

In a similar vein the hypnotherapist can use **Utilisation** skills to integrate whatever feedback the client is providing, by commenting on it (in the form of further Truisms) to help the client in the process of experiencing trance:

'And as your eyelids are blinking and your right leg is twitching...once...and it twitches again...and you move your head to one side...I wonder how you knew that this is exactly what needs to happen for you to develop a deep trance now...'

Truisms About Sensation And Time

<u>The Pattern</u>:

1) 'Many people become aware of gentle feelings of calm or comfort as they go into trance. You'll probably notice this too during certain moments of your trance.'

2) 'Many people find that from time to time they enjoy feeling good about enjoying something new.'

3) 'It's possible that you'll start to notice a certain sensation of peace or harmony or pleasant relaxation.'

4) 'Who knows? Maybe you'll start to notice that you're feeling better at some point in the near future. And maybe you won't even need to consciously analyse why anymore. You'll just be able to get on and enjoy the change.'

5) 'And as one day follows another so it's possible that one good feeling can follow another.'

<u>The Structure</u>:

This pattern nicely links realistic universal statements associated with sensation/feeling to those associated with time in order to compound the efficacy of the concepts being conveyed.

1) 'Many people become aware of gentle feelings of calm or comfort as they go into trance. [Truism of sensation] You'll probably notice this too during certain moments of your trance. [Truism of time]'

2) 'Many people find that from time to time [Truism of time] they enjoy feeling good about enjoying something new [Truism of sensation].'

3) 'It's possible that you'll start [Truism of time] to notice a certain sensation of peace or harmony or pleasant relaxation [Truism of sensation].'

4) 'Who knows? Maybe you'll start [Truism of time] to notice that you're feeling better [Truism of sensation] at some point in the near future [Truism of time]. And maybe you won't even need to consciously analyse why anymore. You'll just be able to get on and enjoy the change.'

5) 'And as one day follows another [Truism of time] so it's possible that one good feeling can follow another [Truism of sensation].'

Try

The Pattern:

1) 'And the amazing thing is even if you try not to consciously think about feeling confident you'll still do so which will be a sign to you that your unconscious is thinking about it more which means that the changes are taking place.'

2) 'Try not to think about being a non-smoker and see what happens.'

3) 'Try not to listen to me and hear what happens.'

4) 'You can try and repeat that old behaviour on one occasion, that's right just you try, but notice what happens instead.'

5) 'And the amazing thing is. You can even try to feel bad about it. That's right, really try, but you won't be able to. Something has changed.'

The Structure:

The use of the word 'try' significantly implies that failure is likely. We've probably all heard someone say: 'I tried my best', in order to explain why they didn't accomplish something. Derren Brown famously used this technique on his popular TV show when he asked some tough, stocky boxers to <u>try and lift</u> a diminutive female volunteer off of the ground. Although these were 'tough guys' who 'worked out' regularly in a boxing gym and, in reality, under normal circumstances, would have easily been able to lift the woman in question, nevertheless, with Derren's skilful use of the word try and the implicit authority in the tone of his voice, suddenly these 'tough guys' found their strength had all but 'evaporated', as they strained, incredulously, <u>trying</u> to lift her.

When used skilfully in therapy, the word try can be used to (a) generate a reversed effect: 'Try not to think about feeling better from time to time.', and (b): suggest the removal of something which is unwanted: 'You just try and get it back and notice how things are different.'

U

Unconscious Association   Conscious   Dissociation

The Pattern:

1) 'And that resource that you have which you're not yet consciously aware of I wonder when your unconscious will start to let you sense it...now?'

2) 'And it could be that that resource which you have somewhere that you are not yet consciously aware of but which is very helpful can just become clear to you now as it helps you feel good...'

3) 'And you could find that a certain helpful feeling which you haven't been thinking about or aware of gently starts to make itself felt for you in ways that let you let yourself feel good as you notice it now...'

4) 'I don't know but you may find that a certain pleasant resourceful emotion which you weren't thinking about or even consciously aware of just then can begin to make itself noticed at the level of conscious awareness as you start to begin to notice what it is and experience more of it now...'

5) 'Some people find that a nice emotion that they weren't even aware of or thinking about at the time just starts to gently work its way into the range of conscious choices that they have about how they

feel so that they notice it and feel good, and this can happen for you too....'

The Structure:

The structure of the Unconscious Conscious Dissociation Association is geared to elicit a resource which is unconscious and dissociated and bring it to conscious associated experience. It can be helpful for introducing the concept of other, hitherto, perhaps, untapped, states and ranges of choices, in indirect ways, and, therefore, it is less likely to elicit resistance or critical analysis on the part of the client. It also helps to contribute to the client's perceptions of their unconscious mind as being a place where a vast range of talents, abilities and greater wherewithal are located and which he/she is now able to draw upon, in a non stressful kind of way (meaning they don't have to 'work up' the resource, it just gently introduces itself).

1)

'And that resource [resource = the focus of the Bind]'

'...that you have which you're not yet consciously aware of [aimed at the unconscious mind in a dissociated way]'

'...I wonder when'

[hypnotic language, if the therapist doesn't know the answer who does? The client at an unconscious level!]

'...your unconscious will start to let you sense it'

[Transferring it from unconscious awareness and a state of dissociation to conscious awareness and a state of association]

'...now?'

[Embedded Command in the form of a question]

2)

'And it could be that that resource [the focus of the pattern] which you have somewhere [dissociated] that you are not yet consciously aware of [unconscious] but which is very helpful can just become clear to you [conscious] now as it helps you feel good [associated]...'

3)

'And you could find that a certain helpful feeling [the focus of the pattern] which you haven't been thinking about [dissociated/unconscious] or aware of [dissociated/unconscious] gently starts to make itself felt [associated] for you in ways that let you let yourself feel good [associated] as you notice it [conscious] now...'

4)

'I don't know but you may find that a certain pleasant resourceful emotion [the focus of the pattern] which you weren't thinking about [unconscious/dissociated] or even consciously aware [unconscious] of just then can begin to make itself noticed [associated] at the level of conscious awareness [conscious] as you start to begin to notice [conscious/associated] what it is and experience more of it [associated] now...'

5)

'Some people find that a nice emotion that they weren't even aware of [dissociated] or thinking about [unconscious] at the time just starts to gently work its way into the range of conscious [conscious] choices that they have about how they feel [associated] so that they notice it [associated/conscious] and feel good [associated], and this can happen for you too...'

Unconscious Conscious Separation

Milton Erickson would often talk to a client about their unconscious mind and/or talk directly to their unconscious mind. This created a different (novel) frame of reference for the client (people don't usually say 'I'm going to talk to your unconscious mind...' in everyday conversation) in which the client's problem could begin to be dealt with at an unconscious level, due to the separation effect, rather than wrestled with at a conscious level. You'll often notice as a result that hypnotherapists who incorporate Ericksonian methods into their work will talk about and/or to the client's unconscious mind too. (See the pattern immediately above for an example.)

Undeniable Non Specifics

The Pattern:

1) 'And you're sitting in the chair...gently breathing in a certain way...and a part of you is thinking about what's going on...'

2) 'And your eyes are closed and you can hear the sound of the music while inwardly you're preparing to make some changes...'

3) 'Your arms are resting on the chair...the muscles in your face have relaxed themselves quite nicely now...and inside you're preparing to do something ...'

The Structure:

This pattern utilises the principle of pacing and leading, by highlighting Truisms, in order to lead to suggestions about non specific behaviours, which can't be denied. The Undeniable Non Specifics that are introduced can then be used as a bridging technique to lead into a further range of suggestions.

1) 'And you're sitting in the chair [Truism]...gently breathing [Truism] in a certain way...and a part of you is thinking about what's going on [Undeniable Non Specific]...'

2) 'And your eyes are closed [Truism] and you can hear the sound of the music [Truism] while inwardly you're preparing to make some changes [Undeniable Non Specific]...'

3) 'Your arms are resting on the chair [Truism] ...the muscles in your face have relaxed themselves [Truism] quite nicely now...and inside you're preparing to do something [Undeniable Non Specific]...'

Here's an example of how the bridging technique can be used to lead into further suggestions, using the first example of this pattern:

1) 'And you're sitting in the chair...gently breathing in a certain way...and a part of you is thinking about what's going on...[bridging to suggestions] and that same part of you which can be thinking about what's going on while you're thinking about it thinking about what's going on can also do many other things while you're wondering like this...after all...think about this...if that part can be thinking about what's going on while you were consciously listening to me talk about the fact that you are sitting in the chair and breathing in a certain way...how much more can that part of you think about like this and how much more powerful is that part and how many wonderful changes do you think it can help you make today while you are consciously thinking elsewhere?'

Universal Deletions

The Pattern:

1) 'And everything that you want to change for the better...can start to work out in all the right ways for you now.'

2) 'Now every time you use those talents which help you…'

3) 'You'll never know how much better things are…'

<u>The Structure</u>:

Universal Deletions combine the Milton Model Universal Quantifier and a Simple Deletion and/or a Comparative Deletion.

1) 'And everything [universal] that you want to change [deleted] for the better [comparative]…can start to work out [deleted] in all the right ways [universal] for you now.'

2) 'Now every time [universal] you use those talents [deleted] which help you…'

3) 'You'll never [universal] know how much better [comparative] things [universal/deleted] are…'

Universal Quantifier

<u>The Pattern</u>:

1) 'Your unconscious always knows how to help you…'

2) 'And now…all the time…you are getting better and better…'

3) 'Every time you do this things improve…'

4) 'Now… your inner self can let you remember these positive suggestions so that you can always

feel different and forever remember that today things have changed for the better for you…'

5) 'Everyone around you will notice this more positive side of your personality emerging…'

6) 'Maybe you used to think that you would never be free of that problem, but here today you are moving beyond it so that things are always, totally, different, forever, for you so that all the most helpful things, which you could ever want to start to become a part of who you are, are always available to you in all the most appropriate, helpful, healthful ways which is why you always notice that now things are all getting better and better…'

The Structure:

Universal Quantifiers, as the name suggests, introduce a 'universal' element to a statement (or question) due to the use of certain types of words. This results in the scope of what's being addressed becoming ratcheted up to infinity. This method can be very helpful when offering suggestions to clients.

1) 'Your unconscious always [universal] knows how to help you…'

2) 'And now… all [universal] the time… you are getting better and better…'

3) 'Every time [universal] you do this things improve…'

4) 'Now… your inner self can let you remember these positive suggestions so that you can always [universal] feel different and forever [universal]

remember that today things have changed for the better for you...'

5) 'Everyone [universal] around you will notice this more positive side of your personality emerging...'

6) 'Maybe you used to think that you would never [universal] be free of that problem, but here today you are moving beyond it so that things are always [universal], totally [universal], different, forever [universal], for you so that all [universal] the most helpful things, which you could ever [universal] want to start to become a part of who you are, are always [universal] available to you in all [universal] the most appropriate, helpful, healthful ways which is why you always [universal] notice that now things are all [universal] getting better and better...

Unpacking

This is an expression that's used when someone is explaining the elements of a language pattern or the principles of an indirect hypnosis / NLP process. For example, this book is about 'unpacking' indirect hypnosis language patterns.

Unspecified Verb

The Pattern:

1) 'As your unconscious helps you change...'

2) 'Your deeper self is going to assist you now...'

3) 'You'll encourage yourself now...'

4) 'You'll make yourself feel good...'

5) 'You're going to improve...'

<u>The Structure</u>:

The Unspecified Verbs pattern introduces verbs which are not clearly defined; they're left 'cloaked', so to speak. As an indirect hypnotherapy principle it's very useful because, in effect, the therapist can leave the actual part which relates to the specificity of the process of 'doing' of the unspecified element up to the unconscious to decide. Meaning that by not saying specifically how something will occur it leaves it up to the ingenuity of the unconscious mind to 'join up the dots' and make it happen. To 'unpack' an Unspecified Verb pattern using the Meta Model (based on the work of Virginia Satir) we could ask 'How specifically will you...?' This has the result of specifying what's missing. However, in the context of indirect hypnotherapy, sometimes it can be useful to leave that part to the client's own wisdom.

1) 'As your unconscious helps you change...'

The 'change' part suggests to the unconscious mind that it will begin to make changes – in a non directive way. A Meta Model question to this, if said in 'non trance' conversation could be: 'What changes?'; or 'How specifically will the change take place?'. However, in the above context the intention is to leave that part 'cloaked' or hidden from obvious conscious consideration so that the unconscious can do what needs to be done.

2) 'Your deeper self is going to assist you now...'

The way in which the assistance will take place is left cloaked.

3) 'You'll encourage yourself now...'

The way in which the client will encourage himself/herself is left cloaked.

4) 'You'll make yourself feel good...'

The way in which the client will make himself/herself feel good is left cloaked.

5) 'You're going to improve...'

The way in which the client will improve is left cloaked.

Until

<u>The Pattern</u>:

1) 'And, what's more, you know you don't even have to start to do this until you sense you're ready.'

2) 'And this will continue until it's all done...'

3) 'And from now until you need to, you will notice this occurring...'

4) 'Turn it up as far as it needs to go until you know you're feeling better...'

5) 'You may even find that this works every day until you have improved so much that it's no longer even necessary...'

The Structure:

The word 'until' can be particularly influential. It sets a definite event moment in time, which is presupposed, by which, when that event moment is reached something will have taken place. That something is specified by the context of the suggestion. In effect, when the event moment is reached it equals (=) an activation of a definite result (specified by the context of the suggestion).

The Pattern:

1) 'And, what's more, you know you don't even have to start to do this until [the client will start to do it at this point] you sense you're ready.'

2) 'And this will continue until [a point at which it's all done will be reached] it's all done...'

3) 'And from now until you need to, you will notice this occurring [a point at which the client no longer needs to do this will be reached...but up until that point they will notice this occurring]...'

4) 'Turn it up as far as it needs to go until you know you're feeling better [the client can 'turn it up' to a point which gives them a biofeedback experience of feeling better]...'

5) 'You may even find that this works every day until you have improved so much that it's no longer even necessary [it will work for a predefined period

of time which is measured in the context that eventually it will no longer need to occur because the positive results will have been so pervasive that a 'quantum leap' will have taken place in which the issue is no longer an issue]...'

Utilisation

The Pattern:

1) 'And as you hear the loud sounds outside you know you are allowed inside to listen and relax as you do...'

2) 'That's right and as you move your head you know you are moving ahead now...'

3) 'And as you arrange your posture you can increase your range of choices...'

4) 'And as you hear the sound of the door closing remember what they say: as one door closes another door opens and I wonder what doors of opportunity are opening for you now?'

5) 'And as you hear the sound from above you know that it's plainly a day for making changes...'

The Structure:

1) 'And as you hear the <u>loud sounds outside</u> you know you are <u>allowed inside</u> to listen and relax as you do...'

2) 'That's right and as you <u>move your head</u> you know you are <u>moving ahead</u> now...'

3) 'And as you <u>arrange your posture</u> you can increase your <u>range of choices</u>...'

4) 'And as you hear the <u>sound of the door closing</u> remember what they say: <u>as one door closes another door opens</u> and I wonder <u>what doors of opportunity are opening for you now</u>?'

5) 'And as you hear the <u>sound from above</u> [a plane] you know that it's <u>plainly</u> a day for making changes...'

I remember when attending my second Unleash The Power Within Fire-walk Seminar with Anthony Robbins, on this occasion at London's Docklands, that during a part of the seminar, in anticipation of our to-be-experienced fire-walk and when Tony was in the process of helping us to shift our mental/emotional states so that we would be 'up for' the fire-walk, he experienced something of a problem, which he overcame with some brilliant Utilisation. He was building our collective response potential [See Building Response Potential] by helping us to positively motivate ourselves (about 3000 people) in the car park at the Docklands venue, where, in just a few hours' time several pits of burning hot coals would be situated, over which we were supposed to walk, unscathed. As he was gearing us up for the big moment however, every few moments he was interrupted by the loud, distracting, sound of the Docklands train system, as an overhead train rumbled by. As someone working in the same field as Tony a part of me was curious as to how he would overcome what, for him was clearly becoming something of a problem. I could tell he was, what I can best describe as I write, perturbed, or perhaps a bit frustrated by what was going on. But he overcame it brilliantly! With some timely Utilisation. After two or three interruptions he started to link the sound of the train powerfully to the state enhancement process he was engineering with us, by saying things like: 'That's it... and now you <u>train</u> yourself...' , and 'This Neuro Associative Conditioning is <u>train</u>ing you to...', etc. Immediately he did this, every time a train rumbled by it actually had the effect of enhancing the suggestions he was making. He tied the sounds of the trains into his desired outcome, to the extent that it actually became conducive to the work he was doing, rather than the original, brief, hindrance it had appeared that it was becoming. In fact, the session actually turned out to be better and more memorable due to the deft Utilisation skills that he employed.

Soon afterwards I was doing several hypnotherapy/NLP treatments on a consultancy basis in a well-known hotel. The hotel was going through some refurbishment work as I was delivering therapy – with lots of construction taking place in the room directly below the treatment room I was using. And the workmen really went to town! At first they started with hammers and chisels during one of the early sessions. Fortunately, like Tony, having been versed in Utilisation, and soon after seeing Tony use it so well at Docklands I tied the sounds into phrases like 'tapping into your unconscious', so that the hammer and chisel sounds became a useful part of the trance. But – the workmen had something else lined up for me that was totally unexpected! Between clients I'd spoken to the manager of the hotel's health club and asked for a different room to use, because, although I was able to utilise what was going on I felt, for all concerned, that ideally another kind of acoustic ambiance would be better in the long run (☺). While he was arranging this for me, nevertheless, I continued to use the original room, due to the scheduled nature of the appointments. The additional surprise took place when I was in the middle of a smoking cessation session. My client was powerfully 'tapping into' her unconscious mind and becoming a happy healthy non-smoker when suddenly a worker downstairs pulled out a pneumatic drill! Bam bam bam bam bam bam uuuuuuuuurrrrrrr rrrrrrr bam bam bam uuuuuurrrrr! The sound was so loud that I had to move so close to my client that I was inches away from her ear, in order for her to be able to continue to hear what I was saying. How was I going to utilise such an intrusive noise? I invited her unconscious mind to rehearse the new behaviour pattern so that it became natural for her to be a non-smoker, to go through a '<u>drill</u>' of the new behaviour, so that 'now and in the future this is how you respond'...(or words with similar intention to those). I consistently tied the word 'drill', used in the context of to 'practice' (here's a bit of irony) and to 'TRAIN', so that, as best I could ensure, the therapy would achieve the desired result. After completing the entire smoking cessation process, with the hammers and chisels and pneumatic drill going on in the room below I 'awakened' my client and 'brought her back to the room'. When she opened her eyes she asked me: 'Did I hear a drill at some point?'. She was actually uncertain about whether or not a drill had been used! When I confirmed that she had heard one she commented by saying that she'd hardly noticed it. What's more - years later she's still a non-smoker! (And it was at this point, for the final two clients, I was moved to a quieter suite in another part of the hotel!)

V

Verb Tenses

<u>The Pattern</u>:

1) 'So... that has been a bit difficult... wasn't it?'

2) 'Okay... you're ready to sort this out... haven't you?'

3) 'Isn't it nice to know that when you have changed things now... you can recall what it used to be like to have that old difficulty... as you consider that now?'

4) 'Okay... so what you used to do is ABC but now because things are different you XYZ... that's right now you XYZ... it just happens this way for you and how much better it is like this... is it not?'

<u>The Structure</u>:

By changing the tenses of verbs conversationally (either when the client is 'in' or 'out' of 'formal' trance – or both) the hypnotherapist can help clients to shift their perceptions regarding the nature of their problem(s).

1) 'So... that has been a bit difficult... wasn't it?'

In this example the therapist has linguistically, twice, put the problem in the past (meaning it's no longer current) and then, with the use of the Tag

Question ('wasn't it?') implied that it's no longer a problem.

2) 'Okay… you're ready to sort this out… haven't you?'

In this example the therapist has met the client in the present tense ('you're ready') and then shifted the problem into the past by ending with ('haven't you?').

3) 'Isn't it nice to know (?) that when you have changed things now… you can recall what it used to be like to have that old difficulty… as you consider that now.'

This example shows how the therapist can orient a client to the future ('when you have changed'), which is then set in the present ('now'), meaning that in the future/now the client can recall what the difficulty (which is now set in the past tense) was, from the present (better) moment ('as you consider this now').

4) 'Okay…so what you used to do is ABC but now because things are different you XYZ… that's right now you XYZ… it just happens this way for you and how much better it is like this… is it not?'

Here a problem behaviour is put into the past ('so what you used to do') while the desired new behaviour replaces it ('things are different you XYZ') now ('how much better it is like this') and in the future (is it not?).

Visual Coordinates

Developing an awareness of subjective Visual Coordinates can support the client in the process of 'looking at' positive images and/or help to alter how the client relates to unwanted subjective visual experiences.

Example: 'And when you say you see a certain image – where specifically is that image?'

W

Wander / Wonder

<u>The Pattern</u>:

1) 'Wandering through trance while you wonder what's happening.'

2) 'And you can wonder as your thoughts wander...'

3) 'I wonder how your thoughts wander or you wonder as I wonder how you can let your thoughts wander and continue to let yourself relax nicely into trance.'

<u>The Structure</u>:

This pattern involves a nice play on two words which sound alike in order to generate trance and (as in examples 2) play down the conscious mind by wrapping the words together in such a way that they will appear confusing...so that the next obvious thing which the speaker says ('continue to let yourself relax nicely into trance') will be readily accepted, because it's easily understood. And by following the obvious suggestion it provides an easy way for the speaker to move from confusion to understanding, which by-so-doing assists the process of therapy to occur.

Weighted Language

<u>The Pattern</u>:

'The people who improve in my experience are the ones who are solution-focussed and who are committed to following through by taking action. What would you rather do, nothing, or take action as well and follow through?'

<u>The Structure</u>:

Weighted Language is used to describe a commentary which is heavily laden with the speaker's own opinion. It can be quite powerful. Based on this opinion, which is 'assumed' to be factual (which of course it may also be) a conclusion can be drawn or a question posed, the answer to which, due to the Weighted Language, is likely to be in agreement with the embedded stance of the speaker.

'The people who improve in my experience [opinion] are the ones who are solution-focussed [opinion] and who are committed to following through by taking action [opinion]. What would you rather do, nothing, or <u>take action as well and follow through</u>?'

WH Words

WH Words are often used to generate 'Open Questions'. This means that by asking a question beginning with '**What**', '**When**', '**Where**', '**Whom**', and '**Why**', a person is more likely to get a detailed response, rather than a one word answer [See also 'Closed Question'].

Some people avoid the use of 'Why Questions' because they say they have the effect of causing the client to 'justify' a behaviour, which can often be unhelpful. However, just as some people say you should 'never' use the word 'but' (because 'everything before 'but' is bullshit'), such polarised beliefs are, I believe, limiting and there is often a timely place to appropriately use all of these words therapeutically.

X

Xenocoding

'Xenocoding' is a word that I 'morphed up' to describe the underlying process of much of what takes place in the process of indirect hypnotherapy. In effect, indirect hypnotherapists code/construct/sequence the language that we use to help our clients to change their behaviours and/or thoughts for new, <u>different</u> and more desirable ones. We therefore use words to 'code difference', in the process helping our clients to experience desired change.

Y

Yes But

The 'Yes But' pattern is one to watch out for in your clients, if you're a practicing therapist. If a client uses this expression too much they can, metaphorically, paint themselves (and their therapist) into a corner from which it can become increasingly difficult to escape. A good way that I have found to bring this to an end is to 'Name The Game'. This means to explain what the client is doing (to the client) and how such continued use of this particular response could sabotage any constructive work that might otherwise take place. I often explain this by using the cycle that's listed in Transactional Analysis books in which a person adopts the role of 'Victim' to someone else's 'Rescuer', eventually becoming the 'Persecutor' of the 'Rescuer'. Like this:

'I want to share something with you now which you probably aren't aware of. I know you want to move forward, so I think you'll find it really useful if I share this with you. In the field of psychology there is a behaviour pattern that's known as the 'Yes But!' pattern. [This implies that the aberrant behaviour is not only noticed but that it's been categorised by an entire field, which adds extensive 'weight' to the explanation being given. It also 'dissociates' it in the sense that, by explaining it this way, the therapist is not 'accusing' the client of a behaviour; he/she is just sharing some evidence from the field of psychology.] Let me give you an example of how it works. A person in an office says to their colleague: 'I can't think of anywhere to go on holiday this year'. So, they're playing, what psychologists call a 'Victim' role [the pattern is noted – by an entire field], because they're implying they're not even able to choose a holiday destination for themselves [this, indirectly, sends some very subtle yet powerful messages to the client]. At which point their colleague adopts what is known as the 'Rescuer' position [highlighting the dynamics of the 'game' and by implication indicating that the therapist is not prepared to adopt this role too] and says something like: 'Have you thought of Malta? Malta is nice.', at which point the 'Victim' says something like: 'YES BUT …I can't go to Malta because I don't like islands'. So the 'Rescuer' says: 'How about Switzerland? It's beautiful there.' To which the 'Victim' replies: 'YES BUT – I can't go there because it will be winter in Switzerland when I'm on holiday and I hate the cold and the snow!'. So the 'Rescuer' says: How about America – America is great, it has everything'. To which the 'Victim' says: 'YES BUT – I can't go there, the flight is too long and I hate long flights!'. So the 'Rescuer' says (with exasperation): 'Well, I can't' think of anywhere to help you then!'. At which point the 'Victim' changes position to become that of 'Persecutor' by saying something like: 'Well – you weren't much help were you?!'.

It's amazing how quickly such a metaphorical exposition of the pattern will help a client shift position and begin to take ownership of the old behaviour - and seek to change it. And, if they (out of habit) repeat it after it's been raised my experience is that they'll likely say 'Oops! There I go again. But at least I caught it this time', or something like that. Of course, by using this principle there are many other implicit messages which are being conveyed by the therapist to the client, but they're being conveyed in a non-confrontational manner and in a sense that provides the client with a way to extricate themselves from the behaviour easily and without perceived blame.

Yes Set

<u>The Pattern</u>:

Client:

'I found you okay. The directions you sent me were very helpful.'

Hypnotherapist:

'So they worked?'

Client:

'Yes.'

Hypnotherapist:

'And you've come along here today because there's something you want to deal with?'

Client:

'Yes!'

Hypnotherapist:

'And it has something to do with what you briefly told me about on the phone?'

Client:

'Yes.'

<u>The Structure</u>:

It's important that the hypnotherapist knows how to help the client feel comfortable at the outset and better still if he/she understands how to elicit agreement with the client quickly too. An existing frame of agreement will more likely help to facilitate the therapeutic work which follows. The above example shows the therapist asking questions which are designed to gain agreement with the client. The more often the client agrees, the stronger the rapport that's generated between the two of them and the more likely the client is to accept the suggestions which take place in the formal trance which will follow.

The golden rule of Yes Sets, generally speaking, is never ask a Yes Set question that you don't already know the answer to. If you do you might receive a 'no' answer and that could set things back (except when that 'no' is a desired 'no', which contextually means 'yes' by agreement; like this: Hypnotherapist: 'So. You didn't expect to get over your problem before hypnotherapy then?'. Client: 'No'...which is an implied 'yes' because they're in agreement with what the hypnotherapist has said).

Yes-Set Pacing And Leading

Hypnotherapist:

'Oh, so you caught the train here today...'

Client:

'Yes.'

Hypnotherapist:

'To get over your problem...'

Client:

'Yes.'

YET

The Pattern:

1) 'Don't make all the changes just yet...'

2) 'Now...some changes can happen now and some not quite yet as everything works into place in all the best ways...but you will know when they are all working right for you...'

3) 'That's it. Think about it. But don't do it right yet. Wait a few more moments to really enjoy getting ready to change and then do it. It's sometimes more pleasurable this way.'

The Structure:

This pattern works much like the Until pattern (See Until). It sets a definite moment in time by which a desired outcome will occur. It can also help to build response potential. Things that we humans want which are withheld seemingly often become more desirable to us. By implying that the outcome is temporarily withheld, while also presupposing that it is a given that it will be experienced, can make the build-up to the experience more significant which can, in turn, make the realisation of the experience itself more powerful than it would have been.

1) 'Don't make all the changes just yet [temporarily withheld, while presupposed that they will be realised]...'

2) 'Now...some changes can happen now and some not quite yet [temporarily withheld, while presupposed that they will be realised] as everything works into place in all the best ways...but you will know when they are all working right for you...'

3) 'That's it. Think about it. But don't do it right yet [temporarily withheld, while presupposed that it will be realised]. Wait a few more moments to really enjoy getting ready to change and then do it. It's sometimes more pleasurable this way.'

You Might

The Pattern:

1) 'You might find that...you feel more positive...'

2) 'You might notice...you're starting to think more positively...'

3) 'You might sense... that things are getting better...'

4) 'You might...experience something good...'

5) 'You might notice a...change right away. I don't know. You might notice a... change gradually. You might even find that you notice a bit of both...but you will find that everything starts to shift in your favour now.'

The Structure:

The expression 'you might' is a nice indirect way of making a suggestion without it appearing too direct. It causes the suggestion to slip under the client's conscious 'radar' (as Carol Lankton MA says) to be received at an unconscious level.

1) 'You might find that...[indirect] you feel more positive...[suggestion]'

2) 'You might notice...[indirect] you're starting to think more positively...[suggestion]'

3) 'You might sense...[indirect] that things are getting better...[suggestion]'

4) 'You might...[indirect] experience something good...[suggestion]'

5) 'You might notice a...[indirect] change right away [suggestion]. I don't know. You might notice a...[indirect] change gradually [suggestion]. You might even find that [indirect] you notice a bit of both...[suggestion] but you will find that... everything starts to shift in your favour now [suggestion].'

Z

Zooming

<u>The Pattern</u>:

1) 'That's right and as you add all of those good thoughts and good feelings and make that picture bigger, brighter... turning the sounds up to a positive level... and bringing it closer and closer and closer until it feels really good. How good is that! That's it.'

2) 'And that old picture...that's it push it away...way over there...over there... while draining the sound right out... so it fades away... over there. Right over there...shrinking smaller aaaannnnddd smaller aaannnnndddd smaller aaaannnnnddd smaller. Going... going... gone!'

<u>The Structure</u>:

Zooming is a term used for rapidly maximizing (or minimizing) submodalities to increase (or decrease) a person's affective response.

Further Information:

Personal

Kerin Webb
www.kerinwebb.com

Gill Webb
www.gill-webb.co.uk

Andrea Lindsay
www.halohypnotherapy.com

Training Courses

Eos Seminars Ltd
www.eosseminars.com
Bournemouth, England.
Phone: 01202 424991

Hypnotherapy CDs & MP3 Downloads

Ultra Hypnosis Ltd
www.ultrahypnosis.co.uk
Bournemouth, England.
Phone: 01202 269247 / 01202 424991

A friend in need is a friend indeed...

Please consider helping any of the following organisations by making a donation(s). Many (if not all) will accept standing orders for £2.00 per month. Every donation helps.

Amnesty International (helping victims of abuse around the planet): www.amnesty.org.uk

DogsTrust (formerly National Canine Defence League): www.dogstrust.org.uk

Dr Hadwen Trust (medical research for humans that doesn't involve harming animals): http://www.crueltyfreeshop.com/drhadwen/

Friends of the Earth (helping to protect our planet and its inhabitants): http://www.foe.co.uk/

Greenpeace (helping to protect our planet and its inhabitants): www.greenpeace.org.uk

Humane Research Trust (medical research for humans that doesn't involve harming animals): http://www.humaneresearch.org.uk/

Oxfam www.oxfam.org.uk

Plan International (supporting needy children in the developing world): http://www.plan-international.org/

PDSA (Peoples Dispensary for Sick Animals): www.pdsa.org.uk

Red Crescent / Red Cross: http://www.ifrc.org/

RSPCA (Royal Society for the Prevention of Cruelty to Animals): www.rspca.org.uk

Salt of the Earth (helping the underprivileged in India): www.salt-of-the-earth.org.uk

WSPA (World Society for the Protection of Animals): www.wspa.org.uk

WWF (World Wide Fund for Nature / World Wildlife Fund): www.wwf.org.uk

UK Membership Organisations

British Board of NLP (BBNLP)
46 Alexander Gate
Stevenage
Herts
SG1 5RG
Phone: 07795 976 458
Email: nlp@bbnlp.com
Web: www.bbnlp.com

✳

Counselling
43 Walker Ave
Wakefield
WF2 0HH
Email: info@counselling.ltd.uk
Web: www.counselling.ltd.uk

✳

Counselling Society (CS)
Suite 7
Bridge House
7 Bridge Street
Taunton
TA1 1TG
Phone: 0870 8503389
Email: info@counsellingsociety.com
Web: www.counsellingsociety.com

✳

General Hypnotherapy Register (GHR)
PO Box 204
Lymington
Hants
UK
SO41 6WP
Phone: 01590 683770
Email: admin@general-hypnotherapy-register.com
Web: www.general-hypnotherapy-register.com

General NLP Register
No1 Witney Chambers
Longbridge Road
Barking
Essex
IG11 8TQ
Phone: 020 8594 7778
Email: enquiries@general-nlp-register.co.uk
Web: www.general-nlp-register.co.uk

✳

The Hypnotherapy Association (HA)
14 Crown St
Chroley
Lancs
PR7 1DX
Phone: 01257 262124
Email: admin@thehypnotherapyassociation.co.uk
Web: www.thehypnotherapyassociation.co.uk

✳

The Hypnotherapy Society (HS)
PO Box 3511
Wells
BA5 2ZR
Phone: 0845 6024585
Email: info@hypnotherapysociety.com
Web: www.hypnotherapysociety.com

Appendix One:

I've mentioned Frank Farrelly A.C.S.W the developer of Provocative Therapy several times in the preceding pages. Copied below is an article that I had published in the British Board of NLP's magazine called The Model in 2005. It highlights some of the principles that I observed Frank Farrelly utilising in his training seminar with us. I'd like to offer my thanks to Dr Jaap Hollander for his permission to quote from the Farrelly Factors which he first codified in this form, based on his own observations of Frank at work, over many years. For a complete listing of the Farrelly Factors you can visit Jaap's website at: http://www.iepdoc.nl .

Here's a copy of the original article.

The Wizard of Wisconsin

Provocative Therapy. What is it? Even the term itself raises questions when the words 'therapy' and 'provocative' are used in a shared context. How does 'it' work? What makes it different from traditional psychotherapy? Where and from whom did it originate? Lot's of questions, so let's get some answers.

The name 'Frank Farrelly' can often be heard spoken (by highly trained psychotherapists) in a state of mixed wonderment and awe, in sentences that are themselves liberally interspersed with the kind of language you'd usually expect to find on some of the wilder football terraces, male-dominated building sites - or even hen nights! How come? Well, it's all because Frank Farrelly A.C.S.W. (past Clinical Professor at the University of

Wisconsin and Assistant Clinical Professor in the Department of Psychiatry at the University of Wisconsin) has developed a most powerful psychotherapeutic approach which actually involves, precision directed 'locker room' language (his definition for the therapeutic expletives that sometimes take place) in order to elicit positive changes in his clients. As Frank Farrelly himself explains, the root meaning of the word 'provoke' means 'to draw out' and that's exactly what Provocative Therapy does. It draws the client out of their self-defeating/dysfunctional patterns by provoking them in such a way that they actually begin to assert their own self-worth. But why would client's in a Provocative Therapy session feel the need to assert their self-worth? After all – isn't it likely that many of them will arrive for therapy feeling that they don't have much in the way of 'self-worth' to account for, let alone enough assertiveness to 'assert' themselves with? Well – let me tell you – you'd be surprised. Very surprised.

Jest a Minute

Farrelly's trademark icon is that of the jester. It's an icon that is aptly chosen. Often you'll see this icon displayed doing a headstand, while simultaneously balancing, on the upturned sole of one foot the 'comedy/tragedy' (or happiness and sadness) theatrical masks that developed in ancient Greece and which have since become the universal symbols for theatre (and role playing). Could they be implying that we (people) collectively spend a lot of time living, perhaps even hiding behind, various masks that we hope the world (others) will perceive to be our 'true' selves? Possibly, maybe, even to the extent that often times a person could even forget what is a mask and what is real? While on the other upturned foot rests that universal symbol of both change and balance – the Yin/Yang. Change - and balance (Hmmnn, maybe there is a deeper meaning to that symbol than is first apparent too?). The jester however, is himself exquisitely poised, while he balances these archetypal symbols and watches the world from his inverted position. But perhaps, just maybe, it's the world that is looking at the jester from the wrong perspective? Perhaps, just maybe, it is the world (meaning most of humanity) which is looking at life from the wrong point of view? You could even suppose that the jester is in actual fact juggling the evocative masks and the Ying/Yang symbol and that too would be quite apt – because one of the meanings of the word 'juggler' is magician. And it is definitely psychotherapeutic magic that takes place when the 'Wizard of Wisconsin' is at work. Curiouser and curiouser! Also of interest to us; while the jester balances the masks, with honed adroitness born of years of experience he isn't himself wearing one. This indicates very much that with Frank 'what you see is what you get', a no hiding, no double talking kind of guy. And in many ways that is exactly what you get when you have an interview with Frank. But, remember, looks can be deceiving – or at least not as revealing as they might be.

The Method to the... Sanity

Every psychotherapist/counsellor should have a copy of Provocative Therapy, by Frank Farrelly and Jeff Brandsma. It's like a breath of fresh air in amongst a, sometimes, sterile, overly clinical, dissociated-from-the-client-as-a-human being field. However, in contrast, Frank Farrelly is above all 'real'. He 'rolls his sleeves up' and, to use a popular phrase of the times 'gets up close and personal'. And, every moment of every moment, every nuance, and every strategy is delivered in a finely tuned manner, in order to develop the right kind of therapeutic response(s) from his client. He doesn't miss a trick, although, one of his strategies is to give the impression that he does!

To watch Frank work (on the surface) is like watching an 'average guy' that you might find in any bar around the world 'shooting the breeze' with someone. Frank can be both your buddy and your adversary at the same time. He, as an adversary (devil's advocate), will 'draw from' his client/interviewee a range of relevant issues that he then, often in seemingly preposterous and/or exaggerated ways, will begin to work upon. For example: if the client's presenting problem is offered as a 'molehill' size case of 'ABC', Frank might get hold of it and suggest (artfully, and in ways that raise helpful questions in the mind of the receiver) that it is in actual fact a proverbial 'mountain' of a problem, maybe even a 'catastrophic' case of the same (...or perhaps not? After all, many clients indulge in 'catastrophising' when dwelling on their problems. So, Frank just does it for them and as a result of this provocation the client is challenged to <u>realistically</u> <u>assess</u> the nature of the situation. This, in turn can result in the seriousness of the original presenting problem diminishing in its destructive seriousness in the client's mind, and therefore becoming much more readily manageable.) This often challenges the client's stereotypical ideas of what psychotherapy is all about. While they may have expected a mollycoddling approach, instead the problem is assessed, even seemingly maximised and then, in effect, given back to the client for them to look at again - albeit from a changed perspective. And so the dance begins. Frank (so it seems) also sometimes attributes deprecating qualities to the client. Often, at first, the client will agree. But within a short while they will usually begin to protest or disagree, sometimes quite loudly (in fact I was once reminded of the phrase, in one situation: 'methinks thou dost protest too loudly', meaning that Frank was acutely precise with his aim in relation to his understanding of the underlying problem and it triggered a powerful response as a result). As things unfold the client continues to assert herself/himself and makes rapid therapeutic value changes, due to the provocative approach and in the process of the dance, magic occurs. Now, this is a very simplified explanation of what takes place. It's likely that no one article could come close to doing justice to the artistry involved; but it does provide something of a 'taster'. Let's then add a bit of seasoning to this taster, by drawing on some explanations written by someone with years' of experience of observing Frank at work. The following descriptions, produced by Dr Jaap Hollander (who has himself hosted Frank Farrelly for training seminars for many years in Europe, and who is a skilled exponent of Provocative Therapy principles) have been delineated from Frank's original book called 'Provocative Therapy', to explain something of the deep structure of what Frank does, and as a result they have since become known as the 'Farrelly Factors'. Below each bullet-pointed Farrelly Factor I have myself taken this opportunity to provide a few additional words that relay my own impressions of them (having seen Frank employing them in our live training seminar). Please bear in mind as you read, that the examples I've added relate to just one possible outcome that each Farrelly Factor could generate. In all likelihood, there are, in each instance, a myriad number of possible related themes that could unfold.

The Farrelly Factors

1)

Don't help the client.

The therapist makes no effort to be helpful; he brings up irrelevant remarks, and wanders off onto side topics, meanders into surrealistic 'dreamscapes'.

Kerin: Often the client will expect the therapist to 'sort it all out' for them. By 'not helping' it can actually help the client to become more determined to find a solution.

2)

Blame the client.

Make the client ludicrously 'responsible' for everything that happened in the past, the present and the future. Give him in a ridiculously humorous way 'responsibility' for <u>all</u> types of things (cf. 'carnival hall of mirrors').

3)

Life is to blame for the client's difficulties.

Everybody and everything else is responsible for what happens to the client. (cf. P.T. 'blame list'.)

Kerin: (Farrelly Factors 2 and 3) the client can start to take a reality check. If he/or she has been blaming others, by attributing blame for 'everything' to everyone and everything <u>other</u> <u>than</u> <u>self</u> it can encourage the client to become more realistic. Or, vice versa, by attributing 'blame' for 'everything' <u>to</u> <u>the</u> <u>client</u> it can achieve the same result.

4)

Idiotic solutions will solve your problem.

Offer totally impossible solutions to the client about how to handle his problem. The more idiotic the solution, the better. The client then makes the effort to find the answer to his problems by himself.

Kerin: As Jaap says, the client begins to 'push' back in the other direction which is the direction that leads to real, workable, solutions.

5)

Imitate the client, mimic the client.

Imitate the client (e.g. his affect), imitate his verbal and non-verbal behavioural patterns. E.G. with the over-intellectual client the therapist becomes more and more abstract and increasingly difficult to understand; or, e.g., with the anxious client, therapist begins to (ineptly) attempt to control his obviously increasing 'panic'.

Kerin: this is another wonderfully helpful approach. By mimicking the client they get the opportunity to see what their behaviours communicate to others. Often, out of misplaced kindness, those closest to a person won't tell them about any 'quirky' behaviour patterns. If a person doesn't know about them - they can't change them. By 'playing them back' for the client to observe it starts to put them in a position of awareness, and this brings choice, and choice can bring change.

6)

Go back and forth.

Play ping-pong. First explain to the client that everything else and everybody else are the reasons for his disaster; then, when he agrees, you begin to explain that he himself is the culprit – then switch back.

Kerin: Set up, upset, set down. A maxim in the field of psychotherapy is: set up, upset and set down. That is to say that you set the therapy situation up, upset the client's rigid dysfunctional system and then help them set down in a better state of being. That's what this principle can achieve. Because a client can arrive with very fixed and rigid beliefs if the therapist 'pushes' in one direction, the client may or may not relax those beliefs. If the client pushes and pulls in all directions it can begin to unravel fixed patterns and allow the client room for new ideas.

7)

Interrupt the client.

To interrupt the client is especially suitable when the client is boringly repetitious. It doesn't' matter how, when or with what topic you interrupt the client.

Kerin: This, to NLPers, can be know as a 'pattern interrupt'. The more lost the client becomes in the same old story of 'woe and misery', the more miserable and woe begotten they are likely to become. By interrupting it shocks/shifts them out of the old, self-draining pattern and allows room for new and better states of being to occur.

8)

What's wrong with that? (More of the same).

The therapist shows the advantages of the client's dysfunctional behaviour and encourages the client: 'do, think, feel more of the same' in an exaggerated manner, giving crazy 'proofs' and 'instant research' to support this.

Kerin: this can cause the client to be even more clear about why they don't like the dysfunctional behaviour and become even more determined to stop/change, etc.

9)

Unifactoral hypothesis to explain everything idiotically.

The therapist gives only <u>one</u> explanation for the symptoms and problems of the client and from then on uses everything the client says to support the hypothesis. E.G. the client says the reason for her problem is that she is becoming old; from then on, the therapist interrupts every client statement as evidence that she is aging rapidly.

Kerin: this can cause the whole issue to become so ludicrous that it's no longer an issue.

10)

Communicate about the client's communication patterns.

E.G.: Client reports in a low voice, how he yells at his children. The therapist ludicrously expresses disbelief in a virtually inaudible tone of voice that the quiet-spoken, gentlemanlike client could possibly yell or scream.

Kerin: in this example the client is not, often 'quiet-spoken' and 'gentlemanlike'. What he is saying and how he is saying it to Frank do not match what he does at home. And Frank mimics his incongruent response (to the presenting problem) issue in such a way that says at a deeper level, 'be real'.

11)

Red-green-colour-blindness.

Find the point where the client is extremely sensitive (often body-image). When the client signals 'STOP!' just keep going (i.e., approach what the client avoids).

Kerin: The client can grow stronger by learning to deal with what they hide from.

12)

Overemphasise the client's assets to the total exclusion of his problem.

When the client has a strong asset (E.G. physical beauty), you can dismiss his problems and say: 'for a handsome guy like you these problems don't even count!'

Kerin: even though what is said is unrealistic, the way it is said can begin to help the client to 'lighten up' and review the problem(s) in a more realistic way. It's likely (as in any interview with Frank) that liberal helpings of humour will have been involved which will support such a change of perspective.

13)

Amuse and amaze.

The therapist acts as if the client's task is to interest and entertain him. He shows marked boredom with the client's story, he barely suppresses yawns, and says, E.G.: 'This problem must bore you to death', or 'you can imagine how tired I get, listening to this crap all the time.'

Kerin: The client will likely have replayed their 'problem' over and over to themselves. Many will have 'done the rounds' and repeated it time-over to many other counsellors and psychotherapists too. It can even become linked to their sense of identity ('my problem is me and I am my problem'). By expressing 'boredom' at the 'crap' the client no longer gets any potential 'secondary gain' from telling the story (Frank 'isn't listening') and it's likely that they will start to shift their own perception of the problem. Something that's so crappy it's boring can't actually be so serious – can it?

14)

Minimize the client's problem.

Therapist: 'Resign yourself to your problem, it's so common and frequent that every second person has it.'

Kerin: I seem to remember that Carl Rogers said something along the lines of: 'what is most private and most personal is often most general'. Many clients think that only they have ever had a problem like 'their' problem. By minimising it (which, in this case, is actually taking a reality check) as in the above example, it can provide an immediate source of relief. After all – if 'every second person has it' then they're pretty normal. This could also be an instance in which Frank would adopt the 'buddy' role. Like he was talking with a pal in a bar over a drink or two. Perhaps along the lines of: 'Hah! Why worry, I mean, every other person has it. All the research says that.'

15)

Maximise the client's problem.

The therapist ineptly anticipates the catastrophic fears of the client. E.G.: 'What you're going through now is nothing. Just wait – the symptoms will increase.' Or the therapist, shocked, gasps 'you did WHAT??!! Or, your catastrophic fears are not so bad – just wait and see how good your wife feels when you are dead!'. Etc.

Kerin: This can generate a: 'Yeah right! I don't believe you.' kind of response. The client knows Frank is joking and, they then begin to do a reality check and in the process, particularly with the introduction of Frank's obvious humour, this helps the client to relate to the issue(s) as more manageable.

16)

Illustrate the impact of the person's behaviour on others (affective, verbal, etc).

If client is aggressive and loud show that you are afraid of his threatening behaviour. If client is seductive, pretend to be overwhelmed by his/her attractiveness.

Kerin: By bringing the affect that the client's behaviour is likely to generate in others to the table, albeit in a directly indirect way, it can enable the client to become aware of what they're doing and this in turn allows for the potential of them making positive changes in the way they behave.

17)

Ludicrously misinterpret the client's weakness and strengths.

Example: If client is timid, humorously suggest that his not responding indicates a serene calmness and self-assurance and compliment him on this.

Kerin: The client could respond by saying: 'No, it's not. And you know it's not. It's because I'm timid. I always have been'. And, in this example, it brings the real issue out into the open, in a way that allows the client to verbalise it. Once this occurs, in effect, 'all the cards are on the table'. What is avoided has been approached (by Frank) in an indirect way, so that the client has made steps to approach it, and then the healing can continue to occur.

The Hyper Factor

Frank Farrelly is an exceptional hypnotherapist. Although, you could be forgiven for thinking that hypnotherapeutic principles have nothing to do with the way he works. However in much the same way that the, now, legendary Dr. Milton Erickson employed hypnosis in ways that people often didn't understand were occurring; so too does Frank. I noticed when watching Frank that he employed what I have called (for want of a better expression) 'hyper themes'. This is to say that Frank works on many levels. There will be the direct level of the 'banter' described above in the Farrelly Factors, relating (or not as the case may be) to the client's presenting problem(s). Then, on another level, there will often be some metaphorical work, which can, without too much difficulty, be consciously noticed and understood. However, often, I detected a theme (akin to a 'life metaphor', directly tailored to the client) which operated at such a global level, that, to the client, it was actually 'too big' to be <u>consciously</u> noticed. In NLP terms we would say Frank 'chunks up'; to the nth degree. And he does it in a way that becomes ever more difficult to detect, but which is increasingly bringing ever more powerful therapeutic elements to the client's unconscious awareness.

Many interviewees commented after their session with Frank that they felt a bit 'spacey', or words to that effect. Almost as if they had been in some kind of Altered State of Consciousness (ASC). Frank, therefore, deserves to be counted amongst the hypnotherapy greats, as well as his special recognition within the field of psychotherapy in general.

But What's He Really Like?

That, then, in short-form, is an introduction to the realm of Provocative Therapy, as developed by Frank Farrelly. But what's Frank like as a person? Well, although my time with him over the seminar was relatively short, over the four days we spent together Gill (my wife) and I did have the opportunity to meet both Frank and his wife June on a social level a number of times. Basically, my opinion of Frank is that he is an approachable, down to earth person. He has genuine empathy and a warm desire to help people get the best out of themselves and their lives. He's highly educated, widely read and full of life experience. He is truly a 'one off'. And he has, almost as a hallmark, a devilish (meant in all the best ways) sense of humour.

Step This Way

In conclusion: wherever you live, if Frank Farrelly is coming to a place near you make sure you take the opportunity of seeing him in action. You'll learn a lot, you'll laugh a lot and you'll have an experience that's akin to an amazing roller coaster ride, through the field of psychotherapeutic wizardry.

Farrelly Factors used with kind permission of Dr Jaap Hollander. Websites: http://www.iepdoc.nl and www.provocatiefcoachen.nl (where a full description of all 39 Farrelly Factors can be found). Provocative Therapy is written by Frank Farrelly A.C.S.W. and Jeff Brandsma and is published by: Meta Publications (ISBN: 0916990036) Frank Farrelly lives with his wife June in Madison, Wisconsin, USA. You can visit Frank's website at: www.provocativetherapy.com

Appendix Two:

In our original training manual I included a script that I had myself written, a number of years ago as course work, for a training programme I attended. Because it was an exposition of Indirect Hypnotherapy principles I added it to our training manual so that delegates would benefit from a detailed 'script' demonstration of how 'Milton Model' language patterns can be employed. For the same reason I have chosen to include it in this book:

Ericksonian Trance – Using The 'Milton Model'

Some Principles – by Kerin Webb

The work of Milton Erickson, MD has become widely acknowledged as containing some of the best examples of how to use a number of hypnotic language patterns in order to facilitate behavioural and psychological change in clients. The purpose of this handout is to highlight a number, out of the many, powerful patterns which can be utilised in trancework, based on some of those utilised by Milton Erickson himself.

First of all, in the process of developing this overview, you will soon be introduced to a number of paragraphs of trance script, within which, you will find interspersed here-and-there explanations of what is taking place, such as why certain phrases are used with reference to the intended outcome which can be generated by their use. The writer's intention is that you will, as a result, become familiar with Ericksonian-style trance material, having participated in this script's linear development, from its start through to its therapeutic conclusion. After you have had the opportunity to consider the script with its stage-by-stage analysis of the underlying patterns which are at work within, you will find, as a follow up, the trance script in its complete form.

Set Up

In line with established principles, the model I shall follow here will be that of: 'Set Up, Up Set, Set Down'. That is to say that before utilising the therapeutic patterns of this script the therapist will first precede doing so by helping the client to become comfortable in order for the trancework to take place. If the client is uncomfortable with the situation it will hinder, if not entirely stymie any trance facilitation. There are a number of ways to do this. The writer's preferred method is to explore the subject of hypnotherapy and hypnosis, uncovering any misconceptions in the process and cementing any useful beliefs which the client may already have. This will almost certainly cover the following issues. The client is likely to have an awareness of what is taking place in the outside world while experiencing trance. For instance, in the writer's locale, they will notice the sound of a clock, some pleasant background music, and, often the breeze gently drifting through the trees. Other things that are of relevance may be the fact that they may notice feelings of warmth, tingling, heaviness, or some other pleasant sensation from time to time. Although it is, of course, also possible to enjoy a good trance while not noticing any such sensations too.

The therapist may like to point out to the client before beginning that they will be able to awaken at any time (and that suggestions will be made to this effect at the start of the induction) so that they will feel more relaxed and in control. It's also often useful to explain to the client that you (the therapist) will suggest that they will **remember everything** that takes place in the trance too (this serves two purposes; 1: it further acts to put the client at ease by underscoring the issue of personal control and, 2: it presupposes that they will experience a trance which they will be able to remember. That presupposition will prove very useful to the process of generating the trance state with the client).

Once the above has been achieved and the client is seated or lying down comfortably you can begin the trancework session.

There are a myriad number of induction techniques. Some favour predominantly a visual bias. Others draw heavily on kinaesthetic sensations. And there are others which aim to generate an auditory rapport. A good trance will incorporate all of these Representational Systems to varying degrees. The trance script below focuses on using an auditory method to gain rapport and in the process utilises a number of visual and kinaesthetic elicitation strategies in the process.

Up Set

The purpose of the trancework in this example is to 'up set' a limiting pattern. In this case it is related to a pattern of perceived 'low self-esteem' (Virginia Satir is reputed to have said that she concluded that all of her clients' problems were generated by a sense of low self-esteem). The Up Set is achieved by using Ericksonian interspersal techniques, during which embedded commands are applied which repeatedly focus on encouraging a developing sense of Personal Power on behalf of the client. Also, a powerful theme within this trance-process is the utilisation of the **confusion technique**. The writer has found this to be an immensely powerful tool for moving beyond conscious doubt, resistance or disbelief. In the process of which, because the conscious mind, in effect 'switches off' due to its inability to deal with the confusional structure of the trance, the therapist is then able to communicate with them at deeper than usual levels.

So, imagine the situation if you will now. The therapist has helped the client to achieve a comfortable attitude and posture. He or she has asked the client to gently close his or her eyes (it's easier doing it that way than with some of the longer persuasion-based techniques) and breathe in a relaxing manner of his or her choosing. And as the therapist gently starts to match his or her rhythm of speech to coincide with that of the client's breathing the utilisation of the language patterns can begin....

....That's right. Just allow yourself to **get into a comfortable position easily now**...in your own time and your own way...and when **you want to relax** more during your **trance...easily**...you can...either by laying **still hear** or when finding you **knew a comfortable position** to take now... and you can...can you not?...and you may want to think about that for a moment....

The reader will notice that this paragraph starts with the therapist commending the client for their behaviour up to this point with a: 'That's right'. Doing so serves to let the client know that what they are doing is okay and it also begins the process of establishing a 'buying set' or 'compliance set' in the client. By commending useful behaviour in the early stages of the therapy it is more likely to produce a similar effect later in the trancework as more therapeutic tools are applied. It is a bit like a sales person 'closing' a customer at various stages of the sales' cycle. The sooner you begin to do so the sooner you will be able to help your client to help himself/herself.

You will also notice an emphasis applied to certain words. For instance: '**get into a comfortable position easily now**…'. This is done gently, sometimes verging on imperceptibly, while at other times it can be attained quite obviously, by changing your intonation levels, upwards or downwards, or by the use of a friendly whisper (care needs to be taken with the whispering technique. It shouldn't be used until a good deal of rapport has been established between client and therapist because, otherwise, it may be deemed to be unusual or even frightening). The reason for using this embedded technique is because evidence has shown that the unconscious mind is far more perceptive that the conscious mind (New Scientist) and because of this, suggestions given in this manner can by-pass the critical self-limiting conscious mind and communicate directly to the unconscious mind. You will also notice what are known as 'permissive' phrases', like: 'and when **you want to relax**' which implies a number of things, the first being that the client can relax if they want to. However, another subtle implication is that the client WILL relax when they want to. This helps the client to feel more at ease, comfortable in the perception that they can do things when and if they want to (that's true), while also having the effect of gently gaining compliance due to the level of secondary (deeper) presupposition that they will relax, which is also, enhanced by the use of an embedded command on the words: 'you want to relax' (which is actually less of a general statement and more of an order). This is followed by a technique that causes the end of one statement to become the beginning of the next, which also has the effect of embedding the command, using confusion to do so. The client may even be wondering: 'Was that the end of the last sentence or the beginning of the next?', and as they are doing so a number of further therapeutic commands can follow, which will by-pass the confused conscious mind and communicate therapeutically with the unconscious instead.

The words: '**Still Hear**' as they appear in the above paragraph are known as a phonological ambiguity. Depending upon the context the same sound can mean two different things. This method refers to both, but just as a double entendre can only truly have one meaning (Ronnie Barker), so too is there one main point of emphasis here, and that is that the client will HEAR what is being said at a deep level.

The '**You knew a comfortable position**' phrase is aimed at using the revivification method of eliciting an experience of relaxation that the client has had in the past and relating it to the now to achieve similar results, rapidly. The additional: '**Can you**

not?' is known as a Tag Question. Tag Questions can be applied when clients are 'resistant', particularly those who have what it known as a Polarity Response (in essence a polarity response happens when a person habitually takes the opposite point of view of the speaker, or responds: 'Yes, but...!', often. In order to deal with such behaviour patterns the therapist can make a statement and add a Tag Question like the above mentioned 'Can you not?' to it. And what this does is depotentiate the polarity response, because the client doesn't know whether to disagree with the original statement or the 'Can you not?' question, which, **being phrased in the negative** sense will lead them to <u>respond</u> <u>in</u> <u>the</u> <u>positive</u>).

The...**'And you may want to think about that.'** is a permissive way of causing the preceding suggestion to be thought about some more, unconsciously and consciously.

> That's it ...**now...** the **nice** thing about **trance....** is that you can do it in **you're unique** way and that may be simply by choosing to **relax more and more deeply**...or just by **listen**-ing to what I say now **consciously and unconsciously**...and as your eyes remain gently closed you can **let** those **deeper learnings** just **happen** as much as **you want them too**, either in a powerful or a profound way...

In this paragraph certain individual words are highlighted to denote embedded commands. By emphasising certain words in this manner it has the effect of linking the embedded words contextually together (the context being the changed pitch) which then creates the effect of causing them to be perceived as a sentence within a sentence, or a sub sentence, for instance:

Now, nice trance

(The use of the word 'Now' often also acts as a command, relating to the phrase which immediately precedes or follows it. In this case it commands a 'nice trance'.)

You're unique (remember we're working on low self-esteem and this phonological ambiguity is designed to help here. So, '**Your unique**' phonologically - and in an embedded way, translates as '**You're Unique**')

Relax more and more deeply – listen – consciously and unconsciously

Let deeper learnings happen, you want them to (or **too** as in '**as well**'. There is also the presupposition here that 'deeper learnings' will take place. Deeper than what? the Meta Model may ask. Deeper in the sense of **meaningful** an unconscious Complex Equivalence can conclude).

And: '**either in a powerful or a profound way...**', powerfully or profoundly both mean similar things, although a choice is implied, but the client is really continuing to be led to the desired state of mind.

Some people choose to explore just how much they can let their body relax in trance too...and you may even want to **recall how you have relaxed** in that way...perhaps by letting the muscles in **your toes relax now**...or in a moment...that's right...just letting the muscles in **your toes relax**...and as **they do** now...you may even notice that you **sense a sensation** of tingling, or warmth, or heaviness, or lightness, or a pleasant coolness in your toes...or even the sensation of no sensation...**everybody does** this...in their own way **which means that** you can **do it** that way too...

By introducing the idea of other people relaxing it serves a number of functions. One is, in effect that a message is conveyed which can be summed up: 'it's okay to do this, lots of others have too'. And then in a very gentle and permissive way a kinaesthetic element is introduced to the process, that of a full body relaxation. Notice the use of:

Sense a sensation....everybody does....which means that....do it

There is also a mind/body reading element at work here too. Many people report noticing such sensations. The fact that you have drawn attention to them can help to mind-read/pace and lead their experience, deepening rapport. The 'sensation of no sensation' (or sometimes 'the sensation of no new sensation') covers all the corners.

And the more you allow those pleasant relaxing feelings or **sensations start to happen**...I don't know what **your unconscious is listening** to now...but I do know that **your unconscious** can **hear many things here** and as you hear here...you can choose to just **let those new**

resources start to build up from **within...without** you consciously having to ...**try** and see if you can **remember at a conscious level** when you notice **your unconscious helps you now**...but sometimes you may be pleased to find that your unconscious has already **let that new helpful behaviour happen** all on it's **own...it** does...because you're unconscious always seeks to **do the best** for you...**know it does**...

Notice here a statement/question is made which is really a command to:

I don't know what **your unconscious is listening** to now....

Which is followed up by a confusional phonological ambiguity:

...can **hear many things here** and as you hear here...

The word 'choose' is used to encourage a permissive self-directed perception on the part of the client, while in actual fact they are being guided to start to choose something they weren't considering choosing before – in our case it's the generation of new resources. Advertisers, cults and the media do not always have ethical purposes in mind when they use such principles.

The use of **'within...without'** reframes the point of reference and adds further conscious confusion to enhance the suggestion process.

And: '**your unconscious helps you now**', starts to further generate the perception of **two levels of consciousness,** one conscious the other (beyond conscious control and more powerful than the conscious mind) unconscious.   Importantly, the suggestion is that the powerful unconscious is focussed on PROVIDING HELP.   What kind of help? The unconscious can choose appropriately.   This is followed by: …'but sometimes you may be pleased to find that your unconscious has already **let that new helpful behaviour happen** all on it's **own…it'.**   Hidden within that sentence is the idea that even when the conscious mind is not thinking about the desired new behaviours the unconscious will be pleasantly surprising the person with demonstrations of them anyway.   That's followed up by a command to 'own' the new behaviour.

And as you <u>feel ready</u> to **let those relaxing feelings** in your feet…gently allow the muscles in your legs to <u>enjoy the process</u> too…you may even find that as you <u>hear the sounds</u> in the outside world now, inside your mind…at a deeper level you can just **allow yourself to relax** with each new sound that your **hear here**…and sometimes you may even **consciously notice a sound** that you've already unconsciously noticed too…which means that **your mind is so powerful** that good <u>things can happen at many levels now</u>…I wonder if you've ever consciously begun to **imagine** just how **many levels of awareness** you have…and the more **you relax** to <u>sense them</u> the more <u>you can use them</u> in your daily life too…and it's good to **do it that way**…all of the <u>successful people</u> **do**…and because they

> know how to **do it** and <u>you know how</u> to **do this** you can **get more good results** too <u>now</u>... <u>and in the future</u> you find that you <u>do it consciously and unconsciously</u> in a very relaxed and natural way...

This paragraph finishes by projecting the unconsciously created aspects forward so that they are both in the here and now (daily life) and in the future for whenever they are needed too. There are a number of embedded commands and confusional techniques; distinctions between different levels of conscious awareness, the appeal to the imagination (I believe it was Emile Coue who explained that when the intellect and imagination 'fight' it is the imagination which will always win. Therefore it is best to have the imagination working towards the desired outcome.) Notice the phrase 'which means that', which uses the Meta Model Complex Equivalence strategy to generate belief that 'good things can happen'.

> ...in fact the less you try to **make this happen** the more it happens and the more **you let it happen** the better it gets...but you already **know this at an unconscious level**...do you not? Don't you?...

The unconscious cannot process a negation (Richard Bandler). By suggesting 'the less you try', it actually facilitates **more unconscious programming** and thoughts focussed to **do exactly** what was, seemingly, suggested that the client shouldn't try to make happen. It's a bit like saying: 'Don't think of Elvis Presley now!'. Then follows an additional confusional/double polarity response technique and an embedded command:

'know this at an unconscious level...do you not? Don't you?...'.

This is added for further affect (the trance can become so profound that it implies, to the conscious mind: 'something different has happened' which in itself can prove to be very therapeutic, at the level of belief. The affect causes a Complex Equivalence related to Cause and Effect. Eg: the trance causes an affect effect, which is equated to meaning that because the client is feeling 'so different' it must mean that the hypnosis is working'. A sort of circular reasoning).

> **And think** for a moment **now** about your unconscious **resources**...and then...in your mind's eye...in a moment...when I say the word 'now'...let yourself notice a situation **now-in-the-future** when **you are doing things well** assisted powerfully from an **unconscious level**...that's it...think about that...**now**...and now...in your mind's eye...over there... **notice yourself** doing that thing...<u>sooooo</u> easily...in fact you may even be pleasantly surprised to **watch how easy this is now**...as you do it from inside **your mind...does it naturally**...that's it watch yourself doing that thing soooo effortlessly...and if there are others around notice how well they **watch yourself doing this now**...notice what you **hear as you do this comfortably**...maybe your own voice...or others positively responding to you...and that feels good doesn't it?...so give yourself permission to enjoy those feelings again now...that's right...

Here, there is an appeal to the visual sense, future pacing the resourceful behaviour. This can help establish the desired responses in advance of the need to use them. There are also suggestions which reframe the 'magnitude' of the situation from one of pre-conceived difficulty or trouble to now-conceived surprising ease and comfort.

Additional reinforcements are offered from 2nd position. This means that whilst the focus has so far been from the client's internal (associated) perspective, you can also reinforce it visually and audibly from the perspective of others who are positively responding to the client's behaviour. Often what creates low self-esteem is a poor perception of how others perceive the self. By perceiving themselves positively **from outside** it can help to greatly reinforce things.

> ...Good and as you **get ready** to let the muscles in **your upper body... can relax...** too...either all in one go, or muscle by muscle or just gently unwinding as you feel **you want to**...you may even choose to allow those important conscious thoughts to continue to happen too as your unconscious goes deeper inside to help you as well...because your unconscious is designed to help you when **you ask your unconscious to do so**...and **I know** that's why you are here now **hear now**...which is why at that deep unconscious level those changes have **already started**...and I wonder how many you have consciously noticed already or if your unconscious is just saving them for later as well...either way **you decide** to do this for yourself...the results are

the same...because when **your unconscious starts to do things**...powerful results occur...to you...

Continuing with the full body relaxation in a permissive way. This is coupled with the suggestion that they actually ask for unconscious support. The writer has found this very helpful in clinical practice. Emphasis is placed on the fact that 'changes have already started', which means that the problem is already being solved.

And then as you let your arms and hands just relax a bit more...just a bit more as much as you like now...think for a moment consciously...or unconsciously if you prefer, about that thing that... **you want to make a change**...now...you know the one...but did you already notice just how much a **change has occurred** because I know that you have been **listen**-ing **deeply** to all of the suggestions which suit **you're unique circumstances**...the obvious ones and all of those embedded ones too and finding ways to **use them right away** whenever **you need to** now...

Which means that as you **allow yourself** to enjoy relaxing **here**...maybe even letting those muscles at the back of your eyes relax too...you may even sense that ...just as **in the past** when you've found that **something is of no use to you any more** and you've **throw**-n **it away**...you're unconscious can throw away any unwanted behaviours too...and... just like when **you've replaced something** with a newer and **improved** way of doing things so now you're unconscious can replace old ways with better ways too...and the good thing about this is that **it's happening now** even as **you relax** and think your conscious thoughts...and even as you **concentrate on this** or just **drift in and out of awareness**...enjoying being able to move between different positive states of being **relaxed at every level**...why don't you take a moment to **do it a bit more**...when **you're ready** too...<u>now</u>... as much as **you like**...

A very veiled metaphor aimed at revivification of a past situation when the client had made a decision to get rid of something which was no longer useful, and as a result anchoring that resource to the present, in order to remove a limiting perception of the self in a similar metaphorical sense.

And think again for a moment **now** about your unconscious **resources**...and then...in your mind's eye...in a moment...once again...when I say the word 'now'...let yourself notice a situation **now-in-the-future** when **you are doing things well** assisted powerfully from an **unconscious level**...and you've done it this way before which means that you can **do it always now**...whenever you need to...that's it...think about that...**now**...and now...in your mind's eye...over there... **notice yourself** doing that thing...<u>sooooo</u> easily again...in fact you may still be pleasantly surprised to **watch how easy this is now**... and it's okay to enjoy doing things well...**naturally**...that's it watch yourself doing that thing soooo effortlessly...and if there are others around notice again how well they **watch yourself doing this now**...watching yourself <u>**doing this so well now**</u>...notice what you are **hearing as you do this comfortably**...maybe hearing your own voice now...or others positively responding to you...and that feels good doesn't it...so give yourself permission to enjoy those feelings again now...that's right...

Further embedded commands and other previously elaborated patterns coupled with additional future pacing in a 'fluffy' manner so that the client can 'fill in the bits' as is most appropriate.

You may even remember just how much you don't consciously remember about what you did last month...until you needed to and then...instantly...naturally and easily...you're unconscious lets you remember...which is the same way that **learning happens in trance**...you don't have to try and **make these changes occur** because you're unconscious will remember to **do it** for you **every time**...just like **you can** <u>remember when you need to</u>...and just relax and enjoy this new **you... knew** you can which is why **you do**...and how much of that did you unconsciously let yourself consciously **be ready** for <u>those good feelings</u> in advance...because you are allowed to **feel good about yourself** at every level...

The above paragraph is structured to introduce the idea of unconscious learning which takes place outside of conscious awareness but which can be brought forward into conscious acquisition when needed with little or no effort.

> You know you should...do you not?...which is why it must happen...because that's the natural way to do things...and I'm wondering whether you will begin now...as you sense how tomorrow is yesterday in the sense that it will be by the next day...which will mean that you are even now in the present **making changes** that will **be with you** <u>in the future too</u>... <u>in the future too</u>...

A modal operator of necessity is coupled with a polarity response depotentiator: You know you should...do you not?', along with a temporal reframing pattern, to introduce the desired behaviours to whenever they are needed.

> And as you **continue to observe** what <u>you notice</u> you may even <u>sense that</u> the more you **see new solutions** just <u>happening naturally</u>...and **don't** try to think about that now...just <u>let it happen anyway</u>...which means that you are finding what you need to do...just like you've always known there are **better ways**....and the more you notice which sounds you are listening to and you are relaxing with each sound that you hear...the more you can...

A comparative deletion is used in the form of: 'better ways'. In Meta Model work a therapist would possibly challenge such a statement. In Milton Model work it is often best to let the client's unconscious mind choose as many 'better ways' as are useful.

Some people like to think about how they will use their new **positive unconscious behaviours** while relaxing in trance...**you can do this** too if you like...think about it...**when** will you let your unconscious step forward and **release those powerful abilities** that you already have deep inside...but this time in ways that you use them consciously too...that's it just take a moment to think about a few of those times when you **will do it this way now**...and you may even be sensing an unconscious difference already?...after all **you are relaxed**...just as your unconscious knew you would...which is why you can now...but remember don't think about too **many new ways** of doing these things now...save some for later... so that your unconscious can **pleasantly surprise** you too....**easily**...and the more easily you do these things the more your unconscious does too...in fact...something that you thought would be difficult turns out to be **ridiculously easy**...**ridiculously easy now** that you **let your unconscious do it for you** instead...while **consciously enjoy doing it together**...

Further emphasis is added here about how easy it will all be, in fact it will be ridiculously easy. There is an appeal to kinaesthetic levels in the sense of 'stepping forward', which implies positive motion (emotion). Asking whether they may have already sensed an unconscious difference will likely generate a response in the client to appropriately create or find a desired response to notice, which will indicate to them that their unconscious is doing things for them. It may be that 'trancey' feeling of relaxation, it may be having responded to the temporal shifts or the 1st and 2nd position, or it may be due to the confusional techniques.

> And in a moment I'll count from 1 to 3 And when I say the number 3 just allow yourself to awaken **remembering everything** that you've noticed consciously or unconsciously so that you can start to **do these better** things **now...and tomorrow** things **get better** even more...**even more**....

And the 'tomorrow things get better even more', is reminiscent of: 'Every day in every way I am getting better and better'.

> 1... Coming on up now.

> 2... Recall the situation in the room.

> 3... Wide awake and fully alert.

Set Down

In this example the Up Set and the Set Down occur during the trance process. As you have noticed, the client is confused, reoriented towards personal power and then future paced to set the new responses in place for when they are desired.

It is possible to add many other language patterns, creative visualisation techniques and command hypnotherapy/classical hypnotherapy patterns to the process too (time does not permit in this example). A point worth mentioning, though, is that John Overdurf and Julie Silverthorn mention in their excellent book Training Trances, that a good time to use classical hypnotherapy is after you have used Ericksonian permissive hypnotherapy to generate a deep trance state. Trance is used to by-pass conscious self-imposed limitation, therefore when the client is in trance and because no such limitations exist at the unconscious level it is quite permissible to be very direct with your suggestions.

For example:

What I'd like you to do in XYZ situation is notice that as soon as ABC starts to happen you will; begin to feel a surge of confidence deep inside...if ....that's okay with you...is it not?

...or something like that, where you explain <u>exactly</u> where, when, and how you want the result to occur. And you will likely find it useful to do so, a number of obvious times, using slightly different words on each occasion. In actual practice I usually divide my trances into several parts:

*Relaxation

*Ericksonian/Meta Language Patterns/Confusional Techniques

*Obvious Suggestions/Command Hypnotherapy

*Further Ericksonian Patterns

*Reorientation to wakefulness
... so the **obvious change work is sandwiched between Ericksonian patterns**. In the above example I have focussed specifically on certain language patterns and confusional techniques which

I use in connection with other methods, depending upon the context.

So, to conclude this overview of Ericksonian Hypnosis, you will notice a number of common themes in the above trance script. The use of Embedded commands and interspersel techniques. Phonological ambiguity. Certain Meta Model violations. Reframing. Reorientation in time and position. And a constant stream of empowering suggestions aimed directly at the unconscious mind with the purpose of facilitating improved self-esteem, by developing an increased sense of personal power coming from deep inside the client.

And here's the script in full.

Ericksonian Trance

….That's right. Just allow yourself to **get into a comfortable position easily now**…in your own time and your own way…and when **you want to relax** more during your **trance…easily**…you can…either by laying **still hear** or when finding you **knew a comfortable position** to take now… and you can…can you not?…and you may want to think about that for a moment….

That's it …**now…** the **nice** thing about **trance….** is that you can do it in **you're unique** way and that may be simply by choosing to **relax more and more deeply**…

…or just by **listen**-ing to what I say now **consciously and unconsciously**…and as your eyes remain gently closed you can **let** those **deeper learnings** just **happen** as much as **you**

want them too, either in a powerful or a profound way...

Some people choose to explore just how much they can let their body relax in trance too...and you may even want to **recall how you have relaxed** in that way...perhaps by letting the muscles in **your toes relax now**...or in a moment...that's right...just letting the muscles in **your toes relax**...and as **they do** now...you may even notice that you **sense a sensation** of tingling, or warmth, or heaviness, or lightness, or a pleasant coolness in your toes...or even the sensation of no sensation...**everybody does** this...in their own way **which means that** you can **do it** that way too...

And the more you allow those pleasant relaxing feelings or **sensations start to happen**...I don't know what **your unconscious is listening** to now...but I do know that **your unconscious** can **hear many things here** and as you hear here...you can choose to just **let those new resources start** to build up from **within...without** you consciously having to ...**try** and see if you can **remember at a conscious level** when you notice **your unconscious helps you now**...but sometimes you may be pleased to find that your unconscious has already **let that new helpful behaviour happen** all on it's **own...it** does...because you're unconscious always seeks to **do the best** for you...**know it does**...

And as you <u>feel ready</u> to **let those relaxing feelings** in your feet...gently allow the muscles in your legs to <u>enjoy the process</u> too...you may even find that as you <u>hear the sounds</u> in the outside world now, inside your mind...at a deeper level you can just **allow yourself to relax** with each new sound that your **hear here**...and sometimes you may even **consciously notice a sound** that you've already unconsciously noticed too...which means that **your mind is so powerful** that good things can happen at many levels now...I wonder if you've ever consciously begun to **imagine** just how **many levels of awareness** you have...and the more **you relax** to sense them the more you can use them in your daily life too...and it's good to **do it that way**...all of the successful people **do**...and because they know how to **do it** and you know how to **do this** you can **get more good results** too now... and in the future you find that you do it consciously and unconsciously in a very relaxed and natural way...

...in fact the less you try to **make this happen** the more it happens and the more **you let it happen** the better it gets...but you already **know this at an unconscious level**...do you not? Don't you?...

And think for a moment **now** about your unconscious **resources**...and then...in your mind's eye...in a moment...when I say the word 'now'...let yourself notice a situation **now-in-the-future** when **you are doing things well** assisted powerfully from an **unconscious level**...that's it...think about that...**now**...and now...in your mind's eye...over there... **notice yourself** doing that thing...sooooo easily...in fact you may even be pleasantly surprised to **watch how easy this is now**...as you do it from inside **your mind...does it naturally**...that's it watch yourself doing that thing soooo effortlessly...

...and if there are others around notice how well they **watch yourself doing this now**...notice what you **hear as you do this comfortably**...maybe your own voice...or others positively responding to you...and that feels good doesn't it...so give yourself permission to enjoy those feelings again now...that's right...

...Good and as you **get ready** to let the muscles in **your upper body... can relax...** too...either all in one go, or muscle by muscle or just gently unwinding as you feel **you want to**...you may even choose to allow those important conscious thoughts to continue to happen too as your unconscious goes deeper inside to help you as well...because your unconscious is designed to help you when **you ask your unconscious to do so**...and **I know** that's why you are here now **hear now**...which is why at that deep unconscious level those changes have **already started**...and I wonder how many you have consciously noticed already or if your unconscious is just saving them for later as well...either way **you decide** to do this for yourself...the results are the same...because when **your unconscious starts to do things**...powerful results occur...to you...

And then as you let your arms and hands just relax a bit more...just a bit more as much as you like now...think for a moment consciously...or unconsciously if you prefer about that thing that... **you want to make a change**...now...you know the one...but did you already notice just how much a **change has occurred** because I know that you have been **listen**-ing **deeply** to all of the suggestions which suit **you're unique circumstances**...the obvious ones and all of those embedded ones too and finding ways to **use them right away** whenever **you need to** <u>now</u>...

Which means that as you **allow yourself** to <u>enjoy relaxing</u> **here**...maybe even letting those muscles at the back of your eyes relax too...you may even sense that ...just as **in the past** when you've found that **something is of no use to you any more** and you've **throw**-n **it way**...you're unconscious can throw away any unwanted behaviours too...and... just like when **you've replaced something** with a <u>newer</u> and **improved** way of doing things so now you're unconscious can replace old ways with better ways too...and the good thing about this is that **it's happening now** even as **you relax** and think your conscious thoughts...and even as you **concentrate on this** or just **drift in and out of awareness**...enjoying being able to move between different positive states of being **relaxed at every level**...why don't you take a moment to **do it a bit more**...when **you're ready** too...<u>now</u>... as much as **you like**...

And think again for a moment **now** about your unconscious **resources**...and then...in your mind's eye...in a moment...once again...when I say the word 'now'...let yourself notice a situation **now-in-the-future** when **you are doing things well** assisted powerfully from an **unconscious level**...and you've done it this way before which means that you can **do it always now**...whenever you need to...that's it...think about that...**now**...and now...in your mind's eye...over there... **notice yourself** doing that thing...<u>sooooo</u> easily again...in fact you may still be pleasantly surprised to **watch how easy this is now**... and it's okay to enjoy doing things well...**naturally**...that's it watch yourself doing that thing soooo effortlessly...and if there are others around notice again how well they **watch yourself doing this now**...watching yourself <u>**doing this so well now**</u>...

...notice what you are **hearing as you do this comfortably**...maybe hearing your own voice now...or others positively responding to you...and that feels good doesn't it...so give yourself permission to enjoy those feelings again now...that's right...

You may even remember just how much you don't consciously remember about what you did last month...until you needed to and then...instantly...naturally and easily...you're unconscious lets you remember...which is the same way that **learning happens in trance**...you don't have to try and **make these changes occur** because you're unconscious will remember to **do it** for you **every time**...just like **you can** <u>remember when you need to</u>...and just relax and enjoy this new **you... knew** you can which is why **you do**...and how much of that did you unconsciously let yourself consciously **be ready** for <u>those good feelings</u> in advance...because you are allowed to **feel good about yourself** at every level...

You know you should...do you not?...which is why it must happen...because that's the natural way to do things...and I'm wondering whether you will begin now...as you sense how tomorrow is yesterday in the sense that it will be by the next day...which will mean that you are even now in the present **making changes** that will **be with you** <u>in the future too</u>... <u>in the future too</u>...

And as you **continue to observe** what you notice you may even sense that the more you **see new solutions** just happening naturally...and **don't** try to think about that now...just let it happen anyway...which means that you are finding what you need to do...just like you've always known there are **better ways**....and the more you notice which sounds you are listening to and you are relaxing with each sound that you hear...the more you can...

Some people like to think about how they will use their new **positive unconscious behaviours** while relaxing in trance...**you can do this** too if you like...think about it...**when** will you let your unconscious step forward and **release those powerful abilities** that you already have deep inside...but this time in ways that you use them consciously too...that's it just take a moment to think about a few of those times when you **will do it this way now**...and you may even be sensing an unconscious difference already?...after all **you are relaxed**...just as your unconscious knew you would...which is why you can now....but remember don't think about too **many new ways** of doing these things now...save some for later... so that your unconscious can **pleasantly surprise** you too....**easily**...and the more easily you do these things the more your unconscious does too...in fact...something that you thought would be difficult turns out to be **ridiculously easy**...**ridiculously easy now** that you **let your unconscious do it for you** instead...while **consciously enjoy doing it** together...

And in a moment I'll count from 1 to 3 And when I say the number 3 just allow yourself to awaken

remembering everything that you've noticed consciously or unconsciously so that you can start to **do these better** things **now...and tomorrow** things **get better** even more...**even more**....

1... Coming on up now.

2... Recall the situation in the room.

3... Wide awake and fully alert.

Appendix Three:

To distinguish specific 'Milton Model' language patterns from Milton's wider range of linguistic skills we coined the term the 'Rossi Model', which we use at Eos Seminars Ltd, in recognition of Dr Ernest Rossi's work with Milton, to denote some of the elements contained within the extended range of Milton's principles. In our manual we included a 'Rossi Model' script to distinguish it from the 'Milton Model' one (above). Of course, while neither of these scripts include all of the patterns detailed elsewhere in this book, when seen 'side by side', they do, nevertheless, highlight many aspects of working with indirect hypnotherapy principles. Here then is a copy of the 'Rossi Model' script that we included in our original manual:

Transcript of a 'Rossi Model' Style Ericksonian Trance

HYP. Would you like to sit is this chair or this chair before you go into a trance?

   [Simple Bind]

CL. Umm...I'll sit here thanks.

HYP. So...you mentioned on the phone that there is something you want to see me about.

CL. Yes.

   [Yes Set]

HYP. And it's to do with a problem.

[Yes Set]

CL. Yes.

[Yes Set]

HYP. And you want to **use hypnotherapy now** to help you.

[Yes Set and Embedded Command]

CL. Yes

[Yes Set]

HYP. But you wouldn't expect it to **be resolved** <u>before</u> we do the trance session would you?

CL. No

[Reverse Yes Set (yes by agreement) – Embedded Command (in bold) - plus Presupposition suggesting (underlined) that the problem will be resolved <u>after</u> the trance has taken place.]

From here we will assume that the hypnotherapist has now gathered enough information to begin the trance session.

Hyp. Okay...before we begin...

[Implication that soon 'we' will begin to do hypnosis]

...I'll tell you something interesting...

[Generating Response Potential]

...about how people...

[Metaphor]

...go into a trance...

[Embedded Command]

...now...

[Embedded Command]

...some people...

[Metaphor]

...like to **relax**...

[Embedded Command]...

...and consciously **try** ...

[The word 'try' carries the implication that they won't be able to consciously follow everything – which can, as a result, produce conscious amnesia]

...to follow everything I say....while other people...

[Metaphor]

...don't bother to consciously listen they just like to **feel comfortable**...

[Embedded Command]

...and **let it happen**...

[Embedded Command]

...and other people...

[Metaphor]

...unconsciously...

[creating unconscious/conscious dissociation in order to 'play the conscious mind down' and activate unrealised unconscious potential]

...**listen**...

[Embedded Command]

...as they give their conscious mind <u>permission</u>...

[Creating a permissive state]

... to **relax**...

[Embedded Command]

...too...

['too' carries the implication that other parts of them have already relaxed]

...and...

[Linking Word]

...you can **do it**...

[Embedded Command]

…. anyway you want to **do it**…

[Embedded Command]

…too…

[citing several ways to relax is an example of Covering All Possible Alternatives - plus the presupposition that they will 'do it too']…

….and as you're considering this…

[Mid-point of a Contingent Suggestion]

…and sensing the sensation…

[Directing Attention inwards]

…of the chair which gently supports you…

[Truism]

…you may be wondering about where you will first…

[Presupposition]

…start to notice…

[Hypnotic Language]

…that **your trance is happening**…

[Embedded Command]

...will you consciously sense your eyelids beginning to flicker more or less...

[Apposition of Opposites]

...as your unconscious mind gently let's you develop a nice comfortable trance...

[Conscious Unconscious Double Bind]

...and will those...

[Dissociation]

...eyes gently close before you consciously sense that the rhythm of your breathing is changing or after you consciously know that it has...

[Conscious Unconscious Double Bind]

...but don't close those...

[Dissociation]

....eyes too quickly...

[Restraint]

...just **let it happen**...

[Embedded Command]

....when your unconscious lets you know **the time is right**...**now**...

[Embedded Command plus Punctuation Ambiguity EG: is the hypnotherapist saying 'the time is right' or 'the time is right now'...or both?]...

CL. Eyes starting to flicker and other NVC.

Hyp. And as your eyes are flickering...

[Truism - Observable]

....and your respiration has become more even....

[Truism - Observable]

....and your hands are resting on the arms of the chair...

[Truism - Observable]

...And...

[Linking Word]

...you're thinking certain thoughts...

[Truism – Non Observable, directing attention inwards]

...I don't know whether...

[If the therapist doesn't 'know' who does? The implication is that the client does]

...whether that flickering will stop <u>as</u> your eyes close or <u>when</u> they close....

[Double Bind – the only way they will find out is when it actually happens. It's also a

Contingent Suggestion because the flickering of the eyes ceasing is contingent upon them closing]...

CL.   Eyes start to close

Hyp. That's right....

[Confirming/Pacing and Leading]

...you're doing really well...

[Confirming/Pacing and Leading]...

CL. Eyes fully close

HYP. Well done...

[Confirming/Pacing and Leading]

...and isn't it amazing...

[Hypnotic Language]

....that those eyes...

[Dissociation]

...knew exactly when **the time is right**...

[Embedded Command]

...to let them **remain closed**...

[Embedded Command]

...in order for your unconscious mind to help you even more...

> [Comparative Deletion – 'even more' than what? Plus a Conscious-Unconscious Dissociation to 'play down' the conscious mind]

Hyp. So that when your unconscious mind begins to let things start to <u>lift</u>...

> [Seeding]

...even more...

> [Comparative Deletion - 'even more' than what?]

... you don't have to consciously make it happen...

> [Not Doing]

...you don't even have to consciously know how it does happen...

> [Not Knowing]

...but it can be really nice, can it not?...

> [Tag Question]

...to begin to experience **higher** feelings...

> [Seeding]

...without even having to try...some people...

[Metaphor]

...dream...

[Hypnotic language]

...about it happening **like this** ...

[Embedded Command]

... while other people...

[Metaphor]

...imagine...

[Hypnotic Language]...

what it will be like...and...

[Linking Word]...

...others...

[Metaphor]

...visualise it...

[Simple Deletion, visualise what?]

...in the back part of their mind...

[Hypnotic Language 'back part' implies the unconscious]

Hyp. But don't...

[Restraint]

...let that hand...

[Dissociation]

...begin to **lift up**...

[Seed Activated]

...of its own accord until **your unconscious**...

[Embedded Command – Phonological Ambiguity 'your unconscious' = 'you're unconscious']

...knows the time is right...

[Implication that the time will be right]

...to find a solution...

[Implication that a solution will be found]

...that works...

[It will 'work']

...for you...

[Tailored Solution]

Hyp.   I wonder whether you will first begin to consciously sense a sensation in your right hand of heaviness or unconsciously sense a sensation in your left hand of lightness...

[Conscious Unconscious Double Bind]

...or will you unconsciously sense a sensation of heaviness in your left hand and consciously sense lightness in your right...

[Conscious Unconscious Double Bind]

...sometimes it can be right to let your left hand lift and sometimes it can be left to your right hand to lift...or while lifting your left hand because it's left... while knowing that it's right for your right hand to feel even more different than you imagined...

[Confusion technique]

CL. Fingers start to twitch on the right hand

Hyp. Excellent. Well done. How did you know that! How did you know your fingers would move **like that** ...

[Embedded Command]

...before...

[Implication that whatever follows the word 'before' will happen]

...your arm begins to **lift**...

[Embedded Command - Seed Activated]

...Isn't it amazing how that hand...

[Dissociation]

...already knew exactly what to do...that's right....you're doing really well...really well...

> [Confirmation and Encouragement – building further Response Potential]

CL. Arm begins to lift higher.

Hyp.   And I wonder...I'm curious to know...how much time will pass before that hand touches your face...

> [Contingent Suggestion: as time passes 'that hand' will touch your face. Presupposition that 'that hand' will touch 'your face']

...and let's face it...

> [Orienting client to continue to focus on raising 'that hand' up to the face with the words 'let's face it']

...the wonderful...

> [Hypnotic Language]

...thing about Trance Time...

> [Implication that there is something that exists that we call Trance Time]

...is that it can happen in unusual ways...

> [Implication that 'unusual' things can take place in trance...such as hand levitation]

...so that a minute of trance time can seem like an hour and an hour of normal time can seem like a minute...

[Time Distortion]

...and whether this happens inside your awareness or outside of your perception...

[Apposition of Opposites]

...you don't have to try to make it happen...

[Not Doing]

...you don't even have to think about it...

[Not Knowing]

...And as this continues to happen...

[Implication that something is happening]

...with each new sound that you hear around you, you can discover yourself relaxing some more...

[Compound Suggestion – the experience of relaxing is Compounded with each sound that is heard]

... and sometimes you can hear things that are not really here or know that they're hear without knowing how you perceive them...

[Illusion of sound]

...or in the back part of your mind you may visualise things which haven't yet existed or know that they exist without knowing that you've seen them...

[Illusion of sight]

....but don't notice too much now...

[Restraint]

...save some...

[Simple Deletion. 'Some' what?]

...for later...excellent. You're doing just fine...just fine. And you can't not ...

[Double Negative = a positive]

...**notice**...

[Embedded Command]

...a certain change starting to happen somewhere...

[Fluff and Super Fluff. A 'certain change' starting to happen 'somewhere']

...because **your unconscious** ...

[Embedded Command]

...mind never can't not...

[Triple Negative = a positive]

...find a solution between now and when you awaken later...

[Time Bind: A solution will be found between 'now' and 'awakening']...

Cl. Arm is very close to face now.

Hyp. And how much time didn't you notice not happening...

[Use of Negatives]

...while that arm quickly moved right up to your face **like this**...

[Embedded Command 'like this', meaning that they will like/enjoy the process, that is employed to help facilitate the therapy]

...it always...

[Universal Quantifier]

...happens this way...and I know that sometimes you are curious...

[Mind Reading]

...and curiosity **like this** can be good...

[Seeding the idea of curiosity and then suggesting that it is here in the present tense and that they will like feeling curious 'like this']...

Hyp. And I wonder which solution...

[Further introduction of the concept of a Solution]

...your unconscious...

[Embedded Command]

...will generate...

[Implication that a solution will be generated]

...first and which will be second and which will be third...

[Implication that three solutions will be generated]

...and will you notice the first one first or will it be the second one that you first notice before you discover...

[Hypnotic Language]

...that you've noticed the first after you've already done it three times ...just after you noticed the third one happening...

[Confusion]

...And...

[Linking word]

...it reminds me of the time when a client once asked me...

[Metaphor]

...how does an unconscious **change now**...

[Embedded Command]

...take place - and I explained that for many clients they don't consciously notice a certain shift of perspective until after it's already happened while for others they unconsciously notice that new perspective before they consciously begin to use it...

[Conscious Unconscious Double Dissociated Double Bind]

... and it may be that you will also notice that you haven't noticed...

[Apposition of Opposites]

...it until after **you've already begun to change now**...

[Embedded Command]

...And I wonder whether 'that hand'...

[Dissociation]

...will touch your face...

[Embedded Command]

...before...

[Implication that they will do what follows]

...you count from one to ten...

[Suggestion to count]

...in your mind or when you just gently think about something else instead...

[or permission not to count and just carry on thinking]

> CL.　Client's hand touches their face. As they do so their eyes demonstrate REM action and their head moves from side to side gently a couple of times...

Hyp.　That's the s..way...

[Pseudo Phonological Ambiguity]

...you and I...

[Phonological Ambiguity: you and eye. Pacing and leading]

...both know that something is happening...

[Truism – something is happening]

....and isn't it wonderful, is it not...

[Tag Question]

...how a positive change like this can take place without you having to make it happen...

[Not Doing]

...or even thinking...

[Not Knowing]

...about how it just occurred...

[Shifted it into the past tense, EG: it has already been achieved: 'it just occurred']...

Hyp. Now eye...

[Phonological Ambiguity]

...want to thank your unconscious mind...

[Phonological Ambiguity – Embedded Command]

...for doing this...

[Lack of Referential Index: doing what?]

...and don't let that hand relax...

[Restraining plus Embedded Command suggesting that 'that hand' will relax]

...back into your lap until **you know**...

[Embedded Command]

...so deeply that you can't consciously know...

[Apposition of Opposites]

...that these changes...

[Nominalisation, Presupposition]

...have been powerfully...

[Hypnotic Language]

...integrated to work for you...

[Personal Solution]

...exactly...

[Precision]

...when...

[Time Contingent]

...you need them...

[Suggestion]

...and in exactly...

[Precision]

...the right ways...

[Situation Contingent]...

CL.   Hand gently rests back into lap.

Hyp. That's right. And isn't it amazing...

[Hypnotic Language]

...that your unconscious knew before you consciously discovered that it was right for your right arm to do it this way while your left arm was left to relax in another way...

[Retrospective Conscious Unconscious Double Bind]

Hyp. And in a moment I'll count from 1-5. When I reach the number 3 you can awaken as a mind and when I reach the number 5 you can fully awaken as a body as well.

[Dissociation]

Hyp. 1, 2, 3. Awakening now as a mind, 4, 5 and fully awakening as a body now as well.

Welcome back!

> [Implied suggestion that they have 'been somewhere' from which they have just 'returned']

'Hyp' = hypnotherapist 'Cl' = client.

Appendix Four:

The following article was published in Issue 2 of the British Board of NLP's magazine, called The Model. There are a number of themes within it that are based on Indirect Hypnotherapy/NLP principles:

Enthusiasm

It's 1968 and he's 33. He looks magnificent. He's dressed in a jet black suit and adorned with his jet black hair and trademark sideburns. The iconic image he presents instantly lets the viewers know who it is they're watching. It's Elvis! He's back. And he's back in style.

The Singer Television Special (now known in the annals of rock n' roll history as the '68 Comeback Special') in which Elvis performed to a television audience, for the first time in years (and in the process reclaimed his crown as the 'king of rock n' roll') is exhilarating to watch. I've seen it many times now and I'm always impressed by the energy and charisma that Elvis radiates throughout this spectacular programme. There's something special about Elvis in this show. It's true his entire career was remarkable, but this particular show stands out at this moment in his life. And you know what I think it is about Elvis that's different? His enthusiasm! After almost a decade in the doldrums of being tied into movie-making contracts making films (many of which) even he didn't like (and he was the star of them!) but which he couldn't extricate himself from, he'd at last found his freedom and re-discovered his first love. Singing to a live audience! And the passion. The excitement.

The enthusiasm is apparent. He is outstanding to watch. Such is the power of enthusiasm.

Follow that dream

Elvis once sang a song called 'Follow That Dream'. In the song he exhorts us by saying: **'When a dream is calling you...there's just one thing that you should do. You've got to follow that dream!'** Anthony Robbins has often cited the dictum which states: **'Success leaves clues'.** That's to say that if we study those who are successful and sincerely replicate the same kind of behaviour we'll generate similar results in our own lives (I call this process 'holistic modelling'. That's to say there's a marked difference between someone who is doing 'plastic modelling', which means they're going through the motions but their heart isn't in it. Whereas in 'holistic modelling' you really put your heart and soul into what you're doing). I like Tony – and I agree with what he says.

Now, back to the song. So Elvis advocates that when a dream is '**calling**' us...we should '**follow**' it. And you know what? If you look at many of the greatest people who've ever lived that's exactly what they did. They had a dream – or a passion which filled them with enthusiasm and that enthusiasm helped energise them so that, whatever life threw at them, they were inexorably on target to do what they wanted to do. To be who they wanted to be.

As one door closes another gate opens

I watched Bill Gates at the global Live 8 concert. You know what I notice about him? He's totally enthusiastic about his work and the projects he's involved in. So's Richard Branson. So was Mother Teresa. So was Dorothy Kerin. Bono is. And we all know Bob Geldof is ******* enthusiastic about his projects too. What's more - all of these people have helped to improve the lives of many others through the power of their enthusiasm. Think about it. If my understanding is correct, back when it seemed an impossible idea to most people, Bill Gates' goal was to have a computer situated on every desk running Microsoft software (or something close to this). And he did it. Now, in today's world, it's a given that most computers are running on Windows. But back then it started as a dream that Bill Gates had - which he 'followed' with enthusiasm. And because of this, now he's probably the biggest philanthropist in history. Sir Richard Branson, as I understand things, started running his business as a youngster from a local phone box. He too had a goal/dream and the enthusiasm to go with it - and he made his dream a reality. Mother Teresa received a message from God which told her she had work to do. So she got started. She got enthusiastic about it, helped thousands and in the process set an example to us all about selflessness. So did Dorothy Kerin. As a desperately ill young person in England in 1912 she encountered a similar experience to Mother Teresa. As a result she had a miraculous recovery from her illness and got enthusiastic about her 'calling'. Due to her lifelong enthusiasm the nursing centre she founded called Burrswood still exists today which provides healing to many, long after Dorothy physically left this world as a, then, elderly lady in the early 1960s. And Bono and Bob Geldof? Well their dedication and enthusiasm is apparent in all that they do. Millions will vouch for that.

Enthusiasm is catching

There's something wonderful about someone who's enthusiastic. Their enthusiasm is catching. It creates a kind of virtuous circle. They behave enthusiastically and their enthusiasm rubs off on those around them. (Dorothy Kerin used to ask: 'What's the good news today?') So those around them start to feel and act enthusiastically too - and everyone benefits! Imagine what it would be like if the whole world lived this way. The way of enthusiasm. If we all looked for the positive potential in our circumstances. And if we enthusiastically found ways together around the challenges that crop up in life from time to time. What a difference that would be.

For instance, just think about what it would be like to work for a company in which enthusiasm was a part of the corporate culture. I'm not talking about 'plastic enthusiasm', the kind that you hear about where people (often under duress) are drilled through a list of daily 'motivational commandments' each morning (that they often don't agree with but have to suffer through) in order to get paid. I'm talking about real heartfelt enthusiasm. The kind that takes a dirt poor child from the streets of Tupelo, Mississippi to a place where he's enthusiastically singing from the heart-of-his-soul for the '68 TV special. The kind that makes life really worth living. How could we begin to do that?

Deliberate acts of enthusiasm

A few years ago someone coined the term 'Random Acts of Kindness' to encourage people to make being kind a part of their day-to-day lives. I like that idea a lot. Of course, in reality, by incorporating such a precept into your life you aren't really practising 'random' acts, in the strict sense of the word. Sure...the time and the place may present itself without premeditation...but the desire to be kind is deliberate. For enthusiasm to fill our lives it also needs to become a deliberate act. That's why I've coined the term 'Deliberate Acts of Enthusiasm'. (I'm not trade marking it ☺ because I thought it might work better if it was placed in the public domain for anyone else who might want to use it to be able to do so too.) I believe that if more people were to get into the habit of practising deliberate acts of enthusiasm in their lives we'd soon notice the difference.

High spirits

Curiously (or not) the word enthusiasm is derived from the Greek word 'enthousiazien' which literally means to be 'possessed by a god'. So this means that, originally, being enthusiastic was considered to be a divine attribute. Maybe it still is? Maybe this means that by being enthusiastic in our lives and in our work we can share a little bit of heaven with those we meet along the way?

If I can dream

The closing song that Elvis sang on the '68 TV Special was a song called 'If I Can Dream'. This time he's dressed in immaculate white. He looks magnificent. And he's filled with passion – with enthusiasm – as he begins singing with the outstanding voice that providence bestowed upon him. At first he sings about the feelings of mistrust and unease that often permeate our global culture. He raises questions which ask, in effect, that if it's possible to dream of a better world...why can't such a dream come true? It's a good question. But then the ebb and flow of the song begins to change as it lifts upwards...the mood shifting higher...becoming hopeful. Moving powerfully towards the crescendo Elvis becomes almost rhetorical in the words that he sings, by effectively answering his own questions, by declaring enthusiastically '**out there in the dark there's a beckoning candle**'. And he's right. Because enthusiasm is like a light that radiates outward bringing illumination and energy to those whom it touches. Elvis continues by singing about the miracles that can take place when we all have the '**strength to dream**', a strength which can itself enable us to '**fly**'. To be lifted above the humdrum. To raise our potential. To move up to another level. Such is the power of enthusiasm.

Possessed by enthusiasm

I never met Elvis personally, but his enduring vitality and enthusiasm have radiated across continents and time and helped to shape my life significantly. Like Elvis, I believe that when we have a dream and when we **follow that dream** with clarity and become possessed by enthusiasm we can enrich our own lives and the lives of those with whom we live. I believe you do too. And maybe...just maybe if we both decide to practice Deliberate Acts of Enthusiasm in our day-to-day lives we'll become a permanent part of that virtuous circle that the great-and-the-good are inviting us to join. And then who knows where that could lead?

Appendix Five:

The following appendix is a reproduction of an article that appears on the Self Help World (www.self-help-world.co.uk) website. It contains information relevant to Indirect Hypnotherapy. Self Help World aims to communicate information to the general public in a contemporary, 'jargon' free, way.

Confidence

Everybody wants it. Those who have it seem to handle life more easily than those who don't. People with confidence are much more self-assured - while those who are not often step back from opportunities when they arise and miss out due to their lack of confidence. So, what is the secret to confidence?

The subject of confidence shares many similarities to that of Positive Thinking (for more about this, see my article on the Positive Thinking page). Confidence is often a matter of perception. And many people are diligently working as hypnotists on themselves – but in the reverse direction! That's to say that they've done a good job of hypnotising themselves into believing that they lack confidence. Often this is achieved by observing others and concluding from the observations that they make – that they are 'not confident' like 'other people'. Talking to you as a therapist, I've met many people who've expressed similar opinions to me. It's as if they think they can read the minds of others and then - based on their (erroneous as it often turns out) interpretation of how they think other people think and feel – they tell themselves that they're part of some group of people who 'lack confidence'. And the more they tell themselves this – the more they start to believe it. It becomes something of a mantra: 'I can't do that – because I lack confidence...I can't do that because I lack confidence'. Actually, it's more than a mantra – it's a form of self-hypnosis.

There's a wonderful book called Trances People Live, in which the author, expert hypnotherapist Stephen Wolinsky Ph.D., explains that most (if not all) clients who present for therapy requesting hypnosis are actually in a self-induced state of hypnosis already! That's right. They're in a self-induced 'problem trance', and the therapist's job, Stephen Wolinsky says...is to first help them OUT of their problem trance! It's after that's taken place that the therapist can help them create a better outlook on life.

So – with this in mind now, let's revisit the subject of confidence again. Now, if you're like others who've assumed that 'other people' are more confident than you – maybe you're wrong? Or at least not as right as you used to think? And maybe, just maybe, the people who think that they supposedly 'lack confidence' actually have just as much confidence as the others – only they haven't realised it? Based on my experience that's often the case. Of that I'm confident (excuse the pun!).

You know, when I've worked with people who are in the public eye. People who rub shoulders, so to speak, with top politicians, celebrities and leading academics I've discovered that most of them are very much like everyone else I meet. They are no 'more' or no 'less' confident than many others. The difference is that they hypnotise themselves, so to speak, in a different way – a better way. That's to say that faced with similar opportunities and challenges, they convince themselves that they can follow through, whereas those who supposedly 'lack confidence' do the opposite. They instead convince themselves that they can't follow through, and then either don't try, or try half-heartedly, and then use the negative experience that they encounter (based on their half-hearted approach) as 'further proof' of their condition.

What's heartening though is that I've also met people, in all walks of life, who have raised their perceptions (and therefore their experience) of their confidence by 'going for it' more often. Because our perception of confidence is often something of a feedback loop, if we get in the habit of 'going for it' more often, chances are, we'll experience more good things in our lives because we follow through regularly, and because we follow through, therefore naturally experiencing more good things, we'll develop a greater sense of confidence in ourselves. It's like a nice mathematical formula: follow through = have more good experiences = feel confident = follow through some more = have more good experiences = feel more confident...and so on.

Let me let you in on another important secret. Confident people still, from time to time, experience moments of doubt. Did that surprise you? But the difference is – they don't let that stop them. They acknowledge their emotions and thoughts – considering what there is to learn from them – and then they continue to move forward.

So – a 'trick' for becoming more confident is to 'go for it' in life, in whichever ways are appropriate for you. If you consistently LIVE UP TO YOUR POTENTIAL you'll experience more experiences reflective of your true self...and the more you do this the more confident you'll feel.

A couple of good books, by other authors on this subject include: Feel The Fear and Do It Anyway (I love that title – it says it all), by Susan Jeffers and The Magic of Thinking Big, by David J. Schwartz. Of course, my own book: Making Your Dreams Your Reality, shares principles for developing more confidence and our Ultra Hypnosis CD, Confidently Confident is specifically designed to help you improve your confidence too.

Remember the formula: follow through = have more good experiences = feel confident = follow through some more = have more good experiences = feel more confident...

...and the more you do the more your confidence will grow!

Kerin Webb 2005.

Appendix Six:

The following appendix is a reproduction of an article that appears on the Self Help World (www.self-help-world.co.uk) website. It contains information relevant to Indirect Hypnotherapy. Self Help World aims to communicate information to the general public in a contemporary, 'jargon' free, way.

Positive Thinking

We all know that there's great power in the skill of positive thinking. Some of us do it naturally - while others have learned how to do it. It doesn't matter whether you've always been a positive thinker or whether it's something you're learning to do now, because the benefits of positive thinking make it one of the most powerful psychological skills in the world - and it starts to work as soon as you start to do it!

Let me share a metaphor with you. One person regularly walks into their garden each morning and scans the sky. At the first sign of a cloud they say: 'I knew it! It's going to be another bad day'. Whereas another person when doing the same says: 'Hardly a cloud in sight - it's a beautiful day', or on an overcast day, perhaps 'We could do with some rain – it'll help the flowers to grow'. One finds the good in a situation (even if, as sometimes happens in life, there are a few clouds around), while the other - at the slightest opportunity to complain - seeks the worst interpretation of the situation.

Notice carefully an important word that I just used. The word 'interpretation'. Because how we interpret life massively affects the way we experience it. And when you look around you – you can see examples of this in your day-to-day life. At work, at home, socially. Some people interpret life in a way that helps them to be positive while others defeat themselves before they start by talking themselves (and those around them) down.

I remember, once, a number of years ago, waiting for a bus at a bus stop. There was a woman at the bus stop who was aged somewhere in her late thirties to early forties. She was talking quite loud to another person at the stop so I couldn't help but over hear what she was saying. The conversation went something like this: 'My sister's children are going to start university soon. They're going to study economics. I think that they're really lucky to have such an opportunity. I'd like to be in their shoes'. Then, I believe, the other person must have said something to her, along the lines of suggesting that she should do a course of study in something that she liked (after all, we live in a world where there are many opportunities these days to train academically and vocationally in a wide range of professional skills at hours to suit our needs). The woman in question responded quickly by saying something along the lines of: 'Oh, I can't do that, I'm too old now. I'm past doing things like that...'. And proceeded to talk herself out of moving forward and into staying in a rut.

As I listened I felt especially moved by her frame of mind – in the sense that I could see her wistfully going through life mourning the opportunities that she'd miss, for the myriad number of reasons that she could manufacture, to hold herself back and...because my mum, then in her late 50s had just gone back to college and was, at that very time, in the process of retraining herself to become an aromatherapist and beauty therapist. (Which she's since turned into a second career that she enjoys very much.)

Two people who arrived at a similar crossroads of opportunity. One turned around and walked away – while the other stepped forward and made the most of it.

The woman at the bus stop 'interpreted' her years as a barrier, whereas my mother interpreted them as an opportunity to do something different with her life.

One of the major keys, therefore, to becoming more positive is learning to manage your thoughts. To choose to interpret things realistically, and with a positive slant. The woman at the bus stop was unrealistic in her thinking and negative in her interpretation.

How can you begin to do this? When faced with opportunities or challenges, aim to think about them in, what we call in the world of NLP/Hypnotherapy a 'solution focused' way. If you look for solutions/positive options, as a matter of habit, things will change for the better. And the more you do this the more powerful your positivity habit will become.

Also – it's always good to create what I call 'positive moments' in your life. You can do this by reading a good book or listening to some pleasant music, or by using some up-beat self-help tapes and CDs. A couple of books I recommend by other authors include: The Success System That Never Fails – by William Clement Stone and Unlimited Power by Anthony Robbins. My own book – Making

Your Dreams Your Reality (by Kerin Webb) is also packed full of useful information on how you can improve your life. And the Ultra Hypnosis 'Positively Positive' CD is especially designed for helping you to improve your positivity levels too.

So – remember – a person's positivity levels are greatly influenced by the way they interpret things. Which means that – now that you know this important principle you can get into the habit of finding the opportunities in life as you become a solution-focused positive thinker.

Appendix Seven:

This appendix is a 'carry over' from our original training manual. It contains various phrases using different indirect hypnotherapy language patterns.

Additional Indirect Language for Therapeutic Interventions

Some examples from the Milton Model

This means that... (Complex Equivalence)

Which is why you will... (Modal Operator of Necessity)

It must... (Modal Operator of Necessity)

Don't think about... (Law of Reversed Effect)

You must... (Modal Operator of Necessity)

It can't happen anymore now that...X...has just happened... (Modal Operator of Possibility and Cause and Effect)

Now as you sit hear in trance...you may begin to sense things are getting better already... (Truism – the client is sitting there so they must agree with the statement which will make them more inclined to agree with what follows. AKA the 'Yes Set')

The amazing thing about...X... is that ......and that it always causes...Y... (Cause and Effect)

I know that sometimes you are... (Mind Reading)

I know that sometimes you do... (Mind Reading)

I know that sometimes you think... (Mind Reading)

I know that sometimes you feel... (Mind Reading)

I know that you must feel curious sometimes... (Mind Reading)

Don't you think it's important for...? (Embedded Suggestion presupposing that what follows is important)

Wouldn't it be better to...? (Comparative Deletion)

Why not let?... (Suggestion phrased as a question, Conversational Postulate)

How many ways can you...? (Solution-focussed – presupposing the client can do whatever follows)

If you had to decide now...what would it be...? (Reframing the client's perspective, with a Modal Operator of Necessity)

You don't have to be sure about this...just think for a moment...what's your best guess...that's all you need to consider now...more certainty can come soon or later...whenever you're ready...right now... ('Best Guess' is always good to use if someone is adamant that they 'don't know', because by simply 'best guessing' they will quite likely feel more at ease to begin thinking about whatever the hypnotherapist is suggesting might be considered).

You know...don't you...that it's good to...? (Tag Question to deal with a Polarity Response)

And you've sensed...haven't you...that it's okay to...? (Mind Reading, Tag Question, Modal Operator of Possibility)

Ask yourself...what would it be like to...? (Reframing)

Have you ever pictured a...? (Question designed to cause the client to start to picture...)

Can you remember a time when you felt X ...what would it be like now...? (Question designed to cause the client to remember a resourceful feeling and re-experience it again now)

You don't have to think about doing it more easily at a conscious level...in fact, if you like you can consciously forget that I just said you can do things more easily now and let your unconscious remember instead...didn't you... ('more easily' = a Comparative Deletion, 'at a conscious level' creates a separation of the perception of the conscious and unconscious state, 'you like you' is a positive Embedded Command... what other patterns can you spot?)

Some more Indirect Language Patterns.

(Can you notice which ones they are?)

I know there must be times when you...

I expect you've wondered...

Now since your unconscious is doing X for you this means that you will begin to notice Y happening sometimes as well...

By the third time your unconscious has done this for you, you will start to notice it consciously too...and that will work even better...because it always happens that way...

I wonder which skills your unconscious will start to develop for you before you notice them happening at a conscious level too...?

The fact that it's better to invite your unconscious to do it for you is demonstrated by the fact that you're here...but then you already know that at some level, which is why you decided to anyway...

You find that your communication and confidence shine brighter than before now...

Your unconscious remembers everything, which is why these changes must happen...

These changes must happen because your unconscious remembers everything...

Don't feel too confident now...save some for later...you can have as much of it as you want now...want it and you can have it...but deep inside you understand that now...

It's a bit like one of those magical stories that you heard as a child...when something wonderful just happened...and everything just got happier and brighter...that's the way it happens in hypnosis now too...

I wouldn't be surprised if you started to notice feeling more X...by tomorrow or even sooner...but you can be pleasantly surprised about it yourself now if you like...

Go down deep into your thoughts and try unsuccessfully to have that problem. It is an unwanted problem wasn't it? It's better now that your unconscious has changed things...hasn't it? I wonder what you'll think when you look back and consider all of the positive changes that happened...haven't they? And how better things have become now... (My thanks to **Alan Jones** for sharing this one with me.)

You don't have to work up confidence all of the time...sometimes you'll also find that your unconscious just helps you to feel calm and more relaxed about things instead...

Would you prefer your unconscious to do it by tomorrow ...or sooner?

Make a decision if you like...do you want this change to happen right away...or quickly?

It's your choice... will you unconsciously cause this to happen right now? Or in a few moments? Think about it... because it must change now...which is why you're here...are you not?

When you think about that problem...what was it about that problem that you didn't like the most?......(pause)............Now in the future what would you prefer to happen now?...

You may have sensed that sometimes when you...X...and that always means that...Y... will follow on naturally...

There must have been a time when you chose to look at something more clearly or in more detail...or listen to something more precisely...or get in touch with something more completely...and you did...and you know that this means that because you did it all of those times before you can do it again whenever you want to now... and in the future...because you already know how to do it...don't you? You know you do...just like you know how to sleep...at the right time...or know how to be more aware at the right time...and sometimes you can be in trance consciously and be very aware and sometimes you are not in trance consciously and you can notice as much as you want to as well...I wonder...don't you? Which new things will you start to notice first now? And how much more will you notice everything that you want to...clearly, precisely and easily...as well?...

Points to remember

Point to remember: I find that it can be useful to employ the words 'please' and 'with great respect' when talking to my clients. I'll often front-load a question, statement, joke or offer some feed-back using either 'please' or 'with great respect' (said with sincerity) so that the client understands that I have their best interests at heart. The words 'thank you' are useful too, particularly when a client (whether in, or not in, 'formal trance') says or does something which is indicative of movement towards improved health.

Point to remember: I believe that a good attitude is more valuable than extensive technical knowledge. We can all always learn more, technically speaking... but a good attitude is an attribute that demonstrates <u>developed character</u>. Clients respond well to high attitudinal competency.

Point to remember: I've found that sometimes one of the best ways to help a client who's trapped in a 'secondary gain loop' (meaning they want to get over their problem, but certain aspects of their problem provide them with unaddressed 'benefits' that they're not prepared to 'lose' as a result of moving toward wellness), is to very directly and very respectfully tell them what secondary gain is and how it works while giving them the opportunity to explore whether or not this subject might be relevant to them, and if it is, how the perceived benefits of having the problem can be obtained in more holistic ways.

Point to remember: Many healers go through a ritual just before working with their clients in which they seek to 'step out' of what remains of their own ego, in order to support the client, free of the 'clutter' that comes with an untamed ego.

...apples of gold in settings of silver.

Proverbs 25:11.

After Word

I'd like to leave you with some important thoughts at this point in the book. It is, I believe, imperative that exponents of language pattern skills use such principles with wisdom and integrity. Brilliant exponents of language pattern skills do so with heart and in all the most appropriate ways. And the mark of an outstanding exponent of language pattern skills is, in my opinion, someone who knows when not to use them.

Best wishes...

Kerin Webb

Author's References (course providers):

(Which includes, in some instances, where relevant, reference to the course manual which accompanied the programme attended.)

Anthony Robbins (The Fire-walk Seminar)

Eos Seminars Ltd (Which includes seminars by Frank Farrelly, Carol Lankton and Stephen Brooks)

International Association of Hypno-Analysts (Neil French)

NLP Learning Company

NLP Northeast

Paul McKenna Training

Proudfoot School of Clinical Hypnosis & Psychotherapy

RSA Counselling Certification (Bournemouth Adult Education Centre)

Training Changes

West Mercia Institute of Counselling & Psychotherapy

Author's References (individuals):

Alan Jones
Andrea Lindsay
Anthony Robbins
Caitlin Walker
Carol Lankton

Colin Saunders
Cricket Kemp
Derek Parker
Dr Richard Bandler
Elizabeth Whitaker
Frank Farrelly
Gill Webb
Guy Barron
Ian Berry
Ken Buck
Mike Treasure
Nick Othen
Pam Webb
Paul McKenna
Peter Webb
Peter Young
Robin Jones
Stephen Brooks
Tom Smith
Wilf Proudfoot

Author's References (audio sets):

Unlimited Power (Anthony Robbins)
Personal Power (Anthony Robbins)

Author's References (books):

A Teaching Seminar With Milton H Erickson
(Edited With Commentary By Jeffrey K. Zeig, PhD)

Analytical Hypnotherapy – Principles And Practice
(E.A. Barnett, MD)

Awaken The Giant Within
(Anthony Robbins)

Chomsky
(John Lyons)

Clinical Practice Of Hypnotherapy
(M. Erik Wright With Beatrice A. Wright)

Collins English Dictionary & Thesaurus
(21st Century Edition)

Combatting Cult Mind Control
(Steven Hassan)

Communication Excellence – Using NLP To Supercharge Your Business Skills
(Ian R. McLaren)

Frogs Into Princes
(Richard Bandler & John Grinder)

Handbook Of Hypnotic Inductions
(George Gafner & Sonja Benson)

Healing In Hypnosis
(Edited By Ernest L. Rossi, Margaret O. Ryan, Florence A. Sharp)

Hypnosis – A Comprehensive Guide
(Tad James, MS, PhD With Lorraine Flores & Jack Schober)

Hypnotherapy – A Practical Handbook
(Hellmut W.A. Karle And Jennifer H. Boys)

Hypnotic Language – Its Structure And Use
(John Burton EdD & Bob G. Bodenhamer DMin)

Hypnotic Realities
(Erickson, Rossi & Rossi)

In Search of Solutions
(William Hudson O'Hanlon, Michele Weiner-Davis)

Magic Demystified
(Byron A. Lewis & Frank Pucelik)

Medical & Dental Hypnosis & Its Clinical Applications
(John Hartland)

Metaphors In Mind
(James Lawley And Penny Tompkins)

Mind Body Therapy
(Ernest L. Rossi, David B. Cheek)

Mind-Lines
(L. Michael Hall And Bobby G. Bodenhamer, D.Min)

Modern Clinical Hypnosis For Habit Control
(Charles M. Citrenbaum, Mark E. King, William I. Cohen)

My Voice Will Go With You
(Edited And With Commentary By Sidney Rosen)

NLP In 21 Days
(Harry Alder And Beryl Heather)

Pattern Of The Hypnotic Techniques Of Milton H. Erickson, MD. Volume 2
(John Grinder, Judith DeLozier And Richard Bandler)

Practical English Usage
(Michael Swann)

Provocative Therapy
(Frank Farrelly And Jeff Brandsma)

Sleight Of Mouth – The Magic Of Conversational Belief Change
(Robert Dilts)

Solution-Oriented Hypnosis
(William Hudson O'Hanlon, Michael Martin)

Taproots – Underlying Principles Of Milton Erickson's Therapy And Hypnosis
(William. O'Hanlon)

The Answer Within – A Clinical Framework Of Ericksonian Hypnotherapy
(Lankton & Lankton)

The Effective Delivery Of Training Using NLP
(Ted Garratt)

The Language Of Change – Elements Of Therapeutic Communication
(Paul Watzlawick)

The Spirit Of NLP
(L. Michael Hall PhD.)

The User's Manual For The Brain
(Bob G. Bodenhamer, D.Min., L. Michael Hall, PhD.)

Time Lining
(Bob G. Bodenhamer And L. Michael Hall)

Training Trances
(Julie Silverthorne & John Overdurf)

Trances People Live
(Stephen Wolinsky, PhD.)

Uncommon Therapy
(Jay Haley)

Understanding NLP – Metaphors And Patterns Of Change
(Peter Young)

Unlimited Power
(Anthony Robbins)

Virginia Satir – The Patterns Of Her Magic
(Steve Andreas)

Whispering In The Wind
(Carmen Bostic St. Clair And John Grinder)

Miscellaneous:

Audio:

Dick Sutphen (via various audio tapes)
Marshall Sylver (via a hypnosis script)
Neil French (via his IAH training course)
Robert Farago (via various CDs)

Websites:

http://www.doyletics.com/art/som1art.htm

http://www.nlpandhypnosis.com/ex1.htm

http://www.semantic-knowledge.com/semantics-2.htm

With Affection:

Anna, Barney, Ben, Bill, Bobby, Buddy, Caesar, Dominic, Fluffy, Hoddy, Jackie, Kim, Millie, Muffin, Robby, Sadie, Sandy, Smokey, Suzie, Tessa, Tetley, Toby, Tristan.

Lightning Source UK Ltd.
Milton Keynes UK
UKOW04f2003250315

248538UK00001B/111/P